Psychological Perspectives on Walking

Psychological Perspectives on Walking provides a comprehensive overview of the benefits of walking and shows how we can encourage people to walk more based on psychological principles. It examines how walking significantly improves health, positively impacts the environment, contributes to resolving social issues, and boosts the local micro-economy. This pioneering book discusses psychological motivations for walking versus not walking and asserts research-based arguments in favour of walking, including both theoretical considerations and everyday concerns.

The book investigates the motivations that can lead to increased walking, advises on how to build walking-conducive habits, and recommends strategies for decision-makers for promoting changes that will allow walking to thrive more easily. The authors include success stories and lessons learned from what have become known as 'walkable' cities to show how interventions and initiatives can succeed on a practical basis.

This accessible, practical book is essential for urban planners; health specialists; policy makers; traffic experts; psychology, civil engineering, and social sciences students; and experts in the field of sustainable mobility. *Psychological Perspectives on Walking* will appeal to anyone in the general population in favour of a sustainable and healthy lifestyle.

Ralf Risser is a visiting professor in the Psychology Department at Palacký University in Olomouc, Czech Republic. He specialises in qualitative survey techniques, behaviour observation, heuristic procedures as workshops, and group-dynamics-based creative and training measures.

Matúš Šucha is an associate professor in the Psychology Department at Palacký University in Olomouc, Czech Republic. He specialises in traffic psychology, and his research focuses on mobility, traffic safety, and sustainable mobility.

'This book covers the psychology behind when and why we choose to walk, from Japan to Jordan, from South Africa to Norway, from Aristotélēs to a future with climate change. You learn about why people walk and why they do not walk from the Kindergartener's perspective as well as from sophisticated scientific models. I have been working with traffic safety for pedestrians for 40 years, and I still learned a lot from reading this book. You will too'. —*Per Gårder, University of Maine, USA*

'Ralf Risser and Matúš Šucha raise critical questions that have long concerned those of us in the field of traffic and mobility. Why is it so that so many people prefer car use over other, especially active traffic modes? What steers these choices and how can one motivate people to walk more? This book offers the reader a comprehensive overview of psychological aspects referring to walking and how to boost walking. It takes up health aspects, climate change issues, equity and social aspects, and safety concerns, among many others. Risser's and Šucha's book is of great interest both for experts in the field – traffic planners, public health professionals, traffic and mobility experts, students, and the general public. In short, it is interesting for everybody who is willing to support sustainable mobility and to learn how to live a more active life'. —*Hector Monterde-i-Bort, University of Valencia, Spain*

'The benefits of walking are well known but still very few cities and towns can be described as truly walkable, i.e. putting pedestrians first. This book offers a range of suggestions for how this goal can be reached, and it will therefore be a valuable addition to other books on walking and sustainable transport. As the title suggests, it has a psychological perspective emphasising the importance of understanding what motivates people to walk. However, in addition to this it clearly demonstrates that the creation of walkable cities is multi-faceted, and the approach is therefore holistic. The result is a comprehensive and stimulating read which will appeal to a wide audience'. —*Sonja Forward, Swedish National Road and Transport Research Institute VTI, Sweden*

'Although various safety measures have enhanced overall traffic safety, pedestrians are still the stepchildren of road traffic experts. Moreover, it's not justified to incorporate pedestrians in an undiscriminating way with bicycles and motorised two-wheelers as "vulnerable road users," as each of them carries different problems and asks for different solutions. Risser and Šucha have supplied a work of merit by giving an unprecedented and conclusive overview of all aspects of pedestrian quality needs in road traffic; among others practical aspects, statistics, psychological modelling for a sustainable mobility, and best practices to reconcile the different traffic modes. And we should give them credit for not proposing the oh-so-modern "renouncing" of other traffic modes in favour of walking. A highly recommended book for all who are seriously willing to know more about walking'. —*Wolfgang Fastenmeier, Berlin Psychological University, Germany*

Psychological Perspectives on Walking

Interventions for Achieving Change

Ralf Risser
Matúš Šucha

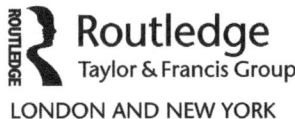

Routledge
Taylor & Francis Group

LONDON AND NEW YORK

First published 2021
by Routledge
2 Park Square, Milton Park, Abingdon, Oxon, OX14 4RN

and by Routledge
605 Third Avenue, New York, NY 10017

Routledge is an imprint of the Taylor & Francis Group, an informa business

British Library Cataloguing-in-Publication Data
A catalogue record for this book is available from the British Library

Library of Congress Cataloging-in-Publication Data
A catalog record has been requested for this book

ISBN: 978-0-367-32259-5 (hbk)
ISBN: 978-0-367-32258-8 (pbk)
ISBN: 978-0-429-31759-0 (ebk)

Typeset in Baskerville
by Nova Techset Private Limited, Bengaluru & Chennai, India

Contents

Introduction

Transport in its present form contributes considerably to a negative climate development. In order to stop this development, the mobility behaviour of people has to change. Societies may want to enhance such a change in the behaviour of their citizens. Among other things, more walking instead of car use where possible will be one goal. For this, a better understanding of the motives lying behind mobility behaviour is needed. Knowledge and methods of the fields of psychology, more specifically social and traffic psychology, will help to achieve this.

The main purpose of writing this book was to deliver a comprehensive overview of psychological knowledge on the issue of walking to readers as the oldest, most basic, and most important transport mode of all. It is written in a way which will, we hope, be understandable for other disciplines than psychology and also for the general population, while at the same time supporting all the conclusions strictly on the basis of empirical knowledge. The motivation for writing the book is, among other things, fuelled by sustainability, health, and public health objectives reflected in many municipal, regional, national, and supra-national master plans and white books.

The central conceptual tenet, thus, is the need to understand the multiple factors that influence walking behaviour, as a prerequisite for achieving change. This is well known in humanistic academic circles, but it remains necessary to continue to make this case more widely appreciated.

Information or knowledge alone will not change behaviour – we need to understand the foundations of behaviour in much greater detail and complexity, including emotions and 'irrational' motives (which hardly ever are irrational). This book is an attempt to describe in complexity and in an easy-to-understand way 'what lies behind the human behaviour', how we can change this behaviour, and how all this is implemented in the choice of a sustainable mode.

The lines of discussion in this book are strictly based on up-to-date research evidence.

THE EUROPEAN CHARTER OF PEDESTRIANS' RIGHTS

This is the full text of legislation adopted by the European Parliament in 1998.

I.   The pedestrian has the right to live in a healthy environment and freely to enjoy the amenities offered by public areas under conditions that adequately safeguard his physical and psychological well-being.

II.   The pedestrian has the right to live in urban or village centres tailored to the needs of human beings and not to the needs of the motor car and to have amenities within walking or cycling distance.

III.   Children, the elderly, and the disabled have the right to expect towns to be places of easy social contact and not places that aggravate their inherent weakness.

IV.   The disabled have the right to specify measures to maximise mobility, such as the elimination of architectural obstacles and the adequate equipping of public means of transport.

V.   The pedestrian has the right to urban areas which are intended exclusively for his use, are as extensive as possible, and are not mere 'pedestrian precincts' but in harmony with the overall organisation of the town.

VI.   The pedestrian has a particular right to expect;
   a.   compliance with chemical and noise emission standards for motor vehicles which scientists consider to be tolerable,
   b.   the introduction into all public transport systems of vehicles that are not a source of either air or noise pollution,
   c.   the creation of 'green lungs', including the planting of trees in urban areas,
   d.   the control of speed limits by modifying the layout of roads and junctions (e.g. by incorporating safety islands, etc.), so that motorists adjust their speed, as a way of safeguarding pedestrian and bicycle traffic effectively,
   e.   the banning of advertising which encourages an improper and dangerous use of the motor car,
   f.   an effective system of road signs whose design also takes into account the needs of the blind and the deaf,
   g.   the adoption of specific measures to ensure that vehicular and pedestrian traffic has ease of access to, and freedom of movement and the possibility of stopping on, roads and pavements respectively (for example: anti-slip pavement surfaces, ramps at kerbs to compensate for the difference

between the levels of the pavement and roadway, roads made wide enough for the traffic they have to carry, special arrangements while building work is in progress, adaptation of the urban street infrastructure to protect motor car traffic, and the provision of parking and rest areas and subways and footbridges),

h. the introduction of a system of risk liability so that the person creating the risk bears the financial consequences thereof (as has been the case in France, for example, since 1985).

VII. The pedestrian has the right to complete and unimpeded mobility, which can be achieved through the integrated use of the means of transport. In particular, he has the right to expect;

a. an extensive and well-equipped public transport service which will meet the needs of all citizens, from the physically fit to the disabled,

b. the provision of bicycle lanes throughout urban areas,

c. the creation of car parks which affect neither the mobility of pedestrians nor their ability to enjoy areas of architectural distinction.

VIII. Each Member State must ensure that comprehensive information on the rights of pedestrians is disseminated through the most appropriate channels and is made available to children from the beginning of their school career.[1]

---

[1] https://visionzero.ca/european-charter-of-pedestrians-rights-1988

1 Setting the scene

The aim of this chapter is to 'set the scene' for readers – to introduce the history of traffic, human needs, and different transport modes and describe what sustainability in transport means and which transport modes are sustainable and why.

The topic of walking is very challenging in times of intensive discussions concerning sustainability. The authors of this book are psychologists and social scientists, and therefore the approach will be via road users: if people do not move, there is no traffic; if people do not walk, there is no walking; and if people do not behave in a sustainable way, traffic will not be sustainable. To make road users – to make ourselves – behave in a sustainable way, we will need behavioural sciences.

What are the problems and challenges of the general situation? Where is the place for pedestrians, and what are the dangers and vulnerabilities they face? What solutions can make people walk more, at least over short distances and instead of short car trips? Just as a reminder, the EU project WALCYNG – Walking and cycling instead of short car trips (Hydén, Nilsson, & Risser) – was finalised in 1998, 20 years ago. So, at that time, there was obviously already the goal of achieving improvements in this respect. Can we say that the situation today is satisfactory? Are things nowadays organised according to the European Charter of Pedestrian Rights? The simple answer is: No, they are not!

But let us start at the beginning.

1.1 The individual has to be addressed

Walking is the first and original way for human beings to move about. Like most other animals, moving about is necessary for them in order to fulfil their needs for nourishment, protection against the weather and enemies, social contacts, and reproduction. This is in contrast to plants, most of which are sedentary in a strict sense – a plant usually does not move away from the place where it is 'planted'.

Without being mobile in the sense of being able to leave the place where we live, we could not exist (unless someone brings all the things that we need to our home or even to the place where we sit or lie), and without the use of our legs (or of a substitute for our legs), we could not even move to our car or to the means of public transport. And, of course, we could not ride a bicycle. Anyone who cannot use his/her legs is handicapped and cannot even manage all the things to be managed indoors, in which case he or she has to be taken care of by other people. We have to move about both indoors and outdoors in order to get the things necessary for our lives done. But this need is not only about getting somewhere or getting something done. One of the curious laws of traffic is that people all over the world spend roughly the same amount of time each day getting to where they need to go. Whether the setting is an African village or an American city, the daily round-trip commute clocks in at about one hour (Vanderbilt, 2008). The noted Italian physicist Cesare Marchetti has taken this idea one step further and pointed out that throughout history, well before the car, humans sought to keep their commute to about one hour. This 'cave instinct', as he calls it, reflects a balance between our desires for mobility (the more territory, the more resources one can acquire and the more mates one can meet) and domesticity (we tend to feel safer and more comfortable at home than on the road). In any case, we are not plants. We were evolved to move from one place to another.

Coming back to the headline: moving from place to place is an inherent human need. But this need does not necessarily have to be satisfied solely by walking. Maybe on some or many occasions some or many of us even want to avoid walking. When looking at Maslow's overview of human needs (Maslow, 1943; see Figure 1.1) we see that there are a lot of needs that push us to look for other mobility modes than walking: comfort, status, the need for achievement, hurry, long distances to be covered, protection (e.g. against adverse weather conditions), safety (by sitting 'safely' in a car in contrast to being exposed as a pedestrian), and so on. Some or all of these needs certainly lie behind the fact that since a very long time ago people have tried to replace walking with other modes and that the portion of walking trips – at least in the industrial world – has constantly gone down in recent decades, when such trips were counted. This aspect will be taken up at several points subsequently.

As we will also see subsequently, there are good reasons to try to stop this trend. Nowadays the following reasons more or less belong to the knowledge base in industrial countries: walking strengthens the heart, it lowers the risk of diabetes and cancer, it helps one lose weight, it prevents dementia, it tones up fitness, it boosts vitamin D (because one is outside), it keeps one young by boosting circulation and increasing the oxygen supply, it has an anti-depressive function, and, last but not least, it has no negative

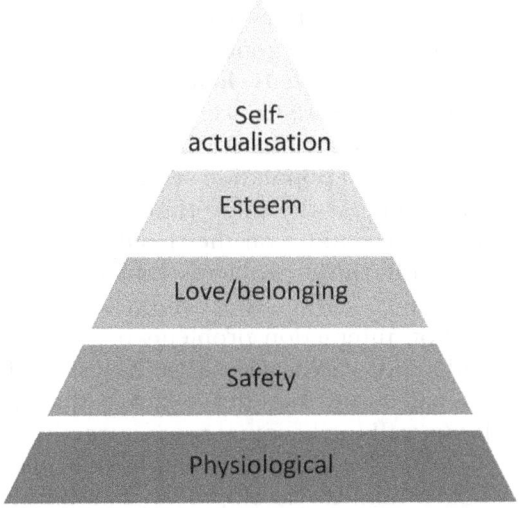

Figure 1.1 Maslow's hierarchy of human needs (Maslow, 1943).

impact on the environment. Physicians may excuse the laymen's wording in this list, but we all know what the wording means. Walking, regularly and for somewhat longer distances (some say 10,000 steps a day; others say 3000 is enough, or half an hour is enough) is healthy and makes us feel good (or at least better). Furthermore, besides health benefits, walking boosts social competences – people who walk more perform better in communication and other social skills. Last but not least, walking helps save money.

More generally, walking is an economically, ecologically, and socially sound mode of transport, as can be seen from the previous list of its advantages (these three criteria of sustainability will be discussed in more detail in Section 1.7 and in Chapter 2). Increasing the share of walking instead of using the car, which is an option for short trips, would certainly contribute to sustainability: it is cheap both for the individual and for society (the economy); it helps to protect the environment – zero emissions, only human energy is needed (ecology); and it supports, among other things, the quality of urban life and both public and individual health (social issues). Recent studies (Martin-Puerta, 2014) have shown that a change in the behaviour of citizens (e.g. the actual use of vehicles – or transport modes) is much more efficient with respect to CO^2 emissions than, for instance, the mere replacement of conventional vehicles with 'low-carb' vehicles. According to different analyses, about ~15%–20% of all car trips are shorter than 2 km (Hydén et al., 1998; Le Vine & Polak, 2009), a distance that can be tackled by walking, and ~50% of all car trips are shorter than 5 km, which can easily be tackled by cycling. In combination with public transport, much longer distances can be covered by environmentally friendly transport modes.

Both safety improvements and changes in the modal split call for a change in the current behaviour of road users (e.g. Groeger & Rothengatter, 1998). Therefore, psychologists or, more generally, social scientists will have to contribute. Strategies to make citizens change their behaviour will be based on know-how from these sciences. Concerning the support of sustainable mode choice, communication measures will have to be the focus, in which thorough analyses of different population segments' needs and exigencies will have to be considered. At the same time, the traffic safety work of the future will have to focus more on the specific traffic safety problems of pedestrians, especially those problems that are connected to their interaction with motorised traffic. More empirical work will be needed in order to find out how interaction problems between road user groups become manifest and in order to develop hypotheses as to how to influence the behaviour of the parties involved in such a way that appropriate safety is guaranteed and thus walking becomes more attractive.

In sum, if one helps to make (more) people walk (more), this means that one supports the sustainable development of mobility, especially if this helps to replace short car trips with walking. Subsequently, theories and models that help provide an understanding of the motives behind mode choice, discussions of ways to enhance walking, and examples that should demonstrate the success of such efforts will be presented.

The advantages of increased amounts of walking by as many citizens as possible can, of course, be seen from a society's point of view. If (more) people walk (more), this will help the health system save money, it will increase citizens' productivity and thus strengthen the economy, and it will generate positive effects for the social climate. At the same time, the costs to society needed for car use (infrastructure, crashes) will decrease. But in order to reach this goal, several of the advantages that were mentioned have to be transformed into arguments that are convincing for different groups of citizens. When personal gains become obvious to people, the probability that they will invest in a certain behaviour increases. The idea of moving to more sustainable mobility only by *renouncing* car use, at least on certain occasions, has no future (see also Kubitzki & Fastenmeier, 2019). Renouncing is nothing that motivates us positively, unless a strong power lies behind it: idealism, faith, superstition, or the like. Usually, we need to see some more concrete positive reinforcement or reward.

To boost fitness and health, to help protect the environment in the easiest way, and others are very good arguments to be used as elements of any convincing communication addressed to the individual. Additionally, the fact that walking is cheap is a good argument, but it has its downsides and is obviously not really convincing. The simplicity of walking and the fact that it is so cheap and without any glamorous characteristics at first sight make it look a poor man's mode of little attraction (also derived from history – walker, wanderer, pilgrim – someone who is so poor that he has nothing but his legs). However, instead of looking at walking as the poor man's mode, one may also argue that walking is the mode of clever people who, for instance, do their daily physical exercise in the most efficient way, not wasting time and money on extra training hours. For anybody whose journey to work is shorter than, say, half an hour, the formula 'I walk to my job because I am a busy person' could be a realistic and at the same time rather witty way to put it.

Thus, from being an inherent human need, for many people, walking could become something that is done with conviction and engagement when they are reminded of its positive aspects with good arguments (see, e.g. Monheim, 2010; Ramos & Alves, 2010). However, as we will see later, under appropriate conditions, walking as a means of transport could also become something that is done with pleasure, as suggested by Sauter (2010), quoting Antoine de Saint-Exupéry. In fact, it should be done with pleasure: walking as the mode of transport of smart and responsible citizens.

1.2   Is it really worthwhile?

Is it worthwhile to enhance walking? Do measures in this direction pay? There will be more discussion of the practical value of enhancing walking later on in this book (Chapter 5), but let us look at some success stories in order to gain an appetite for more talk about enhancing walking. The first example is from New Zealand:

> Notoriously car-centric Auckland in New Zealand recently published a report showing pedestrians as the most economically important transport mode in the city. They estimated that policies which put people off walking on Queen Street, a major shopping area, cost 11,7 million NZ$ a year.
> Shared areas were created in and around Fort Street, a mixed commercial and residential area in the central business district. The city replaced car parking on some streets with trees and outdoor seating, and removed bollards and kerbs that had separated cars from pedestrians. The moves created more space for open-air activities, and made clear accessible routes for the visually impaired.
> This new pedestrian network, at a cost of 23 million NZ$, increased pedestrian volumes by 54% and consumer spending by 47%. Meanwhile, the number of vehicles fell by 25% – and 80% said they felt safer in the area.
> Bruno Royce, who conducted a safety review of the scheme, says shared spaces aren't suitable everywhere, but can be a useful first step towards full pedestrianisation. Despite the changes he says some cars still travelled above 22 kph, higher than the 10-kph ideal. He would like to see the city narrowing or "kinking" the shared space to slow cars, or ban cars completely for part of the day.
> (What would a truly walkable city look like?, 2018)

The next example is from the United States, certainly not the exemplar of a country that supports walking (but we know that in New York, Boston, San Francisco, and other cities, there are areas where walking *is* a pleasure):

> Walkability is both an end and a means, as well as a measure... After several decades spent redesigning pieces of cities, trying to make them more livable, and more successful, I have watched my focus narrow to this topic as the one issue that seems to both influence and embody most of the others. Get walkability right and so much of the rest will follow. The healthiest, wealthiest, most sustainable, and vibrant communities in cities around the world are unique in many ways. But there is one factor above all others that these communities have in common: they are, nearly without fail, highly walkable places.
>
> There is good reason for this. Every day, every one of us is a pedestrian. No matter where we are going or how we choose to get there, every journey begins and ends with a walk. But by creating places that are built for walking, we flick a switch that unlocks the best our cities can offer us and creates communities that are healthier and richer in every way.
>
> (Walkability: Creating great cities by putting pedestrians first, 2015; see also Chapter 5, Success stories)

Let us now stop displaying best practice – this will be a task for later in this book – and let us answer the question whether it is worthwhile to support walking with the words of Stephanie Marino, a Los Angeles designer. She simply states that 'a walkable city is a better city' (LandDesign, 2015) and we hope to be able to demonstrate this in the course of this book.

1.2.1   *The case of captive walkers*

But what is the situation in many non-industrial countries, especially in less developed countries? There, many more people than in most of the richer industrial countries walk, simply because many of them have to walk long distances to fulfil their needs, because they cannot afford a car or any other motorised vehicle, and because there is no public transport available for many trips. Also, much more than in other countries, in less developed countries, the street is a place to live, to spend time, and for children to play. One example that can be mentioned is the situation in many places in South Africa, where people are brought to their townships by minibuses but then have to walk longer distances in order to reach their homes. Sometimes, then, their route leads them along motorways, which they also have to cross at certain points. A situation in which people have to walk longer distances because they have no other options, and where they have to do this under very poor conditions, is of course not something that should be maintained. It has to be added that such cases are more frequent in developing countries, but they are not restricted to those countries. Even in developed countries, there are people who cannot afford a car and who live in areas where public transport is poor and where the infrastructure has developed in such a way that many destinations cannot be reached (easily) by walking (e.g. the countryside in many cases). Such preconditions are even more of a problem for old people who are not able or willing to drive a car anymore and whose ability to walk longer distances is limited by reduced stamina or fragility.

In all these cases, the goal cannot be to convince people to walk (more), and it would be cynical to talk about the advantages of walking concerning health and mood. Rather, politicians and planners have to be convinced to provide better means of transport and better preconditions for walking. When walking is, at least for some citizens, the only mobility option, it has to be ensured that it is safe and reasonably comfortable.

Concerning all the aspects and arguments referred to in this introductory section, there is more to come in the following chapters of this book.

1.3   The history of walking

Walking, or, as Kagge (2019) states in his book *Walking*, 'placing one foot in front of the other', is the most natural form of locomotion for humans, something that we learn as small children and that we do not want to abandon until it is necessary in advanced old age.

Walking – on two legs – can in fact be considered *the* human way of moving about, in contrast to most (other) animals, which usually do not walk on two legs, at least not in an upright position as humans do. Anthropologists assume that the predecessors of modern humans – *Homo erectus* – started to move about on two legs in an upright position three million years ago or even earlier. Donald Johanson found a skeleton of a woman, a predecessor of *Homo sapiens* called *Australopithecus afarensis*, in Ethiopia, which was dated 3.2 million years back. He gave the woman the name Lucy (Johanson & Edey, 1981; Johanson & Shreeve, 1989). He and his colleagues assumed that Lucy had walked upright. This assumption was strongly supported when the researchers found metatarsal bones from other skeletons the same age as Lucy's in the same region of Africa, the shape of which confirmed their assumption. At that time, it seems, moving about on two legs became humans' main mode of mobility. Scientists argue that an upright position and walking not only provided new opportunities of mobility but also that we became what we are (modern civilisations) because we evolved to an upright position. This made it possible to use our hands for other purposes than to move and to see the world from another perspective.

Humans started riding horses (Carr, 2019) in approximately 800 BC, but this was long after humans had started to use wheels, at first for pulling wagons (between ~4000 and 3300 BC). These wagons were first used for transporting goods, but also within the context of warfare, and only later for the transportation of people, most probably often together with goods.

But even then, for many people and still for some thousand years, the main mode of transport was solely by using their legs, although not all would just walk; hunters, people involved in warfare, and sportspeople would often run instead of just walking.

In ancient times, walking was write frequently instead of probably connected with philosophy. Socrates, as is known, could not keep still, always taking strolls in the agora. Aristotle probably owed his nickname 'walker' ('peripatetikos') to the fact that he kept moving on his legs all the time. In the times right after Aristotle (~350 BC) the school of the Peripatetics, a school of philosophers, was founded (~280 BC). The typical characteristic of the members of this group was that they developed their ideas and exchanged their thoughts while walking around in pairs or groups in the *peripatos*, the portico of the philosophers' school. The idea was that the sensory perception of the space would activate the resources of the brain. But in all these cases, walking was limited to within the city walls, one of the (more or less important) motives also being 'to be seen', while the Cynics were forever on the move, shuffling like vagabonds and rambling from city to city (Gros, 2015).

Much later, a long list of philosophers and poets appear to have been confident walkers in the sense that their most important and fruitful thoughts would come to their minds while walking: Rousseau, Kierkegaard, Nietzsche, Rimbaud, or Nerval (Solnit, 2001; Gros, 2015). We also know from Immanuel Kant that he walked along his own special path every day, the same path every day, at exactly the same time every day (from 5 p.m. to 6 p.m. sharp) (Precht, 2011). Kant believed that this rigorous discipline (in addition to others of his habits) was the reason for his long life (he died at the age of 80). According to Heinrich Heine, people would adjust their watches according to the moment when the philosopher passed by rather than according to the bells of the nearby church. Nowhere is it stated explicitly that these walks were occasions on which important thoughts would form. One may assume, though, that Kant attributed great importance to this routine, which he kept up for many years. Last but not least, we have to mention America's first nature writer, David Henry Thoreau, the poet and spokesman of the wild natural world. Thoreau was a radical walker, taking strolls of 4–6 hours each day, with little understanding for those who did not:

> When sometimes I am reminded that the mechanics and shopkeepers stay in their shops not only all the forenoon, but all the afternoon too, sitting with crossed legs, so many of them—as if the legs were made to sit upon, and not to stand or walk upon—I think that they deserve some credit for not having all committed suicide long ago.
>
> (Thoreau, 1994)

Thoreau's books *Walking* and *Walden* became masterpieces of 'nature and walking' literature.

Walking appeals both to the gods, or better to say, to the church (pilgrimage), and to worldly affairs. Important communication by the public or interested groups to decision-makers and representatives of our societies was, and still is, forwarded on foot (e.g. Gandhi's protest walks, Martin Luther King's March to Washington). According to Solnit (2001), there is something symbolic connected to walking in these cases. For instance, people let themselves be brought near to a sanctuary by car, but then a symbolic last part of the pilgrimage is done by walking. It really looks as if it had to be walking, in such cases.

Before the 18th century, dangers seem to have lurked for those who walked on the streets, or the preconditions for walking were not appropriate either technically or socially outside villages and settlements. People who could afford to arranged for walking routes within the limits of their own premises, often shaped as gardens or parks. It was not usual to walk outside those 'protected' areas. Then, in the middle of the 18th century, walking outside those private areas became more common. For instance, public parks were instituted as places where people would walk. In England, those parks would be kept quite natural, resembling a wild natural environment. Later, instead of walking in parks that resembled a wild natural environment, people would start to walk in such an environment itself. Solnit (2001) cites William Wordsworth, who describes his hikes in the Lake District together with his sister. Under such circumstances, the activity of walking became a goal in itself, while where one went was less important. This aspect reflects the fact that walking, or even just being outside, in natural surroundings or in pleasant places designed by men, can be a pleasure. But in most places in Europe, this walking for pleasure was an activity for the aristocracy and other privileged classes; as Gros (2015) notes, public gardens were places much favoured by young girls in the flower of their beauty, married women on the lookout for adventure, and widows seeking consolation. Therefore, associations were founded that were intended to help the less wealthy layers of society to also *savour the joy of walking* in nature, such as, for instance, in 1895, the Naturfreunde (Friends of Nature) in Austria,[1] which for many years also had branches in the United States (Solnit, 2001). The pleasure of walking in natural surroundings is of course still a topic today, though rather dealt with by environmental psychology and not so much in the area of transport. Still, the authors of this book always have their eyes open for texts and information dealing with walking, and when hiking in British Columbia, we found the *Nature Diary of a Quiet Pedestrian*, written and illustrated by Philip Croft, with wonderful descriptions and illustrations of insects, larger animals, and plants, some of which we would then meet and recognise in the course of our wanderings (Croft, 1986).

'To savour the joy of walking' sounds like a good slogan reflecting the pleasure connected to this activity: from a psychological point of view, it is obvious that as soon as pleasure is connected to any activity, this activity will become more frequent, or present high levels of the activity will be preserved. Maybe it turns out that trying to connect walking with pleasure, even in the driest case of fulfilling a duty, is the way to go when we want to convince (more) people – or even just ourselves – to walk (more). *Renouncing* something will not happen, as already stated.

1.4   To work and to school

An important perspective on walking is related to work and education. Back in the times when agriculture was the main source of income for the vast majority of the population, and smaller portions were dealing with crafts and trade and even smaller ones with academic professions (teachers, physicians, lawyers, and also artists and architects), most workplaces were near to people's homes or even in the same building. Most people could, and did, walk to their work. At the beginning of the industrial era, factory owners often provided housing facilities in the vicinity of the factories. Thus, the distances to workplaces were short. Among others, Bryan (1997) writes about Henry Ford's endeavours in this respect. Also well known is Tomáš Bat'a, who always provided housing near his factories for his employees and their families. The appearance and spread of trains, trams, buses, and cars changed things rapidly. It was possible to cover longer distances to get to work, and the necessity to keep the length of the trip to work to an acceptable walking distance became weaker. For many years now, these distances have been increasing. However, the average amount of time we spend on getting to work has remained more or less the same. In Figure 1.2, data from Austria shows that there, faster transport modes have not helped us save time, it seems. We assume that the situation is similar in most other industrial countries, although results from the United States (Santos

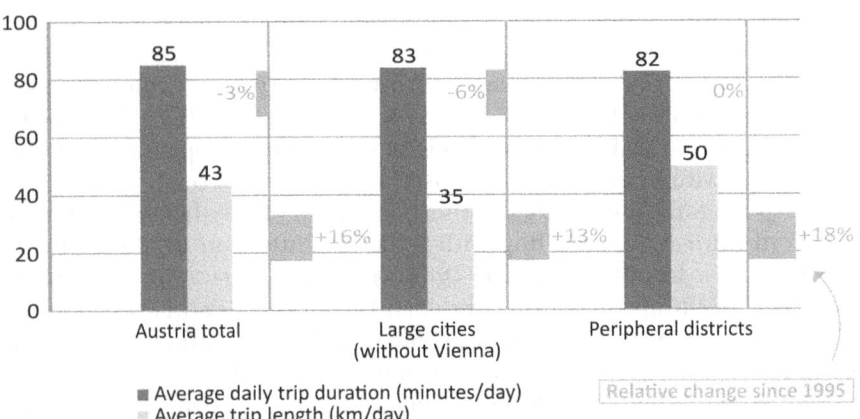

Figure 1.2 Distance covered and time spent on outdoor mobility – 1995 vs. 2013 (Tomschy & Roider, 2015).

et al., 2011) indicate that trip lengths there have been becoming shorter approximately since the turn of the millennium.

In former times, when the distances to work were usually short(er) and could be covered by walking, there was an interesting phenomenon, though. From the end of mediaeval times up to the beginning of industrialisation, many apprentices all over Europe took to walking to other regions and countries for many weeks or months or even years, with the goal being to learn about techniques, mores, and cultures there. For them, this was the precondition for becoming master craftsmen. As they did not have much money, they had to walk, except for the occasional lifts they would sometimes get on wagons or coaches.

Concerning the way to school, there are different stories. In the rural or mountainous regions of Europe, it was quite usual that for decades up to the '50s of the last century, schoolchildren would have to walk for hours in all weather conditions in order to get to school. Chaloupka and Risser (2004) compiled a booklet with reports of colleagues working in the area of transport and mobility who talked about their own mobility during their childhood and youth. In 2019, the list of these reports was completed by 26 more short summaries of other colleagues on the same topic. When reading these contributions (see Chapter 2.4), one realises especially the following: experiences that are remembered and told today are not so different from each other, in spite of stemming from places as distant from each other as Jönköping (Sweden), Delhi (India), Valencia (Spain), Cork (Ireland), Nagoya (Japan), and Moscow (Russia). Leisure trips with parents and relatives and pets and animals play important roles. Walking is a predominant transport mode during childhood and youth. The first trips in different vehicles – from bicycles to cars – left impressions, and accidents caused distress and anxiety in some cases. One does not have the slightest difficulty in understanding either the stories told in the reports received or the emotions expressed directly or indirectly in connection with the reported experiences of walking, of other active modes, of activities outside, with friends or alone. The authors consider these reports a strong motivation to invest energy in research about mobility in the future. Soft mobility may increase without negative global consequences. If the preconditions are appropriate, it is usually perceived positively by the individuals who practise it. We do not depend psychologically on the car as much as we are often led to believe.

However, at the time of the production of this book, in industrial countries, more than three-quarters of the trips to school are made by car, and this portion is increasing internationally. Figure 1.3 shows an example from Austria, where trips by car to accompany children to the kindergarten make up almost 80%, while only 15% of these trips are made by walking, in spite of the fact that in Austria, in most cases, kindergartens are situated a (short) walking distance from people's homes.

Know-how about children as pedestrians, their perception capabilities, and their limits in terms of understanding dangers and safety

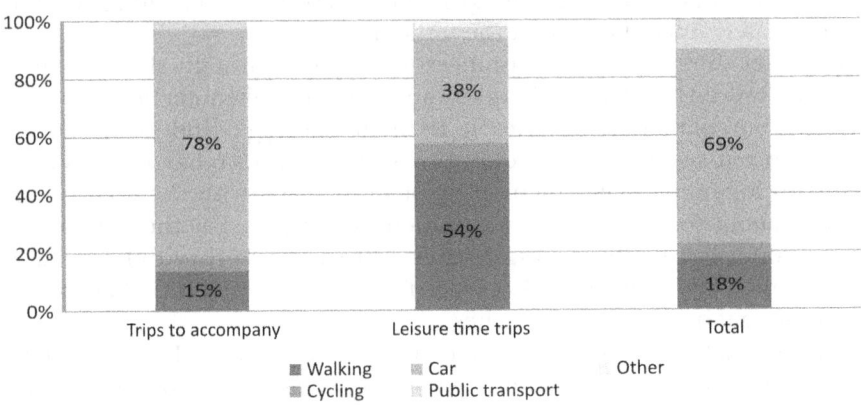

Figure 1.3 Modal split for trips to school and leisure trips in Austria (FFG project ANFANG).[8]

(Ampofo-Boateng & Thomson, 1986) should be central parts of safety and education programmes (Maring & Van Schagen, 1990) for both car drivers and children themselves. This education should not cover only topics dealing with safety, but mobility and mode choice as well. We should make sure that we socialise our children to the world of mode choice, not only to car use.

The other group which needs our special attention is senior citizens. The older we get, the more important walking becomes. Promoting walks and meetings between generations in appropriate streets and spaces will contribute to social well-being (e.g. Bell et al., 2013).

1.5 Efforts to avoid walking?

Some 3000 years or more ago, very powerful individuals – for instance, emperors in China and pharaohs in Egypt – started being transported in litters, while most other people walked in order to fulfil their daily needs. Now, the facts that the pharaohs let themselves be carried around in litters and that people started using horse-drawn wagons some 5000 years ago and riding on horses some 3000 years ago point to one thing: there was a notion that finding alternatives to walking could be advantageous. Because they were quicker? Because travelling like that was perceived as more comfortable? Because not 'having to walk' denoted higher status? Because walking was a tedious activity in most daily routine tasks? Because they – these alternative modes – were more efficient ways of carrying goods? Whatever. Over the millennia and centuries up to today, many different forms of transportation, or mobility modes, came into use. Walking became less important, while during the last centuries the portion of walking trips remained different for different groups or strata of people and in different

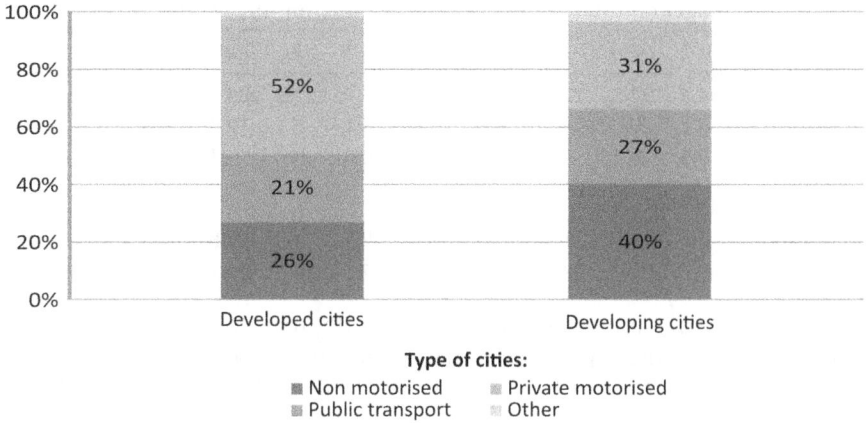

Figure 1.4 Modal split in developed and developing cities (UITP, 2015).

countries. For instance, in African countries, the portions of people who walk are much higher than, for example, in the OECD countries.[2] Figure 1.4 compares cities in developed and developing countries. Walking and public transport play a more important role in developing cities, while car use is preeminent in developed ones.

Can we say that this is a matter of evolution? In some respects, probably yes. In the past (and in some developing countries nowadays), daily physical activity to make a living was quite intense, so it made sense to 'rest' (e.g. ride a horse instead of walking). But nowadays, the situation is quite different. In most developed countries, the daily level of physical activity is well below what is needed. In this respect, we might say that now 'evolution' is naturally leading us back to those transport modes which require physical activity.

We will not go into more detail concerning the history of walking during the last 3000 or more years and by what means walking has been replaced – litters, chariots, coaches, buses, trams, trains, the car, mopeds, or bicycles. However, when looking at the development of the percentage of walking trips in OECD countries, one can see that there has obviously been a constant decrease in recent decades. But there are indications that this might change, although the situation is still unclear, as the graphs and tables subsequently show. For instance, Table 1.1 shows that since 2003, there has been no further reduction of walking trips in Germany.

Figure 1.5 shows that there also seems to be an increase in walking in the United States, both with respect to the number of trips and the distances covered (Santos et al., 2011). We can see that since ~2000, the portions of walking have been increasing in the United States, in Germany, in the Netherlands, and in Denmark, and those of cycling in Germany and the Netherlands, while those figures kept decreasing – in any case until 2008 – in France and the United Kingdom. Further, Figure 1.6 shows that between

Table 1.1 Percentages of different modes in Germany from 1975 to 2015 (MiD, 2019)

	1975	1990	1994	2000	2003	2005	2007	2009	2011	2013	2015
Walks	34.3	27.3	27.2	26.9	23.3	23.0	22.9	23.8	23.3	23.2	23.1
Cycle trips	8.7	9.6	9.8	9.8	8.8	8.7	8.7	9.4	9.8	9.8	9.7
Public transport (cities)	9.5	8.4	8.7	8.7	8.5	9.0	9.2	9.1	9.1	9.1	9.0
Rail transport	1.5	1.6	1.9	2.0	2.0	2.1	2.3	2.3	2.5	2.5	2.6
Private motor transport	46	53.0	52.4	52.5	57.2	57.1	56.9	55.2	55.3	55.3	55.5
Air transport	0.0	0.1	0.1	0.1	0.1	0.1	0.1	0.1	0.1	0.1	0.1
Total	100	100	100	100	100	100	100	100	100	100	100

1995 and 2013, there was a considerable decrease in walking in Austria, while slightly more cycling is taking place.

Have we reached the bottom concerning the portion of walking? In such a case, the end of the chapter on the history of walking could be a blunt statement: that the portion of walking has been going down everywhere in the Western world for a very long time but that we have reached a point where this trend could maybe have stopped. The data presented by Santos

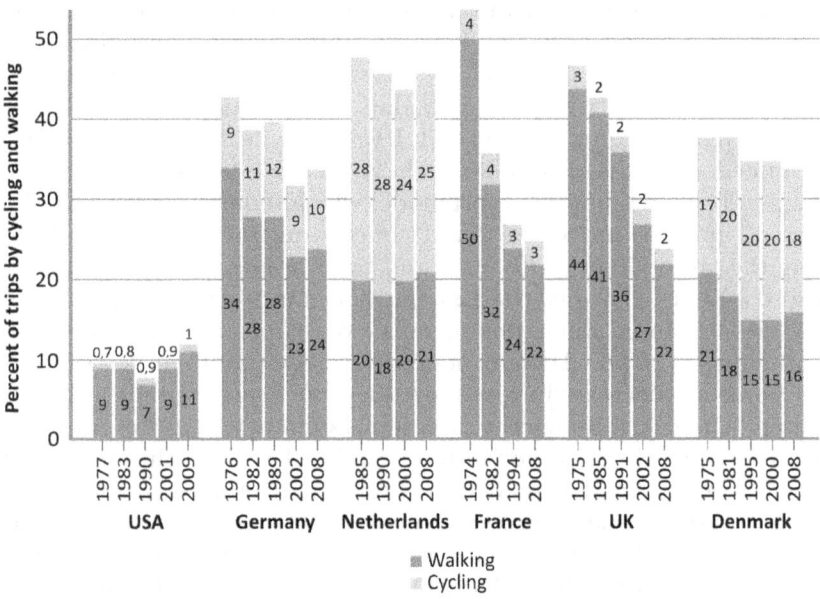

Note: Dissimilarities in data collection methods, timing, and variable definitions limit the comparability of the modal shares shown. The increase reported for the United States in the combined walk and bike share of trips between 1990 and 2001 probably results from a change in methodology that captured previously underreported walk trips.

Figure 1.5 Percentage of trips by cycling and walking in selected countries (Santos et al., 2011).

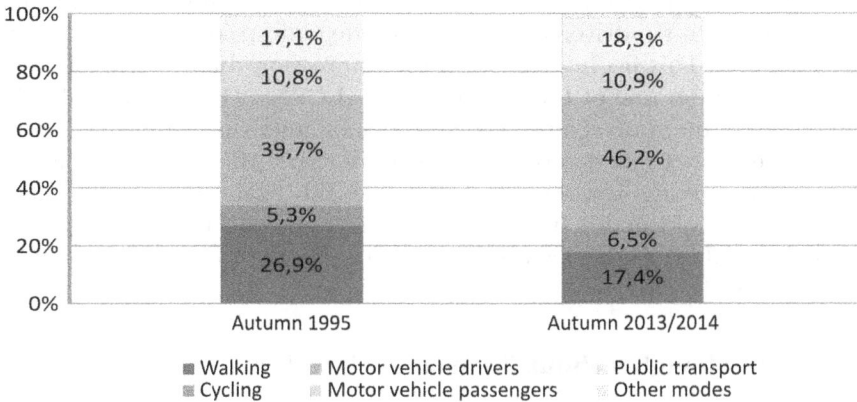

Figure 1.6 Modal split in Austria 1995 and 2013/2014 (Austrian Department of Transport, Innovation, and Infrastructure BMVIT, Österreich Unterwegs 2013/2014).

et al. (2011; see Table 1.2) might also allow such an optimistic assessment concerning the portions of walking.

The fact that much of the media nowadays deals with the topic of walking rather extensively (e.g. https://www.sustrans.org.uk/our-blog/research/all-themes/all/active-travel-in-the-media-exploring-representations-of-walking-and-cycling-in-uk-and-scottish-online-news/) is also encouraging. Thus, maybe the end of the story is not a negative one.

In any case, at the end of this section, we allow ourselves a personal opinion: the image of walking as a transport mode (not as a leisure-time or sport activity) has been low for a very long time. One story that reflects this

Table 1.2 Average annual person trips/household/mode of transport/MSA size (Santos et al., 2011)

Mode of transport							
SMSA or MSA size	*1977*	*1983*	*1990*	*1995*	*2001*	*2009*	*95% CI*
Private							
ALL	2351	2152	2861	3307	3090	2892	30
Public Transport							
ALL	73	60	58	67	58	66	4
Walking							
ALL	261	226	234	205	309	362	13
All Modes							
ALL	2808	2628	3262	3828	3581	3466	32

Abbreviation: (S)MSA = (Standard) Metropolitan Statistical Area.

is about the so-called 'Läufer' (= sprinters) in Vienna, who in former times ran in front of horse-driven coaches and drove pedestrians away with whips (Szegö, 2004). This fits in nicely with the impression that the interviewees gave within the frame of the EU project WALCYNG (Hydén et al., 1997), namely that in many countries and places and on many occasions, pedestrians were treated as second-class road users. Many people, it seems, still look at walking as a second-class mode. But again, there might have been a change of the tide in the last 20 years, especially in the cities of the Western world, where pedestrians could become the prototypes of 'smart and responsible' citizens.

1.6   Some thoughts about ('reasonable') walking distances

Walking is slow, and only relatively short distances can be covered within a reasonable time. What is 'reasonable' depends, of course, on the function and purpose of any walk and on the attitudes of the person involved. Where walking itself is the goal, when wandering, taking strolls, on a pilgrimage, when doing the *paseo* (promenading) on the plaza or in the public garden (Solnit, 2001, p. 66), or when walking as an 'urban flaneur' as described by Walter Benjamin, a 'reasonable' time span is certainly calculated differently from walking on a daily basis with different goals that should be achieved within a limited time connected to the things to be tackled there. Walking 'per se', for its own sake, and walking as a way to get from A to B are very different in this respect. Which length of a walking trip is reasonable is also subject to personal taste. Half an hour's walk may appear acceptable to one person but totally impossible to another one. Anyway, many destinations to be reached within the frame of everyday life (especially in cities), given today's infrastructure that has developed as a result of the technical possibilities available to cover longer distances ad hoc, are too far away to be covered by walking for everybody. We need bicycles, public transport, or cars to reach these goals.

Figure 1.7 shows how many trips are covered by walking (and cycling) and in how many cases other modes are used in cities in Canada, the United States, and selected European countries. The data for such tables is usually gathered with the help of surveys and hardly ever by counting. Likewise, whether walking was counted only for trips from door to door or even as a part of a trip chain is not always clear. Many statistics of the modal split only include the main mode, that is, the one with which the largest part of the trip was covered. For instance, a five-minute walk to the metro might not, and often is not, mentioned or counted, and only the metro trip appears in the statistics. And, in fact, every trip includes some amount of walking, which may vary from a few metres to a few kilometres. We assume that the real amount of walking is severely underestimated in the statistical tables that we get to read. New technologies such as personal pedometers (e.g. as a gadget in smartphones) are very promising for gathering more

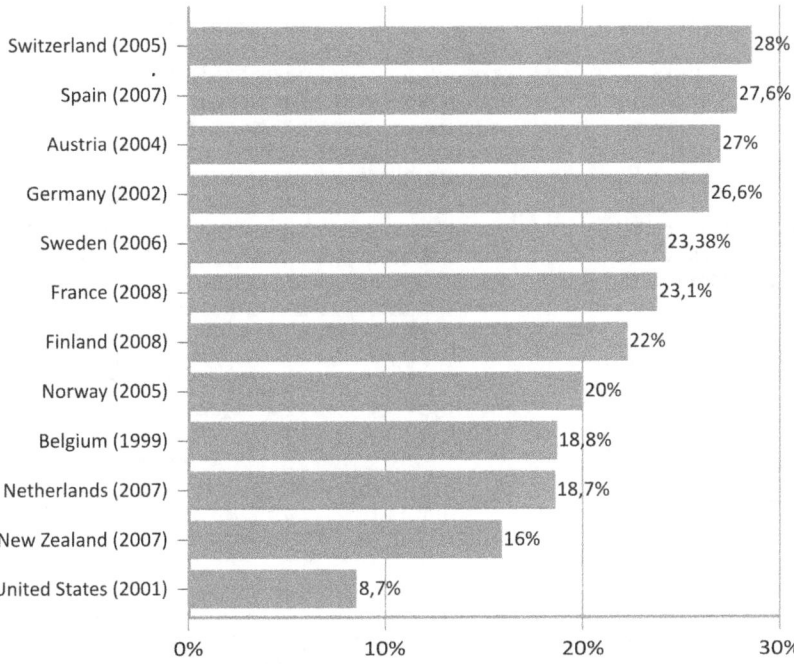

Figure 1.7 Percentage of walking trips of all day trips in the United States, New Zealand, and European countries (Pucher & Dijkstra, 2000).

reasonable data about daily walking distances. The only cases where there is no need to walk in the public space are those when one has a garage at home, at one's workplace, in the shopping mall, and so on. In Europe, this is certainly a rare case. Maybe in Canada and in the United States, this is more usual, but is still probably far from being the case generally. Public transport use is always combined with, at least, very short walks. Those people who probably cover the fewest metres on foot are cyclists. One should maybe also refer to up-and-coming mobility modes, generally called personal e-transporters (PeTs), such as electroscooters, segways, electronically steered mono-wheels, and so on, the portion of daily use of which is still rather unclear: certainly not huge, but growing. Anyway, they do not appear in Figure 1.8.

Quite a lot of walking is done in cities in Sweden, Austria, France, Italy, and Switzerland, followed by Germany and Denmark. The smallest amount of walking in European cities is registered in England and Wales. In the Netherlands, walking is more frequent than in England and Wales but less frequent than in the other mentioned European countries, the reason being that an enormous portion of the population cycles there, followed by Denmark, Germany, Sweden, Switzerland, and Austria. The proportions of cyclists in France, Italy, and England and Wales are lower. Comparably, in

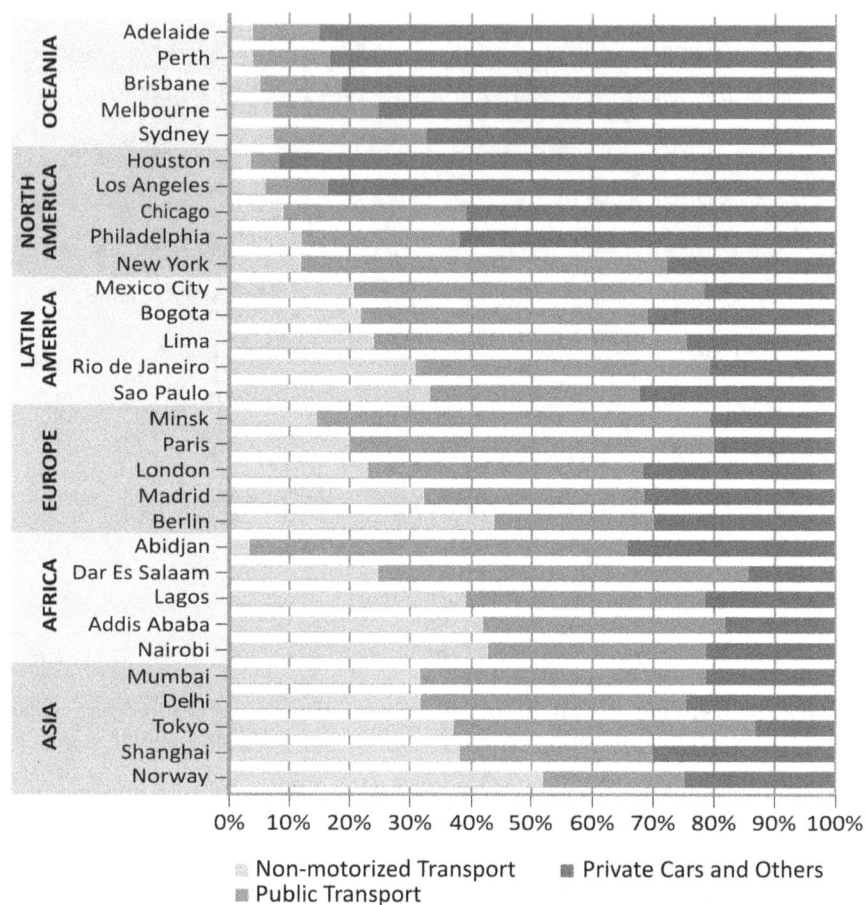

Figure 1.8 Urban walking and cycling (%) in United States, Canada, and selected European countries in 1995 (Pucher & Dijkstra, 2000).

Canada and the United States, walking and cycling do not seem to play any important role at all, although we know that there are cities and/or places there with high proportions of pedestrians. They will be referred to in the last chapter of this book.

In a study carried out by the OECD (Figure 1.9), a look was taken at the percentages of pedestrians for whole countries, that is, the counting was not limited to urban walking. For those countries that are represented in both Tables 1.1 and 1.2, one can compare the percentages. The differences are not too large. In some cases, the percentages are almost the same (Austria, France, the Netherlands), while in Germany, Switzerland, and the United States, the percentage is even larger when one looks at the whole country, and in Sweden, when one looks at trips in the whole

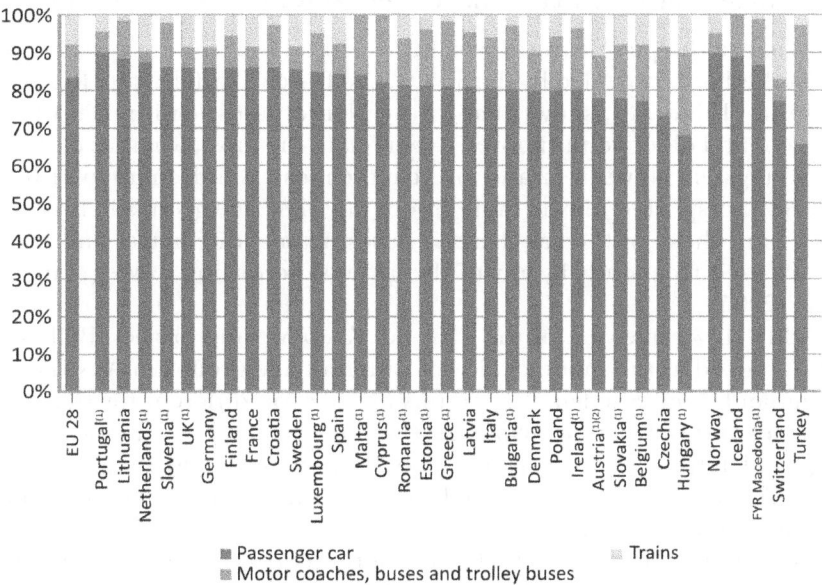

Note: excluding powered two-wheelers. Cyprus, Malta and Iceland: railways not applicable.
(1) Includes estimates or provisional data.
(2) The railway in Liechtenstein is owned and operated by the Austrian ÖBB and included in their statistics.

Figure 1.9 Modal split of inland passenger transport in 2014 of total inland passenger km (Laakso & Heiskanen, 2017).

country, the percentage of walkers is substantially smaller than that of walking trips in cities.

So the question is how well walking is represented in the usual statistics. Figure 1.9, referring to the EU and to associated countries, gives an impression. In spite of the caption stating 'Modal split of inland passenger transport', no trips by walking (nor cycling) are included. This shows clearly that not even researchers automatically think of walking when they discuss 'passenger transport'. This is a serious shortcoming. The reason might be that walking is perceived (correctly) as a basic and natural human activity, something that is so obvious that we 'forget' to deal with it. The problem is that this approach leads to the incorrect assumption that 'walkers always find their way' and that they do not need any relevant infrastructure (unlike cars).

As we have seen in Figure 1.7, the percentages of walking plus cycling, with walking usually being the larger part, in the cities of the highly urbanised European countries, France, Italy, Switzerland, Germany, Austria, and the Netherlands, vary between ~28% and ~45%. Walking is always at around 20% or more. This is certainly not negligible, even if one takes the transport system of the whole country as a reference. The percentages displayed in Figure 1.9 point in the same direction, even if the data collection took place at different points in time and was carried out by different institutes.

1.7   Mode choice: Who are the walkers and what do they need?

But who are the people in these statistics? Who walks (most)? Data from the Netherlands provided by the SWOV, the Dutch Traffic Safety Research Institute (Table 1.3), shows that in the Netherlands, children up to 11 years old and older adults above 75 years walk the most, whereas children and youngsters between 12 and 17 cycle the most. Children up to 11 years are also transported in cars quite frequently. The age groups between 25 and 74 are those of the car drivers. Buses, trams, the metro, and trains are not used frequently by any of the groups, according to Wegman and Aarts (2005).

Within the framework of the ERA-net Keep Moving project, Bell et al. (2010) looked at the mode choice of different age groups in Austria, the Netherlands, and Sweden. The results are not too different for the three countries and show, in principle, that walking increases in importance as we get older, while the importance of other transport modes declines with age. In Austria, for 75% of the people over 80, walking is the most important transport mode (Figure 1.10).

The older people get (above 60), the more frequently they walk, and they probably have to rely on walking and – if we are talking about rural areas – on poor public transport in order to be autonomously mobile. Old and very old people will be captive walkers more often than others, especially in the countryside, if they want to live an autonomous life and not be dependent on others to give them a lift or assist them in other ways.

Table 1.3 Modal split in the Netherlands (2005)

Mode	Age								
	0–11	*12–17*	*18–24*	*25–29*	*30–39*	*40–49*	*50–59*	*60–74*	*75+*
Walking (%)	29	18	20	19	18	17	18	25	34
Cycling (%)	29	52	23	17	20	23	22	24	17
Moped/light moped (%)	0	3	2	1	1	1	1	0	1
Motorcycle/ scooter (%)	0	0	0	0	0	0	0	0	0
Car (%)	40	17	37	56	56	55	54	46	38
Bus (%)	1	5	8	2	1	1	2	2	4
Tram/ metro (%)	0	1	3	2	1	1	1	1	1
Train (%)	0	2	6	3	2	2	1	1	1
Rest (%)	0	1	0	0	0	0	0	1	3
Unknown (%)	0	0	0	0	0	0	0	0	0
Total (%)	100	100	100	100	100	100	100	100	100

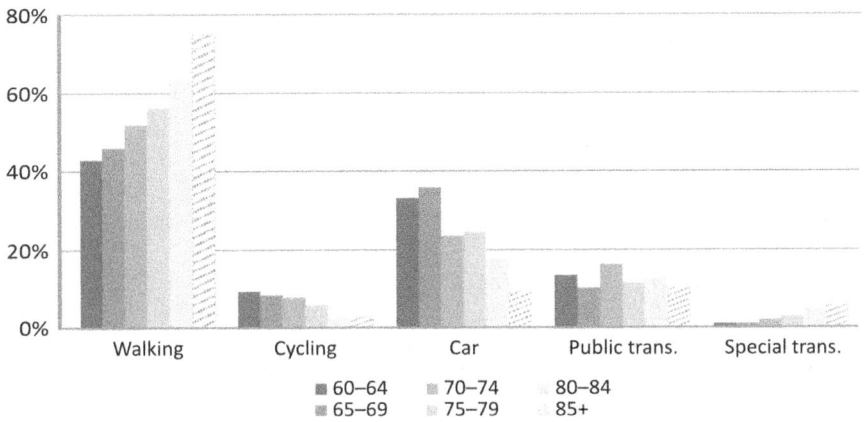

Figure 1.10 Most frequently used transport modes (Bell et al., 2010, SZENAMO).

Other groups of people who have no opportunity to drive a motor vehicle are children and youngsters below 15 years (which is the age from which on in many countries in the world, riding a moped is allowed). Before that age, autonomous mobility – that is, mobility independent of parents or other accompanying persons – is possible only on foot (from school age on, i.e. six years of age in many places), by public transport, if available (from six to seven years upwards in many places), or by bicycle (from 12 years on, usually).

The last group that has to rely on walking, cycling, or public transport consists of those people who do not have a car available to them. These could be citizens from lower socio-economic groups or – quite often – women, in families with only one car, which is mostly used by men (often for work purposes), although this might not frequently be the case in the United States and Canada.

Considering the subtitle of this book, 'Interventions for achieving change', one comes to think that the transport infrastructure of the public spaces all over the world generally does not seem to be well adapted for use by pedestrians, and especially not for children, youngsters, and (very) old people. There is no piece of literature that systematically lists all the shortcomings of traffic infrastructure as far as pedestrians are concerned in a representative and internationally valid way. However, from many studies that deal with the wishes of citizens concerning walking in public spaces – both for getting to destinations and for sojourning – one can deduce what is disturbing walkers or what keeps people from walking (see Figure 1.11).

Figure 1.11 refers to a large sample of interviewees in Vienna, and their wishes reflect the wishes of citizens concerning walking in public spaces: more green areas, better infrastructure for sitting and sojourning, well-illuminated sidewalks at night, clean pavements, more public toilets, shorter

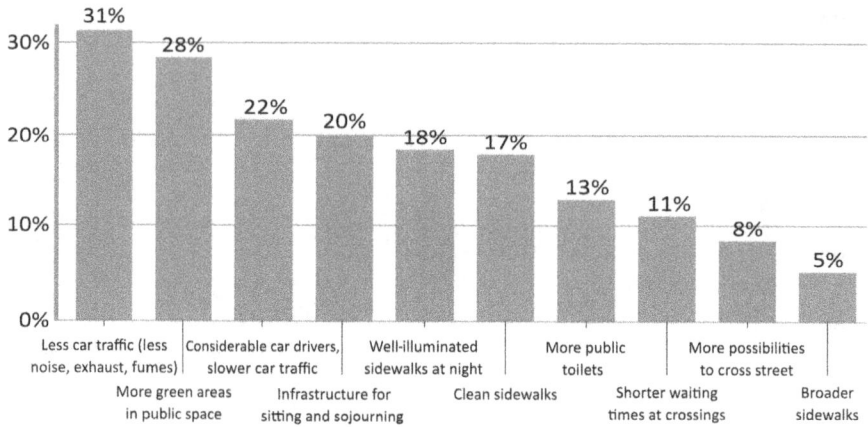

Figure 1.11 Wishes of citizens concerning the infrastructure for walking (Ausserer et al., 2013).

waiting times at crossings, more possibilities for crossing the streets, and broader pavements. Other points that are often criticised are crossings where one has to press a button but then 'nothing happens' (or it takes too long – why not supply sensors?), a lack of refuges in the middle of broader streets, mixed paths for walkers and cyclists providing too little space for the two combined, a lack of connected walking networks, planning and design that requires pedestrians to walk longer distances in order to get from A to B (guard railings labelled as 'traffic safety measures' often have this effect), a lack of coherent signposting, a lack of areas with lower car speeds (30 km/h) or of traffic-quietened zones, and certainly many others, depending on the region, country, or city where one resides or which one is visiting. Even though this data is from Vienna, we can reasonably assume that the wishes of walkers will not differ much in other cities (or at least in other European cities).

Figure 1.12 lists those factors that, according to the Viennese sample of interviewees, keep people from walking and make walking difficult for those who in fact do walk, either voluntarily or as captive walkers:

One can see that dog excrement (on pavements) in the year 2009 was one of the main barriers to walking. Probably, this has changed in the meantime, and probably, this barrier is not as relevant in other cities in the world. But in this table, one also can see that infrastructure aspects are most important for walkers and that distinct features of the infrastructure, again and again, function as barriers to walking. Some aspects have not been mentioned, though, namely those that refer to microstructures such as the height of kerbs and unevenness of the surface, such as bumps and holes, and so on. Those microstructures may contribute to walkers falling, leading to injuries that may be of a severe character, especially as far as older

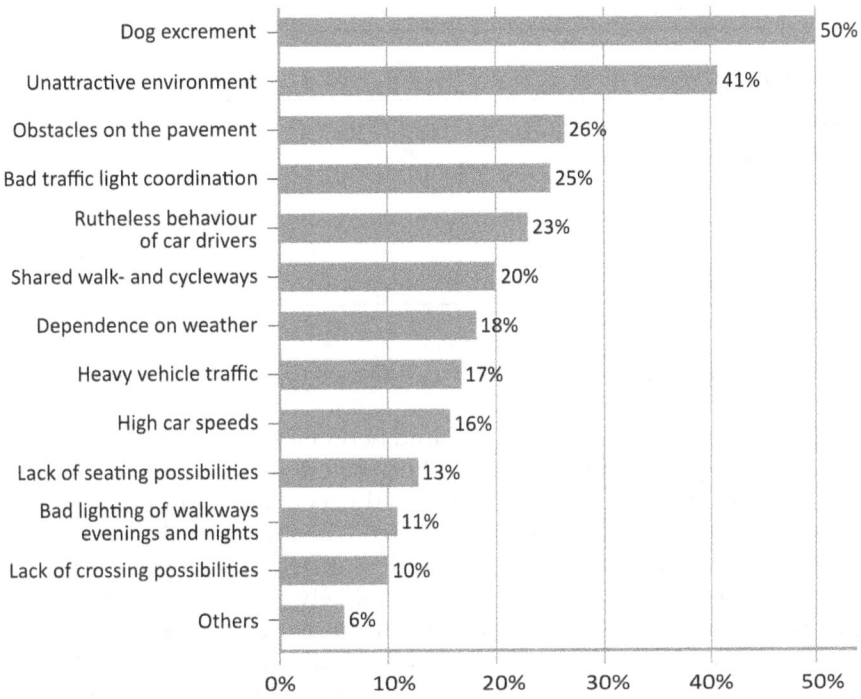

Figure 1.12 Barriers to walking (Ausserer et al., 2009).

citizens are concerned. Methorst et al. (2017) found that pedestrian falls, which are usually not included in the accident statistics in most countries – for some reason, they have never been considered traffic accidents – cost society more money than pedestrian accidents in which (motor) vehicles are involved. This corresponds with recent findings from Olomouc in the Czech Republic, which will be referred to subsequently. In sum, one can state that better adaptation of the infrastructure of the public space to the needs of all groups of pedestrians would certainly be a beneficial intervention.

1.8   Walking quality in Olomouc, Czech Republic

A recent study (2019) involving a cross-cultural comparison of safe and healthy walking behaviours included over 20 countries worldwide. In the Czech Republic, the relevant data was mainly obtained from the population of the city of Olomouc. Therefore, it can be interpreted in the context of a specific municipality.

Regarding the choice of transport mode, the respondents could select from walking, public transport, a private car, train, bicycle, and a personal electric vehicle (skateboard, scooter, etc.). The question was '*What is the primary mode of transport you use?*' Table 1.4 indicates that the most commonly

Table 1.4 Primary mode of transport

Primary mode of transport	Absolute rate	Relative rate (%)
Walking	123	42.7
Public transport	66	22.9
Private car	54	18.8
Train	23	8.0
Bicycle	21	7.3
Personal electric vehicle (skateboard, scooter, etc.)	1	0.3

used mode of transport is walking, followed by public transport and a private car.

No significant differences were found between women and men in terms of their transport mode of choice. The greatest gender-specific difference was identified for the use of trains, which the men in the study sample opted for surprisingly less often than the women (the men were found to be half as likely as the women to choose the train as their primary transport mode). On the other hand, the men were more likely than the women to use a private car as their primary mode of transport (the women were 25% less likely to do so). Variance analysis showed a significant relationship between the age of the respondents and the primarily used mode of transport. The youngest respondents opt for railways the most frequently, while the older ones prefer private cars. This is probably due to the fact that the younger respondents in the sample are generally university students who use the train to commute to their studies. Growing age increases the probability of a person acquiring a car and becoming accustomed to the comfort it provides.

Another question was *'During the last seven days, on how many days did you walk continuously for at least 10 minutes?'* Table 1.5 shows that all the days in the week were indicated with the highest frequency, with the rate decreasing with the number of days. In other words, the majority of the respondents walked continuously for at least 10 minutes every day or almost daily.

Then the daily amount of time people spent walking was asked about. The question read: *'How much time did you usually spend walking on one of these days?'* Table 1.6 indicates that the average time spent walking on a given day was 79 minutes, although the values show significant variability (SD 61). Neither gender-specific nor age-specific significant differences were found regarding the time spent walking. This corresponds nicely with the previous findings concerning the time spent outdoors. This time has not changed for decades.

We also asked about the frequency of the use of public transport. The question read: *'How often do you use public transport?'* Table 1.7 shows that the majority of the respondents use public transport several times per week.

Table 1.5 Number of days on which the respondents walked continuously for at least 10 minutes

Walking days (10+ mins.)	Absolute rate	Relative rate (%)
None	2	0.7
One	3	1.0
Two	18	6.3
Three	23	8.0
Four	25	8.7
Five	37	12.8
Six	30	10.4
Seven	150	52.1

Table 1.6 Number of minutes spent walking on a given day

	Average	Median	Minimum	Maximum	SD
Number of minutes spent walking	79.16	60	0	360	61.09

Table 1.7 Public transport use frequency

Public transport use frequency	Absolute rate	Relative rate (%)
Not at all	20	6.9
Weekly or less	93	32.3
Several times per week	88	30.6
Once a day	14	4.9
More than once a day	73	25.3

No significant gender-specific differences were found in the frequency of the use of public transport. While there were surprisingly more men than women who reported using no public transport at all (women were twice as likely to use it), differences between men and women were completely nonexistent in those respondents who used public transport at least sometimes. Variance analysis showed that there was a significant association between the age of the respondents and the frequency of their use of public transport. Young respondents use public transport several times a week, while the oldest ones do not use it at all. This may be related to the use of a private car, as the most common mode of transport reported by the older respondents in reaction to the previous question.

Similarly to the findings of Methorst et al. (2017), problems with falls in the public space became overt. The question read: '*Within the last three years, how many times have you fallen down while walking along the street or on the pavement/footpath?*' The frequencies of falls are summarised in Table 1.8,

Table 1.8 Number of falls in the last three years

Number of falls	Absolute rate	Relative rate (%)
0	179	62.2
1	42	14.6
2	30	10.4
3	18	6.3
4	3	1.0
5	8	2.8
6	1	0.3

which shows that the majority of the respondents had not fallen down in the last three years – but more than one-third of all the respondents had experienced at least one fall in the last three years.

Interesting significant differences were found in terms of age (the younger, the greater number of falls) but not regarding gender, although the men reported falling down with a slightly higher frequency in comparison to the women. Astonishingly, older people tend to fall significantly less often than younger people (after ten more years of age, only 70% of the present rate of falls is expected). A possible explanation can be that older people do not go outside so often any longer or do not move around on foot as much and thus have far fewer opportunities to fall down in comparison with young people. Another possibility may be that older people are more cautious while walking.

The next section focused on what the respondents would prefer to ban in relation to the protection of pedestrians' health and safety in general. The question was formulated as follows: '*To what extent do you think restrictions should be imposed on the following in order to protect health and safety?*' The respondents were asked to choose between '*complete ban*' and '*no restrictions*'. The following options were considered:

- The use of mobile phones by pedestrians crossing the street
- Pedestrians and alcohol
- The sale of vehicles burning fossil fuel
- Fossil fuel vehicles in city centres
- Municipal public transport vehicles burning fossil fuel
- Vehicles travelling at >40 km/h near pedestrians
- Cyclists on pavements
- Skateboards on pavements

Figure 1.13 outlines the frequencies of the individual responses. It is apparent that pedestrians regard skateboards on pavements as the greatest threat; they see them as being significantly more dangerous than cyclists on pavements. They also find vehicles travelling at high speed and pedestrians using mobile phones while crossing the street dangerous.

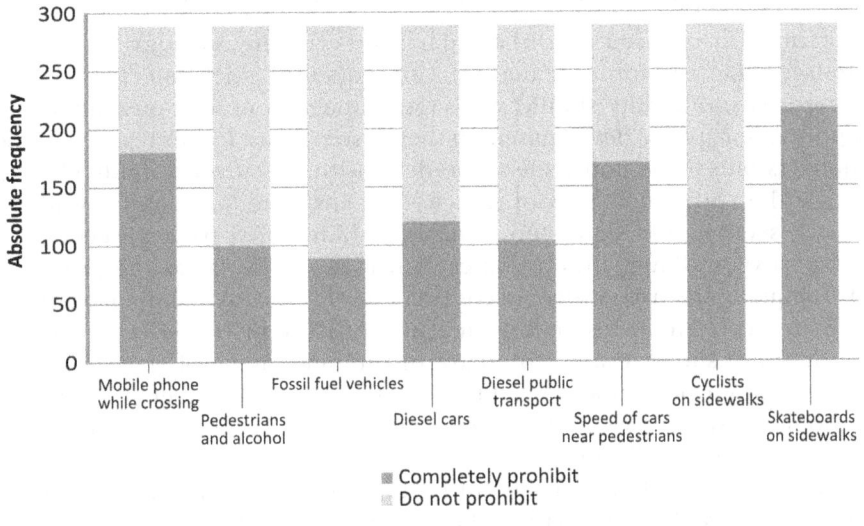

Figure 1.13 Frequencies of activities regarded as dangerous.

To sum up, the citizens of Olomouc generally walk to get around the city, with other common modes of transport being public transport and private cars. In support of these preferences, more than half of all the respondents stated that they walked (for over 10 minutes at a time) every day, spending an average of 80 minutes walking on a weekly basis. Approximately 20% do not use public transport at all, while the remainder use it several times per week. Regarding walking-related falls, it was found that the majority of the respondents had not fallen down at all in the last three years; nevertheless, one-third of the respondents had such experience. Falls were more likely to happen to young people. This was probably due to a higher level of exposure or to their greater representation in the study sample. In addition, the respondents were asked to assess what they considered dangerous for walking and what should be banned. The respondents' differences of opinions on the dangerousness of skateboards on pavements (very dangerous) and bicycles on pavements (rather dangerous) and a potential ban on these practices are noteworthy. Regarding pedestrians' behaviour, two situations were assessed: mobile phone use while crossing the street, which should be banned according to the majority of the respondents, and 'walking under the influence of alcohol', where, on the contrary, the respondents were generally in favour of no restrictions. In addition, the majority of the respondents preferred to restrict the driving speed to a maximum of 40 km/h in areas with heavier pedestrian traffic. In terms of the quality of the air, the majority of the respondents were rather satisfied and rated the air quality as good. In general, the results of this research suggest that Olomouc is a relatively pedestrian- and walking-friendly city.

1.9   Sustainable transport and costs associated with different modes

Sustainability is based on three pillars: the economy, ecology, and social life (see Chapter 2 for more details). Consequently, cities that claim to aim towards sustainability should envisage management and measures that support appropriate development in these three areas. In this respect, mode choice is one important issue to be dealt with, as citizens' mode choices define the traffic demands of the city. For instance, to enhance walking can be seen as one right step towards sustainability: from an economic perspective, walking is the cheapest traffic mode (as far as the provision of adequate infrastructure is concerned). If the provision of walking infrastructure enhances walking, it also appears to be cost effective: recent studies have shown that an increase in the percentage of walkers always boosts the local economy. Walking is, of course, advantageous from an ecological point of view; it produces no exhaust fumes and little noise, and as between 10% and 20% of all car trips could easily be covered on foot, there is considerable room for reducing ecologically disadvantageous car use and replacing it with walking; appropriate measures have to be taken, though. Walking has a positive connection to social life: where there are walkers, there is life, one could say. People feel safe where there are (many) other people and there is thus social control. Moreover, walking allows one to be with, or at least among, other people, without necessarily having to socialise. Not least, walking is healthy, which can be counted as an advantage from all three perspectives: economically, ecologically, and socially speaking.

In any case, walking is in many respects the optimum form of mobility in many cases, and therefore it deserves a special focus. We cannot accept arguments that walking is so natural that we do not need to take care of walkers. In order to meet daily needs, short-distance walks (for work, shopping, free time, etc.) need to be advocated and promoted. If larger parts of the population need to be motivated and inspired to walk (more often), it is necessary to understand the motivation, attitudes, and characteristics of different population groups and what they like and what they dislike in connection with walking. On this basis, appropriate communication and marketing measures have to be taken for each of the relevant groups of citizens. With this knowledge, a sensitive yet progressive road user-oriented approach must be applied when (new) urban spaces are being created, or when old areas are reconstructed, and good design, functionality, and easy accessibility are desired.

Together with cycling, walking has considerable potential to help to achieve better sustainability in transport. Public transport is also usually seen as a mode that is to be preferred to car use from an ecological, economic, and social point of view. A larger study in Vienna (Füssl et al., 2019) showed that public transport use requires quite a lot of physical activity. In this study, public transport in Vienna was called a 'fitness course', because the short trips to and from the public transport stops, boarding the vehicles, negotiating steps and stairs, sometimes standing while travelling, and hurrying if one is late all have the character of physical exercise, at least much more exercise than when one uses a car. In addition, one can walk on the escalators instead of just being transported by the escalator or the lift. One can also use the ordinary stairs, and people do so. Elisabeth Füssl and her colleagues calculated that, on average, when travelling to work and back by public transport, the physical activity is equal to the daily physical activity suggested by the WHO (2011).

As far as the costs of infrastructure for pedestrians or cyclists or the costs for the provision and maintenance of public transport are concerned, there are often complaints that 'those things' cost the taxpayer too much money. But it turns out that if one considers what are called the external costs, in addition to the private expenses one has for the car, car traffic costs the taxpayer much more money per capita per year than public transport (Umweltbundesamt, 2010). In a broadcast of the Second Channel of German Television (ZDF = Zweites Deutsches Fernsehen), the Heute-Show on March 28th 2019, a figure of €2100 uncovered yearly costs for every car registered in Germany was mentioned. 'Uncovered' means that these costs are tax-covered. According to the Statista Institute,[3] there were 47,096,000 cars registered in Germany in 2019. The costs to the taxpayer accrued in this way: 47,096,000 × 2100 = 98,901,600,000, or approximately 99 billion euro. In 2010, the Umweltbundesamt, the German Department for the Environment, produced a much lower figure of 'only' 46.8 billion euro based on calculations for the year 2008. At that time, the number of registered cars was 41,184,000, so this cannot explain the difference between the two figures. Different ways of performing the calculation may lie behind these differences. However, even ~50 billion euro is a tremendous amount of money for a country the size of Germany. A comparison with Austrian data: the Austrian Traffic Club calculated external costs of €120 per 1000 km for a car. The Austrian Traffic Club (Verkehrsclub Österreich) estimated that every Austrian car driver drives 34 km/day on average, resulting in 12,410 km/year.[4] On the basis of €120 being calculated as the costs for 1000 km driven by car, this would lead to yearly costs of €1489.20 per Austrian car driver. All this data, and there are certainly more calculations to be found in other countries, cannot be compared directly because of the different approaches and different calculations (per car, per citizen, etc.). But the size of the costs in Austria and Germany can be roughly estimated as lying somewhere between €1500 and €2000 per car per year. We may assume that these costs will also be roughly the same in other countries.

These costs comprise accident costs (including the costs of loss of human life, reduced health condition, lost income, and material costs), air pollution, climate costs, the noxious effects of noise, environmental costs in connection with the production of cars and the disposal of old cars, costs for damage to the environment and the landscape, negative effects on biodiversity, costs for the quality impairments car transport causes to other modes (time losses, accidents, quality of sojourn), and construction and maintenance costs (which are only partly covered by the specific taxes paid by car owners). Today, when discussing sustainability in connection with car transport, there is often the argument that electro-mobility will solve many problems. It is questionable, though, whether the improvements will be satisfying. Let us look at the ecological factor. Rare earth metals are required for the production of batteries.[5] Another problem with today's car use is its demand for space. This will not change substantially when electric cars are used. Furthermore, nobody knows whether there will be more or fewer cars on the roads then. Maybe the notion that one is driving an ecologically friendly vehicle when driving an electric car will cause more people to buy and use a car instead of other modes. Another question is what electricity is used, whether produced by renewable and clean energy (wind, solar power, clean burning of garbage, etc.) or by electricity that comes from coal-, nuclear-, or oil-fuelled power plants. Furthermore, when one reflects on all these arguments, most of them refer only to the ecological part of mobility. The question is whether electro-mobility will alleviate the economic and social problems connected to car use.

What is more important is that the uncovered costs of the German Railway (DB = Deutsche Bahn), according to a calculation of the Wirtschaftswoche in 2016, were 5 billion euro, compared to uncovered costs for car use of 50–99 billion euro. However, in the Wirtschaftswoche article, the costs for the railways were presented as something 'atrocious'. In Austria, the national financial support for the railways is €17 per 1000-km railway journey[6] (compared to €120 per 1000 km driven by car, as stated previously).

We did not succeed in finding reliable figures concerning walking. We found one interesting calculation of the Austrian cycling lobby (Radlobby Österreich), though, stating that one km of separated cycle path costs as much as 17 m of motorway. One may assume that the costs for pedestrian walkways (boardwalks, etc.) are similar to the costs of cycle paths. Thus, we finish this section by stating with some good reason that driving a car costs society (much) more than walking would cost if really good infrastructure for walking were provided.[7] In the latter case we could also benefit from all the positive economic effects because of the health- and fitness-boosting character of walking, and from the positive economic effects of social life in public spaces.

It really looks as if we will have to see to it to enhance the use of mobility modes that require minimal external energy and resources (energy and resources not stemming from the individual him- or herself) and minimum space per individual and that do not have negative effects on society, such as negative externalities. For shorter distances, walking is, of course, a candidate in this respect, and when thought of in connection with the use of public transport, walking could achieve a substantial improvement in sustainability in the area of human mobility were many car trips to be replaced. The same is valid for cycling, by the way. However, good preconditions are needed to make such mobility acceptable from the citizen's point of view. And if anybody wants to state that 'these things cost too much', just have a look at the previous.

In Chapter 2, we will refer to the sustainable character of walking in more detail.

1.10   We should not have to walk: But love to walk

Taking in a psychological perspective on walking when discussing possible interventions for achieving change always leads us to the individual road user, the individual human being, or small groups of individuals. Striving to achieve change means that in one way or another, the behaviour of individuals has to be changed. Even if, to this end, legal and law enforcement measures will partly be needed, in democratic societies, one will, in the first place, think of informing and convincing (i.e. motivating) citizens. Efforts to achieve behaviour change consist of, for example, awareness raising and social marketing measures (Kotler et al., 2016). Individuals should understand, or remember, or – as the best result – feel that there are a lot of advantages connected to a change to sustainable mobility, both for society and for them personally. The advantages of walking that the individual understands – and that, one hopes, convince him/her – could have different forms; either one has internalised the economic, ecological, and social values connected to walking and is motivated to walk in order to support these values, for example, for idealistic reasons, or because one is a responsible citizen, or one has experienced that walking satisfies other needs that one cannot be conscious of without frequent walking experience. Walking provides feelings of freedom and independence, of fitness and strength, of relaxation and wellbeing. However, such feelings hardly turn to motives that steer behaviour only by being reported by others. It is important that one experiences such feelings oneself, that one has one's own positive sensation.

Thus, a sustainable policy on the part of the authorities, companies where people work, or schools and other educational institutes would include incentive measures to make people walk and thus to make them feel the advantages of walking. The important idea that should function as a leitmotif is: 'We should *not have* to walk – we should *love* to walk'. First, this of course reflects the thought that people should not have to walk distances, or under conditions, that are not acceptable just because there are no alternatives. At the same time, people should not look at walking as something that 'you have to do'. Those who react rather negatively even to short walks should start understanding and feeling the advantages of walking for themselves (fitness, relaxation). At the same time, there is no damage done if they also realise that there is something good for society in it if (more) people walk (more). Such a good thing is something one should actually love even more.

For those who have to walk under difficult conditions, being confronted with facts and arguments showing the advantages of walking could produce some mitigation of their burden. In a certain respect, they could then see some positive aspects connected to the 'limitations' on their mobility. However, the danger of being cynical has to be counteracted, and not only in our book, by working intensely with all kinds of deliberations about how to improve the preconditions for walking for as many people as possible.

SUMMARY

Mobility in its present form contributes to negative climate development. Walking has the potential to replace a considerable percentage of car trips. Between 10% and 20% of all car trips cover only 1 km, a distance that may be seen as an acceptable walking distance for an average grown-up. In combination with well-organised public transport, the portion of trips with individual motor vehicles that could be replaced becomes even higher.

However, even if walking is the most natural way of moving about for human beings, it has continuously been replaced more and more by more comfortable, less tiring, faster, and less environmentally sensitive means. Litters, horses, wheel-based non-motorised vehicles, and, in the end, motor-driven means of transport have gained more and more importance, the car being the most common means of transport today. Such replacement reflects, of course, the satisfaction of needs.

However, people are not so aware of advantages of walking that have the potential to satisfy important needs: to remain healthy, to boost fitness, to feel well, to feel one's body, to enhance creative processes in one's mind. It is proven that walking reduces the probability of becoming afflicted by cancer, depression, dementia, osteoporosis, and many other diseases. Moreover, walking counteracts obesity. When looking at the history of walking, one can see that walking was a much-appreciated leisure-time activity, even if restricted to the more wealthy parts of the population. Philosophers, scientists, and authors underlined the creativity-boosting effects of walking. However, poorer people had no other choice than to walk for their daily errands, without having the time or options for leisure-time walking, similarly to large parts of the population in developing countries.

Nevertheless, the situation is clear, at least theoretically speaking. There are both long-term and short-term advantages that should motivate (more) people to walk (more). However, it seems that the (probabilistic) avoidance of diseases is too abstract to be felt as an immediate advantage, while the immediate advantages – fitness, well-being, and so on – are difficult to perceive for those people who do not usually walk (much). This means that ways to make people aware of the advantages of walking and to convince them to 'go for such advantages' have to be found and applied.

The authors of this book belong among those who do not believe in advocating 'renouncing' something but rather in positive motivation. Walking should be perceived as rewarding and as something that is effective, efficient, and clever. Renouncing car use may be a positive motivation for more fundamental environmentalists, but the majority of the population needs to be reminded of the – more or less – immediate rewards provided by walking and given the opportunity also to experience these advantages.

Notes

1. https://www.naturfreunde.at/ueber-uns/naturfreunde/geschichte/
2. See https://openknowledge.worldbank.org/bitstream from 10 January 2019, Global Mobility Report, 2017
3. https://de.statista.com/statistik/daten/studie/12131/umfrage/pkw-bestand-in-deutschland/
4. https://www.vcoe.at/news/details/vcoe-oesterreichs-autofahrer-fahren-im-schnitt-34-kilometer-pro-tag
5. See https://www.br.de/themen/wissen/seltene-erden-metalle-smartphones-china-100.html and https://www.automobil-produktion.de/hersteller/neue-modelle/wettlauf-um-rohstoffe-fuer-e-mobility-rohstoff-imperialismus-371.html
6. https://www.vcoe.at/themen/ausgeblendete-kosten-des-verkehrs
7. http://ooe.radlobby.at/cms/index.php?id=151
8. https://projekte.ffg.at/projekt/2929330

2 Features and manifestations of walking

The aim of this chapter is to introduce walking from different perspectives and from the points of view of different groups of pedestrians – as listed in the context of the chapter. The emphasis is placed on detailed information, its context, and examples connected with the everyday life of readers. We emphasise the pros and cons of walking under different circumstances and demonstrate how it is all connected.

Currently, 54% of the world's population lives in urban areas, a share that is expected to rise to ∼65% by 2050 (United Nations, 2014). In the EU, around 70% of the population lives in urban areas, and by 2050, this figure will be more than 80% (EPRS, 2014). Urbanisation – a worldwide phenomenon – brings a whole range of problems with it, including those in the transport and mobility domain. The solutions lie in developing a sustainable infrastructure which includes the transport and housing sector, in measures for limiting urban sprawl and individual automobile transportation, and in promoting well-functioning sustainable transport systems, with the main aims being to reduce the amount of traffic – for example, by providing housing, public services, and jobs in the same area – and to provide appropriate mobility options for all citizens.

Walking is in many respects the optimum form of mobility in the city, and therefore it deserves a special focus. In order to meet daily needs, short-distance walks (for work, shopping, free time, etc.) need to be advocated and promoted. In Europe, 15%–20% of all car trips are shorter than 1 km (Rudner & Malone 2011), which takes 10 to 15 minutes by walking. Sixty-six percent of children live at a distance of less than 1 km from their school and 80% at one of less than 2 km (a walk of 20–30 minutes). On many of those trips, children are transported by car (Frey, 2015). If larger parts of the population need to be motivated and inspired to walk (more often), it is necessary to study the motivation, attitudes, and characteristics of different population groups and what they like and dislike in connection with walking. With this knowledge, a sensitive yet progressive road user-oriented approach must be applied when (new) urban spaces are being created, and good design, functionality, and easy accessibility are desired.

2.1   Walking is a sustainable mode of transport

Walking is a sustainable mode of transport: that is what everybody says. Todd Litman (2007) from the Victoria Transport Policy Institute summarised indicators for sustainability which many researchers would consider relevant (see Table 2.1). It is worthwhile to have a look at those indicators and discuss whether walking performs well or not with respect to them. There are three groups of them: economy, social aspects, and the environment.

2.1.1   Economy

Let us have a look at the most important economic indicators according to Table 2.1: per capita mobility is huge, even if not in kilometres but with respect to trips or sections of trips. Virtually everybody walks on a daily basis. The potential to replace short car trips is considerable. Thus, the portion of walking trips could be higher than it is today. In cities in Europe, walking constitutes a substantial portion of all trips from door to door, and in many American cities, it is the goal to achieve higher levels of walking. Travel time for walkers is probably limited at a lower level than, say, would be accepted when sitting in a car. However, the accepted commuting time varies considerably between individuals (on average 45 and 60 minutes per day). But if one has accepted a certain time it takes to walk to selected places, for example, to work, and does so regularly, he or she will find out that this commuting time is utterly stable and reliable, without great variation. The per capita congestion costs are, of course, low, unless one walks through areas where there is a street market or a demonstration or the like, with thousands of people blocking the road. Otherwise, "pedestrian congestion" is not much heard of. The total per capita transport expenditures are as low as they can be. Litman mentions roads and transit services, meaning building and maintenance of walking facilities, and for walkers, these are definitely lower than for all other transport modes (though not zero, as some might suggest by arguing that "walkers will always find their way and do not need special infrastructure").

Other indicators for economic features that Litman considers helpful are availability, speed, safety, and prestige relative to automobile travel. Availability is, of course, given for all people who are able to walk, that is, all those without motor impairments. Speed is, of course, low if one is speaking of longer distances. Over short distances, say, up to one kilometre, walking as measured from door to door can be faster – or it will at least not be much slower – than a trip with public transport, or even than a car trip, just because it is the most direct mode and there are no waiting times,

Table 2.1 Recommended transport indicator set by VTPI (Litman, 2007)

	Economic	Social	Environmental
Most important (Should usually be used)	• Per capita mobility (daily or annual person-miles or trips) • Mode split (personal travel: non-motorised, automobile, and public transport; freight: truck, rail, ship, and air) • Average commute travel time and reliability • Per capita congestion costs • Total per capita transport expenditures (vehicles, parking, roads, and transit services)	• Per capita traffic crashes and fatalities • Quality of transport for disadvantaged people (disabled, low incomes, children, etc.) • Affordability (portion of household budgets devoted to transport) • Overall satisfaction rating of transport system (based on objective user surveys) • Universal design (consideration of disabled people's needs in transport planning)	• Per capita energy consumption, disaggregated by mode • Energy consumption per freight ton-mile • Per capita air pollution emissions (various types), disaggregated by mode • Per capita land devoted to transport facilities (roads, parking, ports, and airports) • Air and noise pollution exposure and damage to health • Impervious surface coverage and storm water management practices
Helpful (Should be used if possible)	• Relative quality (availability, speed, reliability, safety, and prestige) of non-automobile modes (walking, cycling, ridesharing, and public transit) relative to automobile travel • Number of public services within a 10-minute walk and job opportunities within a 30-minute commute for residents	• Portion of residents who walk or cycle sufficiently for health (15 minutes or more daily) • Portion of children walking or cycling to school • Community cohesion (quality of interactions among neighbours) • Degree to which cultural resources are considered in transport planning	• Community liveability ratings • Water pollution emissions • Habitat preservation • Use of renewable fuels • Transport facility resource efficiency (such as use of renewable materials and energy-efficient lighting)
Specialised (Use to address particular needs or objectives)	• Percentage of households with internet access • Change in property values	Transit affordability • Housing affordability in accessible locations	Impacts on special habitats and environmental resources • Heat island effects
Planning process	Comprehensive (takes into account all significant impacts, using best current evaluation practices). Inclusive (substantial involvement of people who are affected, with special efforts to ensure that disadvantaged and vulnerable groups are involved). Based on accessibility rather than mobility. Application of smart growth land use policies.		
Market efficiency	Percentage of total transportation costs that are efficiently priced. Neutrality (public policies do not arbitrarily favour a particular mode or group) in transport pricing, taxes, planning, investment, etc. Applies least cost planning.		

no starting times, and no search times for a parking space. The number of public services within a 10-minute walk means services within a radius of just below one kilometre, which it takes 12 minutes to walk (calculated on the basis of an average walking speed of 5 km/h). One kilometre is not really a narrow radius, and we may assume that most people living in cities in developed countries – more than three-quarters of the total population in Europe, much more than that in Japan, Canada, and the United States – have most of the public services they need within this radius. In some developing countries – China, Indonesia, India, the Philippines, all of Africa – and in smaller villages in the countryside in developed countries, things might be a little more difficult. Similar arguments are valid concerning job opportunities within a 30-minute radius. This equals 2.5 km at a walking speed of 5 km/h and actually covers quite a huge area of 19.6 square kilometres, which is almost the same as the area of Vienna's 2nd district, Leopoldstadt (19.3 km²), and more than the average area of the 23 districts of Vienna (18).

The dimensions of cities in Europe are not too different, so this comparison is certainly valid in Europe, meaning that job opportunities within a 30-minute walking distance would probably be available for quite many people in Europe.

However, today's situation is certainly such that because of the availability of a car for a large part of the population, for quite a number of years, many people have accepted jobs that are out of reach for walking. Establishing institutions with many workplaces – industrial sites, shopping malls, outlets, and so on – on the outskirts of cities far away from centres or in the notorious "middle of nowhere" – was facilitated by this; not many people or authorities would have objected to this development until lately. Nowadays, in major European cities, any company or enterprise that wants to install larger complexes anywhere within or outside the city has to show that they can be reached by some high-potential public transport means. However, at this moment (2019), many people have workplaces that are more distant from their homes than a 30-minute walking distance. By this argument, we do not want to argue that citizens should look for jobs close to where they live in the first place, although this might be a good idea. What we want to suggest is that one should also consider how the time on the way to work and back from it is spent. Depending on the mode of travel, this could be more relaxing or more stressful.

Concerning the percentage of households with internet access and the change in property values, there is a relationship between the quality and the walkability of the area.[1] If the area is attractive for walkers, then usually the property values increase, and in such a case, the internet connection will also be good.

We do not discuss the planning process and market efficiency here, as they belong among those tasks of the authorities by which all three pillars of sustainability are moderated.

2.1.2   Social aspects

Concerning social aspects, the per capita traffic crashes and fatalities are most relevant variables. Pedestrians, especially children and the elderly, are the most vulnerable road users (VRUs). The US Federal Highway Administration (2014) stated that 12% of the fatalities in road crashes are pedestrians (4000 annually) and that around 59,000 pedestrians are injured every year in the United States alone. In 2016, 5320 pedestrians were killed in road accidents in the EU, which is 21% of all road fatalities. The percentage of pedestrian fatalities out of total road fatalities is lowest in the Netherlands (8%), Finland (11%), and Belgium (12%), compared to Romania (37%), Estonia (36%), and Latvia (35%). The percentage of pedestrian fatalities is high for children, as well as for the elderly. Age and gender are crucial factors in road users' behaviour and their safety; children, as well as elderly people, are at high risk of pedestrian injury (Niebuhr et al., 2016). Children under 14 have many limitations as pedestrians, since their physiological, motor, cognitive, and emotional abilities have yet to fully mature. Young children usually fail to determine the safe timing of crossing the road (Rosenbloom & Wolf, 2002); furthermore, children's appraisal of the prospective danger and sensation of fear in road crossing scenarios are low compared to adults (Rosenbloom et al., 2008). Similarly, the deterioration of sensory, motor, and cognitive abilities in elderly people has an adverse effect on their road crossing abilities (Bian & Andersen, 2008). In addition, the elderly are not always aware of their age-related limitations, leading to misconceptions and overestimation of their actual road crossing performance (Zivotofsky et al., 2012). Moreover, they tend to rely on the correct crossing behaviour of younger pedestrians, and while following them at crossings without checking twice, because of their visual and motor limitations, they often do not manage to reach the other side of the road safely. The main reason for the high fatality rate of old people lies in their higher frailty (European Commission, 2018).

Research often points at multiple factors associated with pedestrians' safe behaviour, such as distraction, fatigue, situational variables, and more. But when considering that pedestrians are killed by car drivers and never the other way round, it seems a little odd to blame pedestrians for not taking care while "forgetting" that cars are steered by people who should be held responsible for the damage they do to others.

Walking can be considered a sustainable mode only if it is safe and comfortable to walk. By "safe", we mean that the relative chance of being injured or killed is the same as, or lower than, for most other transport modes. By comfortable, we mean that people will be motivated to walk because walking itself is a joyful activity. The average grown-up can theoretically see to him- or herself that he or she can walk under safe conditions (although ruthless car drivers can do unexpected things that are beyond the control of a single pedestrian). The problem is much bigger for disadvantaged persons. Senior citizens do in many cases have problems with the traffic system, as far as subjective safety is concerned. They tend to feel disturbed by how other road users behave. Children are endangered as well, because they lack several abilities that would allow them to assess traffic situations appropriately. Grown-ups sitting in cars could be expected to take care of children and to pay special attention to them when they are out walking, cycling, or playing. We hear a lot of stories – and have data to show – that obviously grown-ups do not always assume this responsibility. The quality of transport for disadvantaged people (disabled, low incomes, children, etc.) is at risk in many other respects, as well; crossing times provided by traffic lights are in many cases too short for people with motor problems, of whom many belong to the group of old or very old citizens. For low-income families, the risk factor is that their children spend more time in the streets (often playing) than others, and thus their exposure to risk is bigger. In many countries, motor vehicles that turn left or right at intersections have a green light at the same time as pedestrians and cyclists coming from the same direction have a green light for going straight on and going through the intersection. Long ago, Pasanen (2001) demonstrated in a very convincing way that car drivers "are not afraid of vulnerable road users" and thus do not consider them sufficiently. Figure 2.1 shows that car drivers make sure that there will mainly be no critical interaction with those road users that represent a danger for them – that is, all vehicles in the motor vehicle lane that approach from the left – while they do not look thoroughly in the direction from which vulnerable road users might appear. In the case displayed in Figure 2.1, cyclists should be expected from the right.

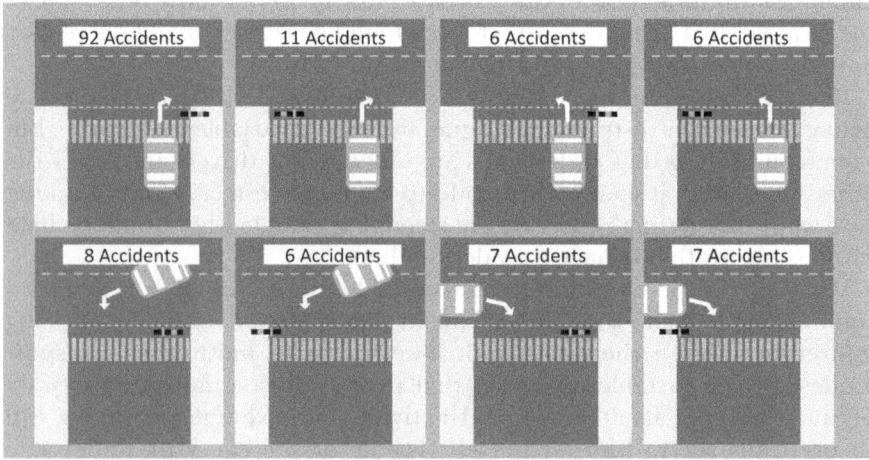

Figure 2.1 Accident types at non-signalised crossings of two-way cycle paths and minor streets (Pasanen, 2001).

Many parents are afraid for the safety of their children when they are moving in the public space. They decide to bring them to school by car instead of allowing them to go to school by themselves, walking or cycling, together with peers. As walking is not perceived as a convenient and safe mode by many – maybe because it has become a bad habit not to walk, but probably also because the infrastructure for walking does not work well or is not pleasant or safe – often, not even short distances are covered by walking when parents and children go to kindergarten or school together. We can observe a paradox here: people who take their children to school by car say that they do so because there are too many cars outside the school and that therefore it is not safe to let the children walk to school. Concerning both safety and comfort, the study by Knoblauch et al. (1996) is interesting. They showed that the environment at the time when they carried out their study did not meet the needs of older pedestrians. They studied 16 pedestrian crossings in four US cities, and the results showed that the 15th-percentile walking speed of pedestrians between 14 and 64 of age was 4.5 km/h (1.25 m/sec), while that for pedestrians aged 65 years and over was only 3.5 km/h (0.97 m/sec). They therefore suggested that for design purposes, the values should actually be 4.4 km/h (1.22 m/sec), and 3.3 km/h (0.91 m/sec) for older pedestrians, which is obviously lower than is usual in OECD countries. The authors of this study, however, did not mention the usual design or crossing speeds that are envisaged by the time spans provided at intersections. What they say is that those times are usually too short. In fact, it is a truism among experts discussed at many meetings that deal with walking that the crossing times that are provided are usually too short, while the times that pedestrians have to wait at red lights are (too) long.

2.1.2.1 Holistic approach: Diamond model

A systematic look at the disadvantages for pedestrians with the help of the diamond model (Risser, 2000; see Figure 2.2) maybe provides a better insight into the problems that both walkers and societies that want to enhance walking are confronted with. It considers individual features, communication among road users, societal aspects, infrastructure characteristics, and the features of the mode itself. According to this model, attitudes, motives, emotions, cognitions, habits, and performance, that is, individual characteristics, influence our behaviour as underlying features. However, these individual characteristics are shaped in the course of our socialisation in our interaction with the outside world, and they undergo a continuous influence by the outside world. Thus, whether we like and practise regular walking depends on those individual features but also on the influence from the other areas that are displayed in Figure 2.2.

Communication between road users goes on at all places where they meet. Communication – synonymous with interaction – between pedestrians and

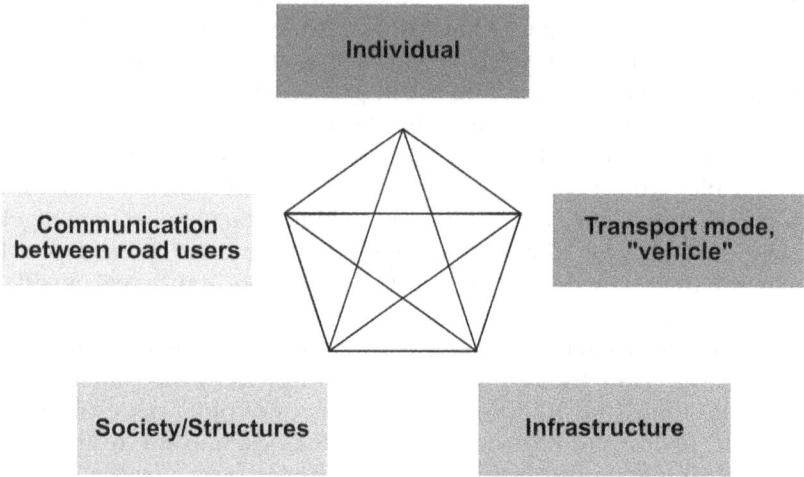

Figure 2.2 The diamond model (Risser, 2000).

car drivers frequently has characteristics that undermine the willingness to walk of many road users. Interviews with pedestrians, especially with older ones, indicate that, for example, high speeds of cars, a lack of abiding by the rules by car drivers, and ruthless behaviour on the part of car drivers cause difficulties for pedestrians and reduce the quality of travel for pedestrians.

The societal preconditions set the value of walking. How is walking treated in the media, by decision makers, and by politicians, or is it treated at all? What does the family and what do peers think and express about walking, what is discussed in the pub: is walking there a topic at all? Everybody is affected by such aspects; it is part of our socialisation, which never ends throughout our life. When looking at research work in the area of transport, one also gets an impression about what value is attributed to walking. The same is true for laws and informal norms, characteristics of the public discussion and traffic culture. People in official positions set the scene for walking with their decisions, for instance, by the infrastructure they have implemented. The general conclusion is that the value attributed to walking is low, concerning all the aspects mentioned.

The infrastructure of public spaces, too, frequently and in many places gives the impression that walkers are not very highly esteemed. Apart from pedestrian zones or urban parks, walking facilities are often poor, boardwalks are too narrow and often absent, crossing facilities prioritise car traffic, and the safety of pedestrians is often at risk there, while waiting times are long and crossing times are short, kerbs are irregular, and surfaces are uneven. In the Netherlands, data from the whole province of Groningen shows that pedestrian falls cause more societal costs than accidents between pedestrians and motor vehicles (Methorts et al., 2010). It is legitimate to assume that the quality and maintenance of infrastructure contribute substantially to such results.

The **"walking" vehicle**, our body, gets tired easily; is susceptible to physical efforts, long distances, and steep flights of steps; and is easily injured. Therefore, in order to make walking attractive and thus exploit its full potential for sustainability, the preconditions for walking should be adapted accordingly. Walkers – not all of them, but many, for example, older people – need places to rest, and the network of walking facilities should be finely meshed in order to avoid inappropriately long walking distances from A to B; flights of steps, underpasses, and the kerbs of boardwalks should meet the needs of weaker walkers, and pedestrian safety should be seen to. The latter, however, is often aimed at by implementing barriers and by expecting pedestrians to accept long waiting times and detours. So far, not much weight has been put on these exigencies of walkers, nor has much creativity been invested with respect to practical and technological support for everyday activities, such as shoes (not as fashion products but as "vehicles"), rucksacks and other assets for shopping, and so on. They do exist, but their marketing and design are mostly far from fancy (besides sport equipment – which is, by the way, also very often used by regular walkers in the city, as it is of good quality and comfortable). Without the possibility of measuring this, one could probably say that this is improving, including changes on the technological side, such as path finders and other support apps based on the use of nomadic devices. Is the future bright? Optimists say that walking is still not very attractive for industry, but this will change.

Getting back to Litman's indicators (Table 2.1), the next in the list is affordability. There, walking is, of course, the winner, except for people who have physical difficulties with walking and for those who live too far away from any destination for it to be reached by walking. Those who can cover many of their daily distances by walking will in any case save a lot of money by using up only a small part of their household budget. When turning things around by looking at people who have to walk because the household budget is so small that no other modes can be afforded, we have, of course, a different type of problem – the situation for those people is certainly not sustainable: walking should be an option, not a must.

Overall satisfaction with walking is next on the list. Litman regrets that ratings of the transport system by users (walkers) based on objective user surveys are difficult to find. The most comprehensive study was carried out within the frame of the EU Project WALCYNG (Hydén et al., 1997). One main result from that large European study was that many pedestrians feel like second-class road users, a role that nobody likes to take on. Later, on a smaller scale, road users were interviewed within the frame of the COST project Pedestrian Quality Needs (PQN) (Methorst et al., 2010). In the opinion of road users, the assessment of the preconditions for walking and of the activity itself is, on the one hand, influenced by individual abilities and one's own health, and, on the other hand, by the distribution and the distance to places to go to. Whether the built environment makes walking easy or provides barriers is essential, as is the availability of public transport and information for walkers for navigation and the fulfilling of tasks, such as for shopping, cultural activities, and other services. Last but not least, societal issues play a role, as do income (does one have to walk or does one walk voluntarily?), level of education, and how society looks at walking, that is, the status of walkers.

The work within the frame of the EU project SIZE (Life quality of senior citizens in relation to mobility conditions; Amann et al., 2006) was oriented towards older people (over 65), and the questions were not strictly limited to walking but rather to the use of the public space more generally. However, from the character of the answers, one can understand that in many cases, the people who were interviewed speak in their role as walkers. Interviews concerning the appraisal of mobility conditions were conducted with 3309 senior citizens in eight different countries in Europe: Austria, the Czech Republic, Germany, Ireland, Italy, Poland, Spain, and Sweden. The interviewees identified difficult technical, physical, and social conditions. Many of them feared victimisation. Ruthlessness on the part of car drivers was felt to be a problem, including the fact that speed limits are not respected. Other problems mentioned were the lack of toilets in the public space, bad maintenance of pavements, and vehicles on footpaths, but also a decrease in their own senses. The results showed that there were interpersonal, international, and gender-related differences in the answers. For example, women showed more fear. They were less satisfied with their mobility conditions and attributed greater urgency to their improvement.

2.1.2.2   *The public space and quality of life*

Walking has a strong potential to be associated with positive emotions and a good quality of life (e.g. Silva 2011, FHWA, 2014). Thus, promoting walking has the potential to enhance the quality of life. In any case, the character of the public space, more specifically design elements on the micro level (e.g. kerbs, the quality of the pavement, etc.), the meso level (e.g. the layout of intersections, programmed waiting and crossing times at intersections), and the macro level (e.g. the network of walking paths and facilities and length of routes to relevant places) is most relevant concerning the resulting perceived quality for walkers. In Table 2.2, a universal design is listed, not least in order to consider disabled people's needs in transport planning. But it is easy to imagine that universal design elements will provide advantages for all types of people who walk if we consider only the needs of pedestrians. Problems may arise if planners also have to consider the interests of drivers of motor vehicles, for whom design elements that are advantageous for walkers could mean the loss of advantages they have so far been able to benefit from. The behaviour of people as vehicle drivers would then have

Table 2.2 What is generally important for QoL – population vs. experts
(EU project HOTEL, Risser et al., 2004)

Importance of certain aspects	Population (n = 184)		Experts (n = 17)	
	Unimportant %	Important %	Unimportant %	Important %
Usability for elderly & disabled	1	95.6	0	100
Smooth flow of traffic for drivers	11.5	65.6	5.9	76.5
Smooth flow of traffic for cyclists	9.4	82.6	0	100
Smooth flow of traffic for pedestrians	1.1	93.9	0	100
Equity between different traffic groups (cyclists, drivers, pedestrians)	8.8	80.3	5.9	88.2
Ease and convenience for car drivers	12.6	61.0	17.6	41.2
Ease and convenience for cyclists	3.3	80.9	0	94.1
Ease and convenience for pedestrians	0	88.5	9	100
Beauty & aesthetics	6.0	75.2	0	100
Environment (noise/air)	1.7	92.2	0	100
Children's safety/security	0	99.5	0	100
Elderly and disabled persons' safety/security	1.0	97.3	0	100
Your own safety/security	5.4	94.5	0	88.2
Traffic safety	6.5	93.4	0	100
Quality of life	3.8	96.2	0	100

to be controlled more thoroughly (e.g. speed choice), less space would be allocated to them (parking and driving into centres would have to be limited), they would have to cope with longer waiting times at intersections, and so on. On the other hand, to find compromises in order to satisfy the needs of both walkers and cyclists would become easier if more space were allocated to walkers and cyclists as a result of reduced consumption of space by motor vehicles.

An indicator that is certainly helpful for assessing the social aspects of walking is the percentage of residents who walk or cycle sufficiently for their health (15 minutes or more daily), as this enhances public health and thus helps societies to save money. At an individual level, regular walking or cycling will lead to better health, better fitness, and a better mood. Of course, as mentioned previously, the problem is that those who do not walk or cycle cannot perceive these advantages. The portion of children walking or cycling to school is another indicator that to a certain degree reflects how the quality of walkways is perceived by parents. If they judge and feel that walkways are safe, the probability that they will let their children walk or cycle to school will be higher (Ausserer et al., 2012).

But the quality of walkways or the quality of sites, routes, and places for walkers is not only important for children. In the EU project HOTEL (How to analyse life quality), a clear relationship between the attractiveness of public spaces and the perceived quality of life could be established (Risser et al., 2004). Roadside interviews were carried out within the frame of a pilot study in Kristianstad, a Swedish city with about 40,000 inhabitants. Interviewees were addressed randomly at the roadside. One selection criterion was familiarity with the place. In addition to 184 citizens at the roadside, 17 experts from the Municipality of Kristianstad were interviewed. All these interviews were carried out after a larger re-designing of the central city square. Improvements to walking facilities and barrier-free access to as many facilities as possible were among the goals of these changes. Other aspects touched by the changes are listed in Table 2.2.

Both the experts and the citizens assess the changes as important in most respects, except for good conditions for car drivers. Where the figures do not add up to 100%, some of the respondents did not know any answer or were undecided.

The results in Table 2.3 show that perceived changes in quality of life (QoL) and in all the other variables that relate to walking correlate highly.

The correlations in Table 2.3 indicate that the aspects in Table 2.2 that were elaborated and formulated within the frame of the interviews with pedestrians and with the help of expert interviews are relevant contributors to life quality. As is shown in Table 2.4, especially comfort for pedestrians, the usability of the area for elderly and disabled persons, feeling safe – that is, perceived traffic safety – and social interaction with other people showed high correlations with the perceived quality of life. So did the perceived safety of children, the fact that the traffic flow for pedestrians was smoother after the changes had been implemented, the beauty and aesthetics that made dwelling in the modified area more enjoyable, and the perceived safety of the elderly and disabled.

On a more moderate significance level, even perceived increased equity between road users, improved environmental quality concerning air and noise levels, a smoother traffic flow for cyclists, and greater ease of use of the area by walkers are experienced as contributors to an improved level of the quality of life on this modified central square in the Swedish city of Kristianstad.

Analysis of the answers given by different road user groups (besides pedestrians) showed that even frequent car drivers identified those improvements in the perceived quality of life, in spite of the fact that for them, the situation rather deteriorated (Bein et al., 2004). Support for walking from that side is definitely pleasing.

Table 2.3 Correlations between perceived changes (EU project HOTEL, Risser et al., 2004)

Item		Var1 Traffic Safety	Var2 Child Safety	Var3 Feeling Safe	Var4 Usabil. of eld. & dis.	Var5 Smooth traffic flow pedestr.	Var6 Smooth traffic flow cyclists	Var7 Smooth traffic flow car driv.	Var8 Equity b/w traffic groups	Var9 Ease and comfort pedestr.	Var10 Ease and comfort car driv.	Var11 Ease and comfort cyclists	Var12 Safety of eld. & dis.	Var13 Environ. (air, noise)	Var14 Social interact. with other	**Var15 QoL**	Var16 District more beautif.	Var17 Nice to be here
	Has improved:																	
Var1	Traffic safety	1.00																
Var2	Children's safety	0.73	1.00															
Var3	Feeling safe	0.96	0.65	1.00														
Var4	Usability for elderly & disabled persons	0.69	0.75	0.62	1.00													
Var5	Smooth traffic flow for pedestrians	0.52	0.44	0.42	0.52	1.00												
Var6	Smooth traffic flow for cyclists	0.41	0.44	0.32	0.44	0.48	1.00											
Var7	Smooth traffic flow car drivers	0.10	0.80	0.15	0.05	0.05	0.18	1.00										
Var8	Equity between traffic groups	0.45	0.48	0.39	0.45	0.40	0.37	0.25	1.00									
Var9	Ease and comfort for pedestrians	0.51	0.50	0.47	0.52	0.60	0.40	0.32	0.41	1.00								
Var10	Ease and comfort for car drivers	0.97	0.03	0.13	-0.01	0.00	0.13	0.76	0.25	-0.01	1.00							
Var11	Ease and comfort for cyclists	0.33	0.40	0.30	0.39	0.42	0.68	0.26	0.47	0.43	0.31	1.00						
Var12	Safety of elderly & disabled persons	0.47	0.46	0.41	0.61	0.48	0.45	0.06	0.35	0.59	0.06	0.50	1.00					
Var13	Environment (air, noise, ...)	0.31	0.35	0.28	0.40	0.28	0.29	0.30	0.32	0.38	-0.07	0.23	0.28	1.00				
Var14	Social interaction with other persons	0.35	0.31	0.28	0.26	0.30	0.26	-0.20	0.32	0.34	-0.11	0.23	0.22	0.36	1.00			
Var15	**Quality of life**	**0.45**	**0.44**	**0.47**	**0.48**	**0.44**	0.36	0.15	0.38	**0.50**	0.02	0.34	**0.40**	0.38	0.47	1.00		
Var16	The district is more beautiful now	0.43	0.39	0.37	0.44	0.34	0.42	0.38	0.29	0.37	0.42	0.41	0.41	0.32	0.29	**0.43**	1.00	
Var17	It is nicer to be here now	0.41	0.35	0.38	0.40	0.47	0.36	0.60	0.37	0.41	0.05	0.44	0.44	0.34	0.29	**0.42**	0.70	1.00

Table 2.4 Factors that enhance life quality (EU project HOTEL, Risser et al., 2004)

Improvements –> Improvements in QoL?	*Correlation with QoL*	
Comfort for pedestrians	0.50	high
Usability for elderly and disabled people	0.48	high
Feeling safe	0.47	high
Social interaction with other people	0.47	high
Traffic safety	**0.45**	**high**
Children's safety	0.44	high
Smooth traffic flow for pedestrians	0.44	high
Beauty and aesthetics of the urban space	0.43	high
Dwelling in this area is more enjoyable than before	0.42	high
Safety of elderly and disabled people	0.40	high
Equity between road users	0.38	moderate
Environmental quality (air, noise)	0.38	moderate
Smooth traffic flow for cyclists	0.36	moderate
Ease and comfort for pedestrians	0.34	moderate
Smooth traffic flow for car drivers	0.15	no
Comfort for car drivers	0.02	no

Almost ten years later than Bein et al. (2004), Ausserer et al. (2013) asked Viennese citizens what they considered the most disturbing preconditions in the public space that kept them – and that would keep others – from walking (more), in other words, what the barriers to walking were. When one looks at Figure 2.3, it is fully clear that the most relevant hindrances to walking in the city of Vienna in the year 2013 stemmed from car use, from

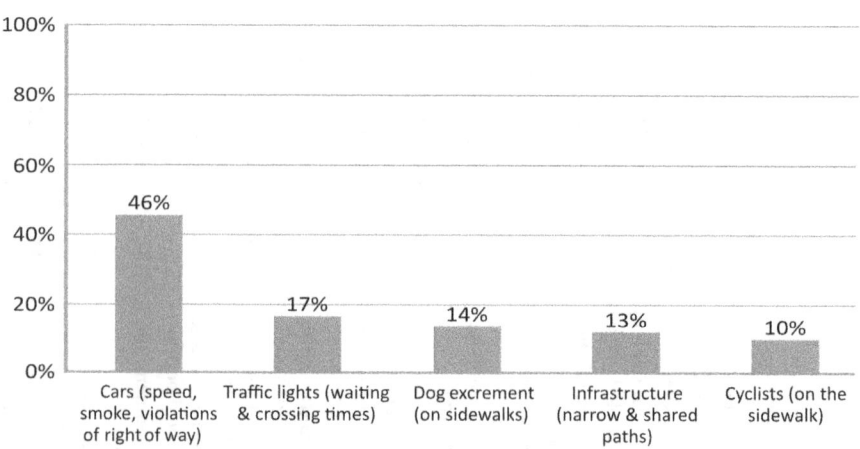

Figure 2.3 Factors that keep people in Vienna from walking (Ausserer et al., 2013).

car traffic, from how cars were used by drivers, and from an infrastructure that was tailor-made for cars. Problems with cyclists, which are very often presented as the greatest problem for pedestrians – we suspect, by supporters of car traffic – do not appear as being that important when considering the results of the study by Ausserer et al. (2013).

Walking makes people visible to other people. People can thus communicate with each other if they want, or at least they can greet each other. Direct communication is not so easy, if possible at all, when people are sitting in their cars. To assume that personal relationships – the glue of community cohesion – are fostered if people are outside and "expose" themselves is legitimate. We do know that not every communication process is necessarily a pleasant one, but in any case, having the opportunity to communicate allows people to learn about other people and, if possible and necessary, to adapt. According to Skynner and Cleese (1993), communication with others helps us find out that "the others" are usually friendly, easy to handle, and "just like us". It is more probable that a stronger sense of togetherness arises than that more communication with each other generates adverse effects. In any case, heavy car traffic affects togetherness negatively, and less car traffic allows more communication across the street (which is obviously on foot; see Figure 2.4).

But even if we just imagine people outside, in a public space, without directly communicating with each other, this may have positive effects concerning the quality of the places: *"By creating spaces that make it easy for people to give way to each other, to stop and chat, we can enhance the social use and enjoyment of our public spaces. And stress reduction through urban design is not only*

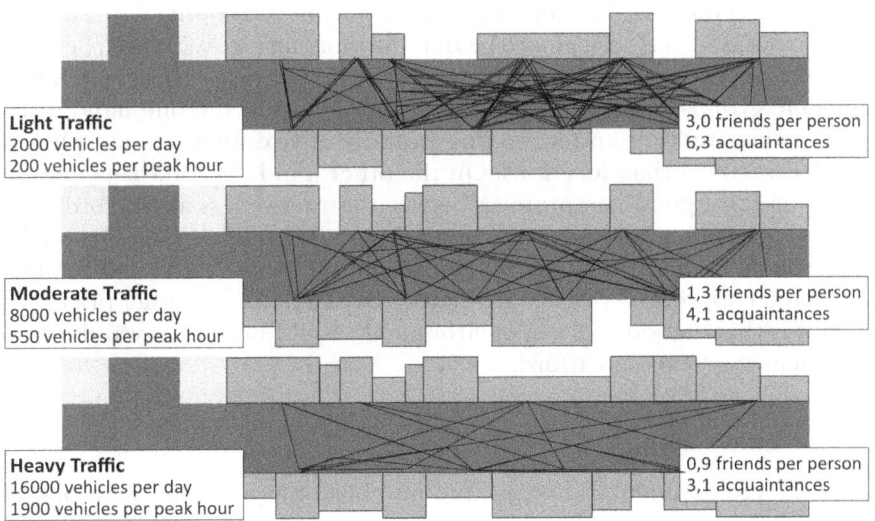

Figure 2.4 Influence of car traffic on social contacts (Appleyard, Gerson, & Lintell, 1981).

desirable – it's also achievable. We can see the success of schemes designed to encourage lingering in spaces such as Campo di Siena, Broadway in New York, the Lungomare in Naples. In places such as these, people are encouraged to stop, look around, enjoy a coffee, chat, absorb the atmosphere," says Nick Tyler in *The Conversation.*[2] What he says is that, of course, people walking in the street are not enough – we also need to strive for a pleasant and well usable infrastructure – but such an infrastructure is nothing when there are no people outside. However, an appropriate infrastructure will make people be there, and then there will be the desired effect – a good social climate in any such place. Cultural attractions will also contribute to the quality of the environment. Being able to walk in an attractive environment where there is also the possibility of visiting museums or historic sites will be a pleasure for many, not only for tourists but also for those who live there or in the vicinity. Additionally, walking to a concert, to the cinema, or to the theatre are activities one easily associates with a city that has good life quality. Cultural heritage lends a sense of place and attracts people. If planners succeed in combining walking and culture, walking will unfold its sustainable character even more.

Except for people with motor impairments, walking is affordable for everybody. Thus, when taking transit affordability as an indicator concerning the social issues pillar of sustainability, walking is definitely sustainable. However, a problem could arise in connection with the affordability of housing. There seems to be a relationship between the attractiveness of places, not least mirrored by their good preconditions for walking, and housing prices. The consequence could be, and in many cases is, that inhabited areas – not parks – that attract many walkers become too expensive for people, including walkers, with lower incomes. One cannot say that it is walking that impairs sustainability in this connection. However, the paradoxical effect seems to be that the more attractive an area becomes, the more expensive housing becomes as well, and in the end, only higher-income groups can afford to live in such areas. On the one hand, this is proof that walking and a walking-friendly environment create pleasant and attractive urban locations. On the other hand, "the market" does not provide for a good compromise between attractiveness and affordability. Clearly, the aim must be that locations that are friendly to walkers should be affordable for all income groups of citizens. Of course, there will be always a "market approach" (higher attractiveness of a place → higher price). The point is that a good walking environment should become a standard that all income groups can afford.

2.1.3   Environment

On the environmental side, a large number of aspects are mentioned in Table 2.1 that are considered important for the assessment of the degree of sustainability of any transport mode. Firstly, per capita energy consumption is listed. There is no difficulty at all and no long list of studies is needed to decide that walking does not consume much energy, generally, nor per freight ton-mile. There is no need to say that the distances that walkers can cover, and the tons that they can transport, are limited. On the other hand, it is sufficiently well known by now that many car trips only cover short distances that one also manage by walking, given an attitude that does not make walking something abominable. Nor does one transport heavy goods every day, a frequent reason given by people when explaining why they use the car regularly. A lot of shopping is done on foot,[3] often by those members of the household that do not use the family car regularly, and still more often women. It is difficult to calculate how many tons are brought home by walkers all over the world, or only just in any country that one wants to have a look at, in this respect. We suspect that here we are talking about a substantial tonnage, and when calculating the performance of walking – in fact, energy consumption per freight ton-mile – we probably find out that walking is doing very well. A study in the Austrian federal country of Vorarlberg by the VCÖ (the Austrian Traffic Club Verkehrsclub Österreich) showed that 1.15 million shopping trips (33% of all shopping trips) are done on foot or by bicycle and 1.6 million (50%) by car, the rest in combination with public transport. The analysis also showed that three out of ten shopping trips by car are shorter than 1 km, 50% are shorter than 2.5 km, and 70% shorter than 5 km. Thus, there is considerable potential for replacing shopping trips done by car and increasing the number of those done in a climate-friendly way. With an average pedestrian speed of 5 km/h, a distance of 1 km can be covered in 12 minutes on foot. However, it is important to note that, according to the same study, the majority of shopping trips are done on foot or by bike if the shops lie in the centre of town, while up to 90% of those to shops on the outskirts of town are carried out by car,[4] which apparently has something to do with the distance needed to travel to reach the shop.

As far as per capita air pollution emissions are concerned, we may be sure that walking is the champion, ex aequo with bicycling. Although their emission of harmful substances is not totally zero, it is probably very near to that; in any case, we found no studies concerning this question. Walking and cycling are definitely environmentally friendly in this respect, as is the per capita land devoted to transport facilities (roads, parking, etc.). Pedestrians need little space, the least of all modes, in fact. Still, in many cases, not even that little space they need is conceded to them. A more negative point concerning the sustainability of walking in the "environment" pillar is walkers' exposure to air pollution. Walkers are exposed, as cyclists are, but still, car drivers inhale the worst air (e.g. Freeland et al., 2017).[5] Still, even if car drivers are worse off, the problem remains that bad air in places with dense motor vehicle traffic is a serious drawback concerning the sustainability of walking. Even if air pollution does not lead to more serious health problems for walkers than for other groups, it definitely reduces the attractiveness of walking.

Concerning exposure to noise pollution, it is known that especially people who live near to larger roads or to railway lines suffer. Actually, the noise pollution from traffic is the most disturbing of all noise sources in cities. Figure 2.5[6] refers to citizens in general. The exposure of pedestrians

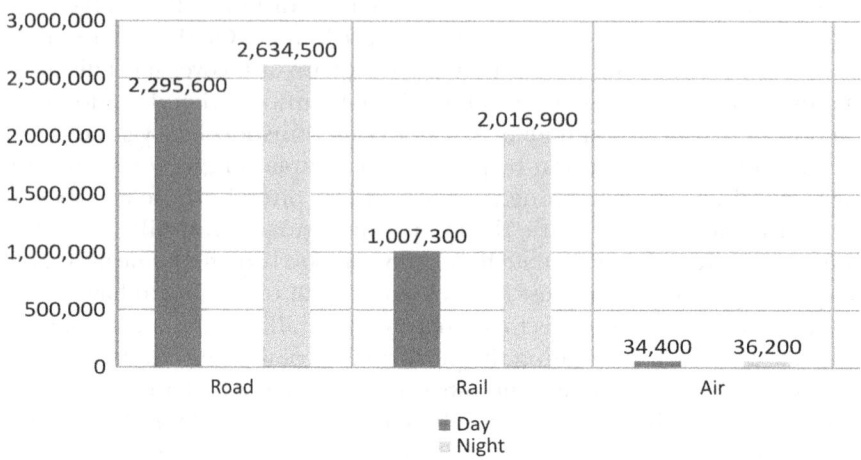

Figure 2.5 Subjective disturbance by noise stemming from road, rail, and air traffic (Umweltbundesamt, 2019).

to noise has not been studied much. We could not find any research work on that topic, though one may speculate that walkers are frequently disturbed by noise stemming from car traffic, much more so than people sitting in their cars and isolated from noise to a certain degree.

For all land transport, the sealing of the surface, producing impervious surface areas, is necessary to a greater or lesser degree. Very little sealing happens as a result of rail traffic infrastructure and walking, somewhat more for cycling, but very much more for motorised road transport. Concerning walking, in the countryside, there are not many asphalt or concrete roads just for pedestrians, so the sealing for the sake of walking is near to zero, we dare say. In cities, the largest areas are covered mostly for cars and less for cyclists and pedestrians. Thus, concerning land use, the sealing of the ground and, consequently, problems with storm and water management are hardly exacerbated by walking; quite the contrary: the replacement of car transport by soft modes, including walking, would allow for fewer square kilometres to be to allocated to transport and, for example, for more green areas in cities, which the citizens usually highly appreciate (Ausserer & Risser, 2018).

2.2   Walking as a health issue

When health is affected, this has both economic and social consequences, and thus this issue belongs to two of the pillars of sustainability, and it is related to the environmental area as well because environmental preconditions affect health. We have already mentioned the health consequences of air and noise pollution at the beginning of this book, and walking does not contribute to those. Traffic safety is definitely a public health issue and will be taken up further subsequently, pointing out that traffic crashes constitute one of the major problem areas in connection with walking, seriously undermining its otherwise positive sustainability balance.

When surfing through different web pages that pop up in connection with the combined keywords walking and health, one ends up with at least 11 big health advantages that are commented on there.[7]

1. For instance, they refer to medical journals that have calculated that 150 minutes of brisk walking per week can add 3.4 years to one's lifespan.
2. Regular walking also helps people to maintain their weight, though this is, of course, not independent of what and how much they eat.
3. At the same time, keeping one's blood pressure under good control functions much better if one walks regularly and appropriately – which varies among studies between the previously mentioned 150 minutes per week, that is, ~21.5 minutes per day, and up to 10,000 steps a day, that is, ~7.5 kilometres or 1.5 hours – which may appear more than it really is because there you count every step indoors and outdoors, to the bathroom, in the garden, and so on. Still, to do 10,000 steps a day will not be possible without some outdoor walking, for example, shopping or walking to a public transport stop.
4. Studies have also shown that walking reduces the probability of developing dementia, the reason being that it boosts the blood flow in the brain.
5. Additionally, walking helps to protect the health of one's bones, and it reduces the risk of bone thinning and other types of bone degeneration, labelled with the Latin words osteoporosis and osteoarthritis. *"Walkers have the healthiest knees,"* as it is usually said.
6. The reduction of the risk of cancer is mentioned by almost any author who discusses walking and health. There seems to be no doubt that walking reduces the risk of at least some types of cancer, such as cancer of the intestines, of the breast, and of the prostate, on the basis of the assumption of walking between three and seven hours a week.
7. The control of diabetes will also be more easy and efficient when one walks regularly and sufficiently much.
8. Another very important health effect is that walking reduces the cholesterol level, and thus the risk of heart disease is reduced substantially.
9. The fact that a reduction of the risk of stroke has also been identified is attributed to the lowering of blood pressure by regular walking.
10. Walking for one hour per day – which is equal to ~6000 steps – is also said to help reduce arthritic pain, although people who have such pain might feel reluctant to walk. It seems that if one overcomes that reluctance with controlled bodily exercise such as walking, this will do one good.
11. Last but not least, and very importantly, walking improves one's mood, which can be considered a general overarching health effect and is a remedy for depression.

Of course, this is not a complete list but rather refers to the advantages which are stressed the most. In reality, the lifestyle of "walkers" is also connected to many other positive factors.

2.3   Walking and traffic safety

Worldwide, more than 400,000 people annually die as pedestrians. The OECD estimates that there are 20,000 pedestrian fatalities annually in the OECD member countries, with a considerable variation between countries (Figure 2.6).

In Figure 2.7, we can see the percentage change in pedestrian fatalities between 2010 and 2016 in the selected countries (ITF, 2018). The trends are rather mixed; we can see sharp drops of up to 38% in the case of Norway on the one hand and, astonishingly, on the other hand a sharp increase of up to 36% in the case of Sweden, which is otherwise considered a very safe country, and 39% in the United States.

As for the United States, a total of 5977 pedestrian deaths occurred in 2017. Pedestrian fatalities decreased by 2% compared to 2016, which was the highest level since 1990. Although pedestrian deaths were 20% lower in 2017 than in 1975, they had increased by 45% since they reached their lowest point in 2009 (FARS, 2018).

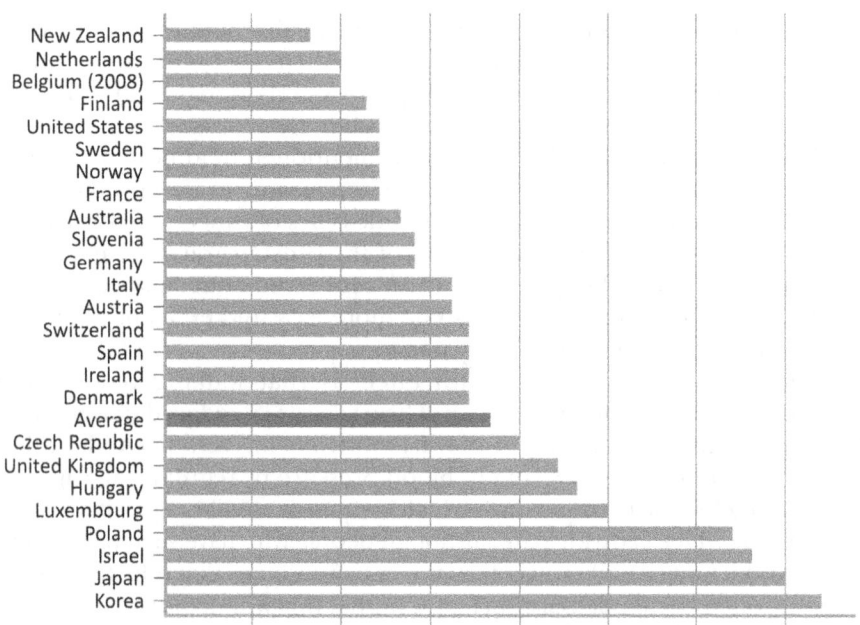

Figure 2.6 Pedestrian fatalities as a percentage of all road fatalities in 26 OECD countries (ITF, 2011).

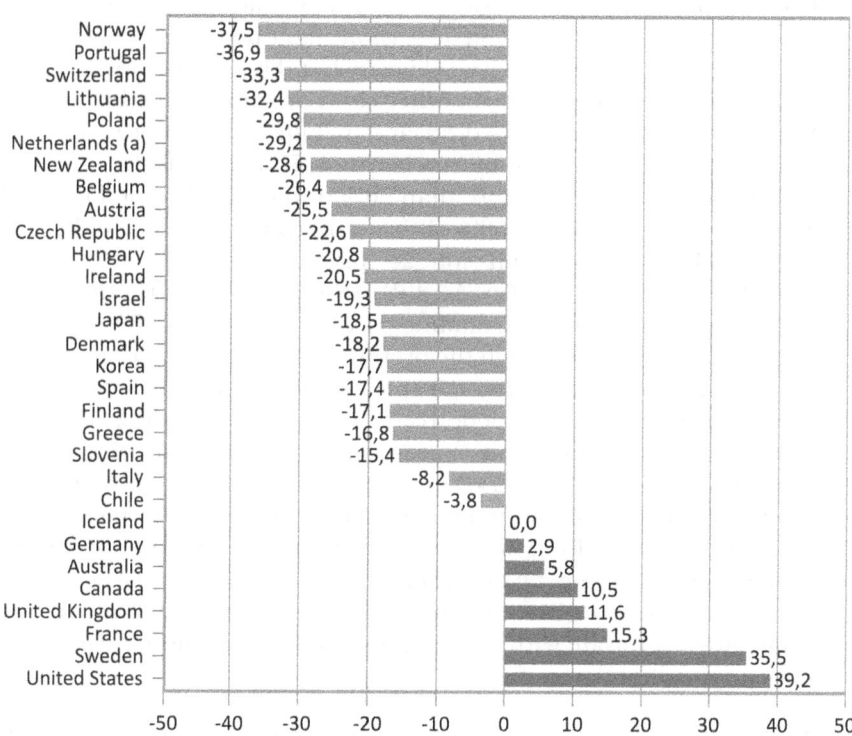

Figure 2.7 The percentage change in pedestrian fatalities between 2010 and 2016 in the selected countries (ITF, 2018).

Pedestrians are called vulnerable road users – together with cyclists and motorcyclists – because they have no protective coachwork around their body. At the same time, traffic conditions are often uncomfortable and difficult to cope with and experienced as being unsafe, which keeps many people from walking. This is especially the case for older people, people with impairments, and children. According to the ITF (2011), around 30% of pedestrians have impaired mobility at any given time as a result of temporary or permanent health impairments or because they are carrying bags or other objects or, for example, when walking with a pram. Concerning children, parents are often reluctant to let them walk or cycle to school because they fear for their safety.

Some statements and truisms may help to give a more colourful picture of traffic safety issues in connection with walking:

- According to our own estimates, 50% of the population are not able, or have no chance, to use a car as a driver; that is, they have to move about as vulnerable road users more than the others (in many cases as pedestrians).

- Fatal injuries result almost only from other road users, mostly motor vehicles. In Vienna (2004), in 75% of all fatal pedestrian accidents, a car was the other party involved (Figure 2.8). This figure most probably does not differ too much from other cities or countries in Europe.
- When involved in crashes, pedestrians are killed much more often than other road users (except motorcycle riders; Hakkert, 2010).
- In urban environments, more than 50% of the people killed in traffic are pedestrians and 50%–60% of the pedestrians killed are older than 65 years (European Commission, 2018).
- Data for the EU-19 (DaCoTA, 2012) shows that the proportion of pedestrian fatalities in total fatalities is around 20% (data for the EU-28 is not available). Even though the overall number of pedestrian fatalities is constantly decreasing (though this is not true for all EU countries, as shown in Figure 2.7), pedestrian fatalities as a proportion of all fatalities are remaining stable or are even increasing slightly (Figure 2.9). Similarly, despite the decrease in the total number of fatalities, trends in the United States show an unexplained increase in pedestrian fatalities (Patek & Thoma, 2013). The trend in recent years seems to be continuing in the direction of the data shown here.
- Pedestrians have to live with broken taboos: for example, they are systematically unsafe with green lights at crossings where turning cars have a green light as well.

Additionally, there is one topic that is not appropriately dealt with in the literature, and that concerns pedestrian falls, as already mentioned before. According to Methorst et al. (2017), in the Netherlands, slightly more than

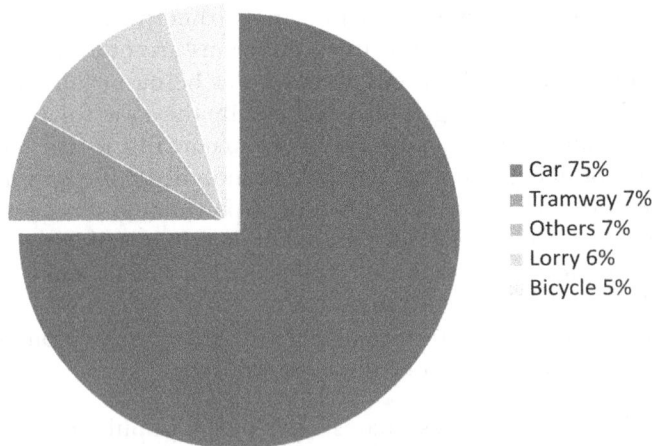

Figure 2.8 Other parties involved in fatal accidents involving pedestrians (City of Vienna 2011, in Walkspace, 2012).

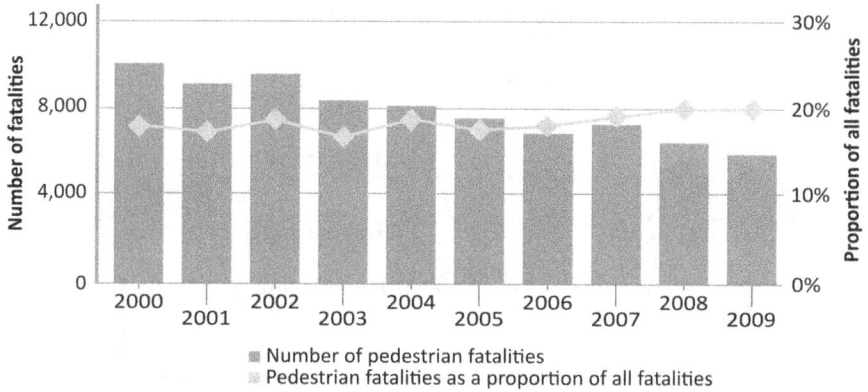

Figure 2.9 Number of pedestrian fatalities and proportion of total fatalities in the EU-19, 2000–2009 (CARE Database 2012, in DaCoTA, 2012).

50% of all pedestrian deaths and the majority of injured pedestrians result from pedestrians falling, the awkward aspect being that nowhere are those falls treated as traffic casualties (as no motor vehicle is involved). Thus, the statistical data concerning this type of mishap is very poor, while there is certainly a relationship between such accidents and shortcomings in the traffic environment, both concerning design and maintenance.

From a psychological perspective, traffic safety has to be discussed as an issue of individual interest. That means that it is important how safety is perceived by road users themselves. Objective safety is not necessarily reflected at an equivalent scale by our subjective assessment. For instance, the commonsense notion is that the hazards connected to high speeds are usually underestimated by drivers, while the dangers posed to one's children, represented in the traffic environment by cars going fast, are usually estimated as being very high (while the word "overestimated" sounds wrong in this connection). The latter example points to the fact that perceived lacks of safety definitely influence the propensity of people to walk. Accordingly, Rehbein (2014), citing Gifford (2007a and b) and Brunswick (1956), looks at traffic safety as one important quality factor influencing satisfaction with a traffic mode and consequently affecting mode choice (see Figure 2.10).

Fyhri et al. (2010), who dealt with the question of what elements constitute comfort in traffic, with a special focus on children, came to the same conclusion. When traffic safety is perceived as being low, comfort is perceived as being poor. This plays a certain role in connection with mode choice according to many studies, but seems to have its strongest effects when children and their safety (as perceived by parents) are concerned.

The Swedish artist Karl Jilg produced some wonderful drawings trying to depict how the public space might be perceived by different types of road

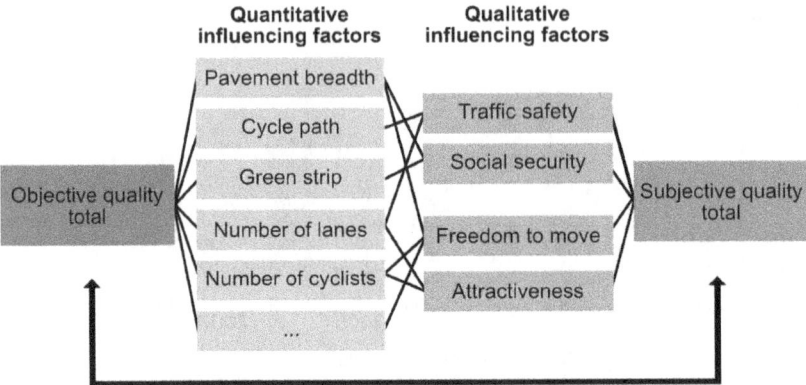

Figure 2.10 Quantitative and qualitative factors for the assessment of walking routes (Rehbein, 2014).

users and how much of the public space is dedicated to cars. Figure 2.11 subsequently imagines the world of the pedestrian in an urban environment. It provides an impression of how one might feel when out in the public space. We can only cope with this situation because we have become so used to it that we do not realise any more how appalling the situation really is.

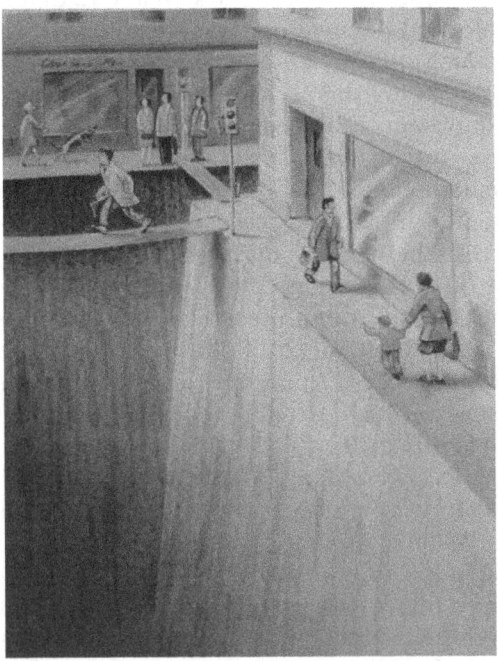

Figure 2.11 How walking in the city might feel (illustration by Karl Jilg).

In sum, for the promotion of walking, it is crucial to provide preconditions for pedestrians that are safe both objectively and also subjectively, that is, that are perceived as being safe. However, the data available all around the world shows that pedestrians are at risk of being injured or killed in traffic more often than all other road users except motorcyclists.

Studies on selected road sections in different countries revealed a systematic relation between average speeds on road sections or in road networks and the number of accidents and people killed. This was examined in empirical studies in Sweden, Denmark, the United States, Australia, the Netherlands, and others (see, e.g. Elvik et al., 2004; Elvik, 2009; Rosén et al., 2011). A significant percentage of pedestrian accidents occur at secured crossings, with the main contributor to the accidents being motor vehicle speed. A Swedish study with observations at pedestrian crossings showed that very often, drivers make pedestrians renounce their right of way by not reducing speed when approaching a crossing; instead of this, some even accelerate before a pedestrian crossing, thus making it evident that they will not stop (Várhelyi, 1996). This study also showed a direct relationship between speed and preparedness to yield: the higher the initial approaching speed, the lower the preparedness to yield. Summing up, this means that one of the most important measures to make walking more attractive is to dramatically reduce car speeds (to 30 km per hour, as is often suggested) and to enforce speed rules seriously, so that the social norm becomes the same as, or close to, the speed limit.

2.4 Children and walking

When discussing children and traffic in combination, we usually refer to their safety, or to a lack of safety, either perceived – usually by the parents rather than the children – or reflected in accident statistics. Concerning their mobility, small children play only a minor role in research. Hardly any statistical data on the mobility behaviour of children can be found. Especially children younger than six years old, that is, usually pre-school children, are badly treated in this respect. But in fact, socialisation starts with personal experience from early childhood on. One's later "mobility life" is not least shaped by one's mobility in the time of one's early childhood. If people are used to walking as children, they will probably also walk more (often) as adults. In two Austrian studies about the mobility situation of pre-school and primary school children in Vienna and in the surroundings of Vienna (Ausserer et al., 2011, 2012), data on their mobility was analysed, focusing on trips to and from kindergarten and primary school. More than 2000 parents in Vienna and Lower Austria were asked about the way their children travelled to kindergarten and to school. They were also asked to estimate the share of car trips which could be replaced by alternative modes. The pre-school children were asked to sketch in drawings how they would like to go to kindergarten, and the primary school pupils answered questions in groups, in order to give an impression of what they themselves would prefer. The results showed that walking was still the main mobility mode on the way to kindergarten, and, less pronouncedly, to primary school. However, one-third of all trips to kindergartens and primary schools in Vienna and in the surroundings of Vienna are done by car. The interesting thing is that more than half of these trips take no more than five minutes, while the longest distance in the sample that was analysed was ~2 km, that is, ~30 minutes on foot at a reasonably low speed, as will be the case with children. This means that there is significant potential to replace car trips by walking on the way to kindergarten. Studies like these are also common in other European countries, usually under the label "Ways to school", with similar results to those in Vienna.

The parents who were interviewed did see the positive aspect of walking together. *"You have more time for each other,"* a father of a four-year-old girl said, for instance. But experienced road safety problems are one important reason for taking children to kindergarten and to primary school by car instead of walking together and letting them walk alone as soon as they have reached a certain age. Of course, practical reasons play an important role, as well: in the morning, parents go to work by car, and it does not cost much time to take their children to kindergarten and primary school on their way, thereby not having to be afraid for the safety of their children. Walking together is to be considered less practical when one has to continue to one's workplace after having accompanied one's child, unless there is an efficient public transport system available to proceed – which is rarely the case in rural areas – or if one's workplace is also within walking distance of one's children's kindergarten or primary school.

2.4.1   Children's safety in traffic

Figure 2.12, subsequently, from the Netherlands indicates that the risk of children in kindergarten and primary school getting killed in traffic is rather low compared to the age groups above 10 years. Moreover, the numbers of children killed and injured in Europe are decreasing, among other things as a result of a decrease in birth rates and the improved safety of modern cars. Still, most of the children who are killed or injured are passengers in cars, followed by pedestrians and cyclists. It is difficult to state clearly, though, which mode is more "dangerous", because reliable exposure data is lacking. The studies of Ausserer et al. (2011, 2012) presented such data, but only for Vienna and its surroundings, and it cannot simply be taken as generally valid. What can be said, though, is that in recent decades, car use, including accompanying trips to school and other destinations, has been steadily increasing. The results of the study of Fyhri et al. (2010) indicate, though, that many parents frequently perceive the traffic situation as being unsafe and thus are afraid for the safety of their children. As a result, which is also supported by habit, parents prefer to transport

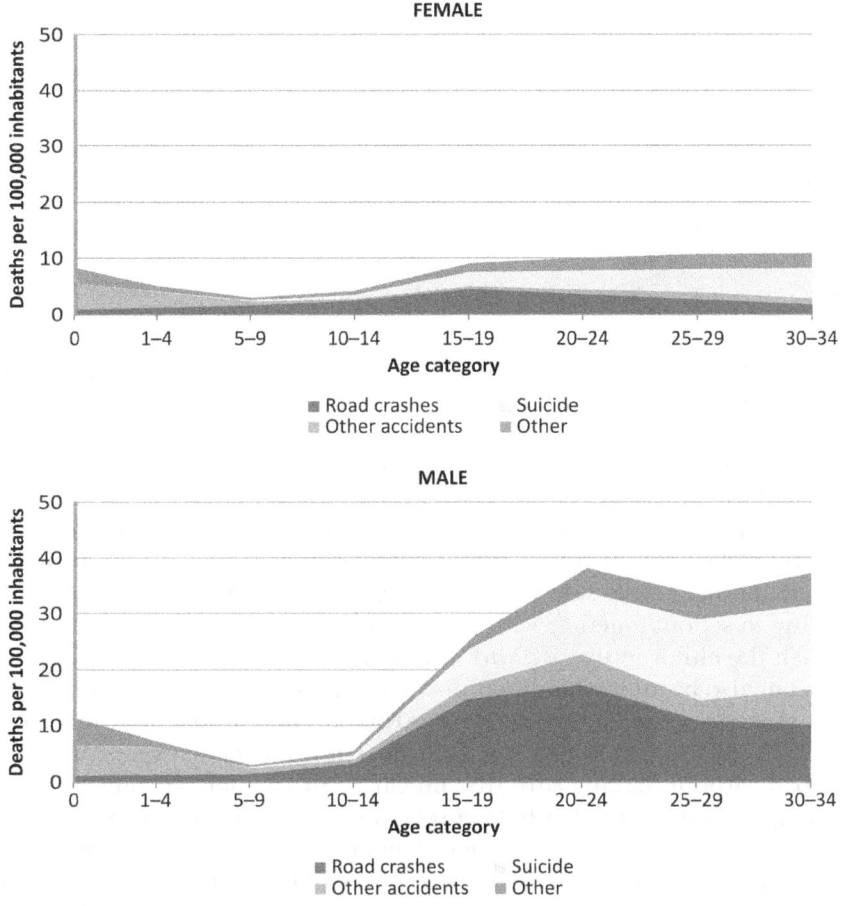

Figure 2.12 Unnatural deaths per 100,000 inhabitants by cause, age, and gender during the period 1999–2008 in the Netherlands (SWOV, 2012).

their children to kindergarten or to school by the "safest mode", the car, obviously not knowing, or ignoring the fact, that children are killed much more often as car passengers than as pedestrians. Satisfactory exposure data is not available, so one cannot say that it is safer to walk than to be a car passenger, but it should be pointed out that transporting children by car does not make their trips fully safe, either (https://www.iihs.org/topics/fatality-statistics/detail/children).

In any case, there is a general increase in the number of parents who bring their children to school by car, which in turn increases the risk to those outside cars – children or other pedestrians – and subsequently a decrease in the number of those children who (still) walk to school. The "collateral damage" of this is that by increasingly transporting their children in the

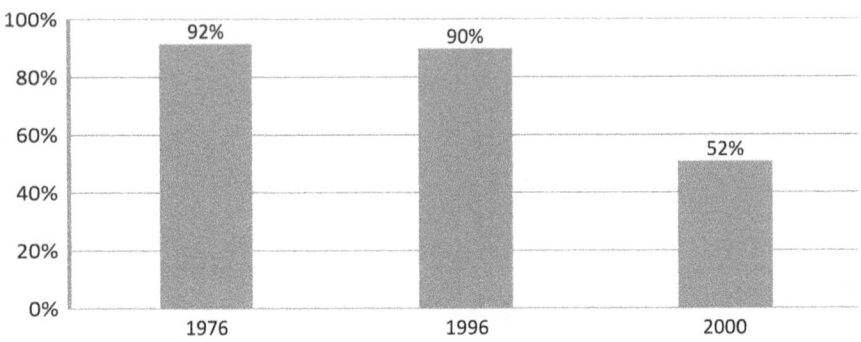

Figure 2.13 Unaccompanied school trips of six-to-seven-year-old children in Germany 1976–2000 (Funk & Fassmann, 2002).

car during the last 30–40 years (see Figure 2.13 for Germany), parents have restricted the independent mobility of their children.

Alas, traffic safety problems are not solved by such decisions. Rather, the contrary is the case. Accident numbers are probably not reduced. Instead, there is another severe safety shortcoming connected to this development. Walking to school together with one's children would provide the chance to teach the children to cope with traffic, not only by learning the official rules, but also by understanding informal norms and how to communicate in an efficient and safe way with other road users. For instance, it is most important to learn that a green light does not mean that one can cross the road without making sure that no car is turning left or right, thereby crossing one's path, or that having seen a car does not mean that the car driver has seen you, and many others. Generally speaking, experience with the traffic environment is not gathered by avoiding the use of the public space, thus preventing them from learning to use it autonomously. However, in the beginning, trips on foot or by bicycle have to be guided by parents or other accompanying persons, which could be one of the reasons transport by car is preferred. The first vicious cycle resulting from this has been pointed out previously – increasing car use and a decreasing number of children walking – and has a negative impact on the per capita safety of the "remaining" walkers (see Figure 2.14). The other vicious cycle, connected to the first one, is that children do not learn to handle traffic in the way that children and youngsters could do autonomously, namely as walkers. What this means is, of course, that in case they do walk on one occasion or another, their risk of getting involved in an accident will be higher because of their lack of exercise and experience.

2.4.1.1   Development of skills

The differences in children's physical and psychological skills depend on their age but also on other influencing factors. In fact, greater levels of

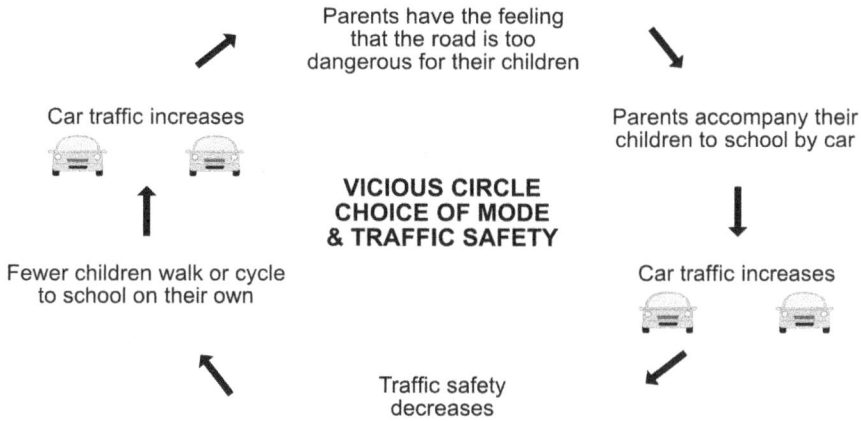

Figure 2.14 Choice of mode and traffic safety (Rauh, 2001).

physical activity diminish the risk of falling or other injuries related to motion. Children who travel mainly by car have lower levels of physical activity, and because of their lack of experience, they are less successful in negotiating road traffic as pedestrians, public transport users, or cyclists. Additionally, their ability to develop risk awareness and therefore to perceive traffic situations as dangerous is influenced by such experience (though age is the dominant factor here). A general disadvantage of low motion levels that is not related to traffic safety is that inactive children are less healthy, and their psychomotor development and also their attentiveness are negatively affected (DaCoTA, 2012). In sum, physical activity is important, not only for children, but especially for children. A very easy way to provide a certain amount of physical exercise is to walk to kindergarten and to school, together with accompanying persons or – as soon as this is possible – alone. As Figure 2.15 subsequently shows, walking can also easily be combined with other activities that provide fun. When we talk of skills, we also refer to the more general skills of coping with one's living environment; finding one's way; and learning and knowing more and more details about the streets, the buildings, the places where one can play, and where it is dangerous because of traffic or because *"there is a big dog around that house"*.

In short, children are empowered by being allowed and given the opportunity to move autonomously outdoors, which they actually seem to like. When children were asked about their preferred mode of transport, they provided an interesting picture (Umweltamt Stadt Karlsruhe, 2003): 950 schoolchildren were asked about how they would like to go to school, and the discrepancy between their wishes and the reality was demonstrated impressively: in this case, not in support of walking but in support of cycling and using scooters. In any case, they wanted to use the car less (see Figure 2.16 subsequently). The figures of Rudner & Malone (2011) for Australia show a similar picture: almost 70% of children wanted to walk or cycle; only

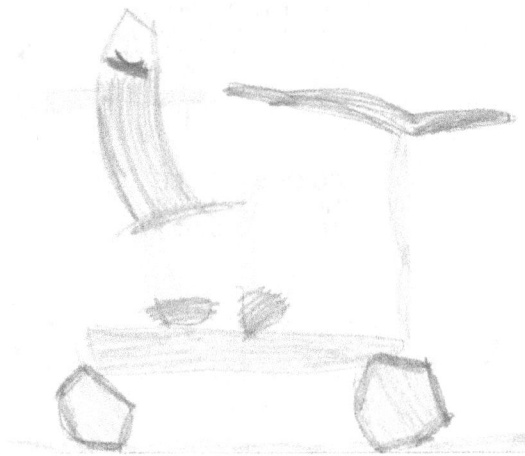

"This is how I would like to go to the Kindergarten"
(Bernhard, 5 years)

Figure 2.15 'This is how I would like to go to the kindergarten' (Ausserer et al., 2010).

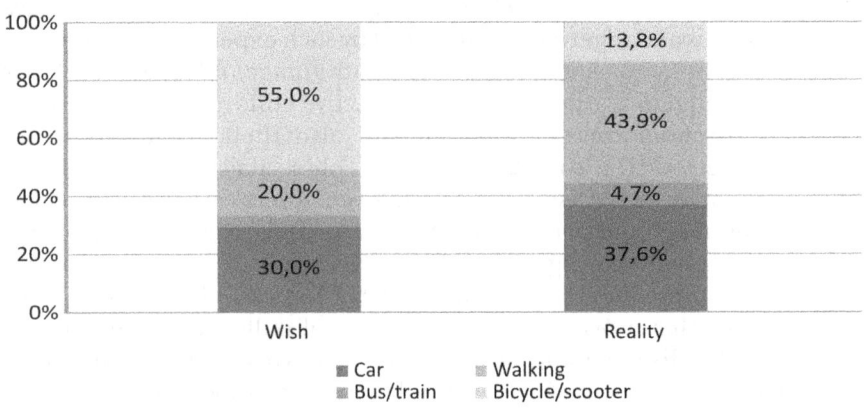

Figure 2.16 Preferred transport mode of 950 children (Umweltamt Stadt Karlsruhe, 2003).

18% preferred a car ride. Good travel and traffic conditions for children and young people can help to change and shape the traffic behaviour of future generations in a positive and sustainable way.

Of course, it is the duty of grown-ups to see to it that all the necessary safety provisions are considered and taken, but with a sense of proportion. Not letting children walk alone in the public space when this would generally be possible and taking them to virtually every destination by car, with the *"parents' taxi"*, reflects the absence of this sense and interferes with the sensible development of our children. Again, and this cannot be repeated too often, the best way to get a thorough impression of the possible hazards that one's children can come across on their daily trips and how well children are able to cope with these hazards is to walk together as often as possible, thereby observing the children, and to give feedback where necessary. The same principle is used (and well evaluated) within the frame of what is called a graduated driving licence, where a period of driving accompanied by a parent or another significant person is part of the process.

Much of what has been written previously about children and walking is connected to the character of both the traffic infrastructure and of traffic itself, clearly the result of the ever-increasing car traffic over the decades, where many other issues that should have been considered appropriately have been neglected. Among other things, children themselves and their needs have been neglected. Children need interaction with their parents; their parents are models for them so that they learn to develop clever and appropriate ways to cope with both their physical and social environment. Parents should let children do things – jump, run, play, generally use their bodies – and they should teach children to do things. Handing children over to the car as transportable goods is certainly not the way to teach them how to use and appreciate the public space both in the vicinity of their homes and at greater distances from them, on the way to school, to their mates' homes, to training sessions, and to cultural events.

On the following pages, we introduce some examples of their own mobility during childhood and youth given by colleagues working with transport and mobility from all over the world. These examples are anonymised, and they are written in the reporters' own words. They had the maximum freedom for those texts. The instruction was to write approximately half a page to one page of text; it could be more but should not be less. Here come their stories.

2.4.2   Tales about mobility in childhood and youth all around the world

Subsequently, a number of short tales by traffic and mobility researchers about their own mobility during their childhood and youth are reported. In 2004, Chaloupka and Risser compiled a booklet with such reports of colleagues from all over the world. In 2019, the list of these reports was completed with 26 more short summaries of other colleagues on the same topic. When reading these contributions, one realises that experiences that are remembered and told about today are not so different from each other, in spite of originating from countries as distant from each other as Sweden, India, Spain, Ireland, Japan, Ghana, or Russia. Walking is a predominant travel mode during childhood and youth. The first trips with different vehicles – from bicycles to cars – have left impressions, and accidents have caused distress and anxiety in some cases. One does not have the slightest difficulty in understanding both the stories told in the reports received and the emotions expressed directly or indirectly in connection with the reported experiences of walking, of other active modes, of activities outside, with friends or alone.

BRAZIL (*1975)

My earliest recollection: I spent my childhood in a medium-sized city (about 250,000 inhabitants) located in the Southern part of the country. I always comment in the plural – us – because it was me and my brother. We used to go to school on foot since the distance was less than 1000 m. For tours, we used the family car. During our teens, we began to ride bicycles more for some journeys, since using the local transport demanded a certain maturity that we did not have in childhood. The city had a high rate of motorisation and rugged topography.

Our journeys were mainly to school, language courses, and visits to family and friends. When we were left alone, we would walk; when we were accompanied by our parents, by car.

At the end of our adolescence, when we entered the university, the use of public transport by bus became part of our routine, given the distance from the centre of the city to the campus, approximately 25 km.

CANADA (*1955)

My earliest recollection of my mobility involved very short walking trips to the homes of neighbourhood friends who lived within 150 metres from my home. These trips were restricted to sidewalks next to low-volume local roads and these trips were probably closely monitored by a watchful parent. Upon entering elementary school at age five, I was able to walk to school, as it was located approximately 350 metres from my home. As a very young student, I was either accompanied by a parent on my journey to school or by my older brother who was instructed to ensure my journey to and from school was safe. I attended my elementary school until grade 8 and all of my trips involved walking to school, since trips by bicycle and public transport were generally not necessary.

After school and at weekends, most of my trips (i.e. without my parents) during my elementary years (i.e., up to grade 8, or approximately age 13) were made either on foot as a pedestrian, by bicycle, or motorised transport, including private vehicles or public transport. The choice of mode generally depended on three things: (1) the length of the journey, (2) the purpose of the journey, and (3) the weather conditions at the time of the journey. Short trips were usually made on foot, whereas longer trips were made by bicycle. However, growing up in a mid-sized Canadian city with adverse weather conditions during the winter months sometimes did not allow for pedestrian or cycling trips.

When I consider the trips that I made with my family, these were almost entirely made in a private vehicle. There was (is) a distinct lack of compact urban form in the Canadian city where I grew up, which reduced the ability to walk or cycle in a meaningful way. The reliance on private vehicles was very normal for me when growing up.

When I entered high school in grade 9 (age 14), the school was now located approximately 2.5 kilometres away from my home. Each morning, my brother and I would be driven to our high school by our father on his way to work. At the end of the school day, we were required to find our own way home. When the weather was reasonable, this trip was made on foot as a pedestrian but if the weather was poor, then this trip would be made by public transport or possibly by getting a ride with an older student with a car. The day that I turned 16 years old, I obtained my driver's licence and immediately purchased a vehicle. After this date (i.e. grades 11 and 12), my trips to school were made in my own private vehicle. I can generally state that once I owned a vehicle, walking, cycling, and public transport trips were reduced significantly – or were virtually eliminated.

In summary, I would state that most of my trips up to age 16 (i.e., my personal trips not involving my family) involved walking (70%), followed by cycling (20%), with public transport representing 10%. However, this changed significantly at age 16, where I would suggest that my trips were almost entirely made by private vehicle (90%), with all other transportation modes (walking, cycling, or public transport) representing 10%.

CZECH REPUBLIC (*1989)

I spent most of my childhood (counting up to 18 years of age) either in the capital city (1.5 million residents) or – mostly during holidays – with my aunt in a small city (<15,000 residents) near the North-Western border of the republic. Considering my mobility at that time, the patterns differed slightly between the two places:

a. With my aunt, I went out for a walk in the surroundings practically on a daily basis. We also took many trips by train or bus, going camping or visiting other places in the republic, and walking was our main mode of transport as soon as we arrived at our destination. The same was true when I was going to summer camps on my own (three weeks in July/ August ever since I was 11). When I was around 10, I also got a new bike and we took longer cycling trips, too. All in all, when I was with my aunt, I sure walked a lot;

b. In the city, I had to travel to school across the whole city (ca. one hour). Up until the third grade, I managed this via the mother of one of my classmates who lived nearby, and she took us both to and from school by car. From the third grade, I started to go to school on my own, by tram, subway, and bus. I remember enjoying trying different routes, as there were different combinations of traffic modes possible. (Once I even tried to cross the whole city on foot, just to see how long it would take and whether I could find safe passages across the points I usually crossed with a tram or a bus – such as the river near the train station, or the highway along the river. I did it and it took me for about 3.5 hours, and I was very proud of myself.) When I was older, I also frequently stopped in the city to take a walk, read a book in a mall, or just do a little "window-shopping". After school or at weekends, I was usually playing outside, as there was a forest near where I lived, and sometimes we went cycling, too.

To sum it up, in my childhood and youth, I think I definitely spent a lot of time walking and taking public transport. This was partly due to the fact that our own car was stolen before I entered third grade, and we did not get a new one until I was… way older. But I think of it as a great time which gave me a lot of freedom and I really enjoyed it.

ENGLAND (*1952)

Travelling to school in the '50 s and '60s: I started at our Yorkshire village primary school when I was five years old. It was 1957. My brother and I walked to school. Almost no-one went by car. Those that lived more than walking distance away went by bus. It was quite a walk for me as a five-year-old: about one kilometre, and I did it there and back twice every day because I went home for lunch. So I walked at least four kilometres a day… plus any sports and other activities during and after school. But it was normal in those days, and other kids walked a good deal further than we did!

When I was about nine I noticed that a couple of other kids in our neighbourhood were taking the bus to school. I decided that I'd had enough of all the walking and decided to take the bus too. The fare from our nearest bus stop to school was a penny. There were 240 pennies in a British pound in those days before decimalisation, so even at that time it was a cheap ride! I got to know the other kids who rode the bus, and we decided that in the time we spent waiting for the bus it would be almost quicker to walk. So we started keeping the pennies that our parents gave us for the fare and spent them on sweets instead. A few pennies bought quite a handful of "goodies", as we called them. Of course, we eventually got found out and the bus money stopped!

I went to a boys' grammar school in 1963, when I was 11. It was an 11-km bus journey every day, so there was no more coming home for lunch. Several double-decker buses passed through our village, taking kids from other neighbouring villages to our school in the market town of Beverley. The bus journeys to and from school were certainly much more fun than what happened at school! Typically, kids were singing, fighting, throwing things out of the window, and being cheeky to the bus conductor. What was less enjoyable in the morning was trying to finish neglected homework that needed to be handed in that morning! The senior boys always sat on the front seats upstairs. None of us younger kids would dare to sit there! They all smoked. Smoking was allowed on the upper deck and considered very cool. On a cold wet day the windows would steam up and the air quality on the upper deck of the bus reached danger levels! We all had a bus pass that gave us free transport to school. Of course, there was always someone who had either lost or forgotten their pass. Me too occasionally. The conductor had to take our name and address and a bill was sent to our home. It was hardly worth the administration costs for such a small amount of money, but rules were rules! The bus home was even more riotous. Perhaps it was the proverbial "being let out of school" syndrome. When the bus approached our village the most courageous amongst us would attempt to jump off before the bus had stopped. There were no doors at the back of the bus so it was common practice to jump off anywhere one cared to. It was quite a sport and some boys were experts, but there were also a few casualties!

In the final years at school, when we were 16+, some of us had motorbikes or scooters. We weren't allowed to travel to school on them for reasons best known to the headmaster, so those that did needed to find a hiding place near the school, and wear a disguise so as not to be recognised. One of my friends had an old BSA 650 with a double sidecar. It could accommodate four people: two on the bike and two in the sidecar. We had some interesting and memorable adventures on that bike! Happy days!

FINLAND (*1951)

I spent my youth in a small town with about 20,000 inhabitants. Ever since I was about six, a bicycle was my main mode of transport and mobility, complemented with walking during the winter months. There were two bus routes in the town, but neither of them passed close to our home, so public transport was never an option for travel inside the town.

We did have a summer cottage about 20 km away, and we usually travelled there by bus as the cottage was close to the main road connecting Turku and Helsinki, and the bus also had a stop close (200 m) to our home. My parents bought a car when I was 13, so then the trips to the cottage were made by car. My parents normally used a bike for commuting, and very seldom the car.

I was never enthusiastic about a moped, although that would have been an option from age 15 onwards. We lived close to the school (about 200 m at primary school, then perhaps 1.2 km to the lyceum). So it was quick by bicycle, and not too far for walking, either. In addition, I have always liked walking a lot. Most of my friends also lived in the town, only one perhaps 2 km outside, but that was well reachable by bicycle.

Everything changed when I became 18, and got a driver's licence. I never used it to go to school, but it was the evening vehicle, riding along the main street with a few friends, back and forth, always the same two end points, where we turned. And tens of others doing the same. We did not always use our car; sometimes my friends had their parents' car. And two of my classmates had cars of their own. During the first months that I had a driving licence I always volunteered at home when a driver was being sought. The novelty wore off quite quickly, though.

I think I was 19 when I bought a cheap 12-year-old 125-cc MZ motorcycle, with classic "elephant ear" seats, from a farmer. That then became my personal cottage vehicle, and also the vehicle for riding along the main street, for a while. After a year I had a crash with a car on the main street with the car driving out from a parking place to the street, looking in my direction, leading to my conclusion that he had seen me, but after the crash he claimed he did not see me at all. Then I realised that motorcycling was too risky, and abandoned it. My brother was more courageous and took it up – he had already been using a moped since he was 15.

FRANCE (*1979)

I grew up in a suburb of Paris, Le Raincy, which is quite walkable and dense.

As far as I remember, I walked to the "maternelle" (3–5 y) or elementary school (6–10 y), but I don't know if I ever went alone.

For college (11–14), I was walking 800 m from home, and I think I was going alone from some age, but I don't remember which. It was about the same distance for the next step (lycee, high school, 15–18 yo) and I went there alone. We did not ride bikes much in the streets; it was not encouraged (I don't remember why). I used to go to play at my friends' houses in the same city, within similar ranges. I did not go to many other activities that I can remember. The main street did provide some interesting shopping for kids, some games or a bakery for food, but I don't remember strolling much on my own. We would go to the public market with my parents, again within 1 km of home.

I was actually one year ahead from age seven so I finished high school (in French: baccalaureat) at 17 to go to study for two years in the "classes preparatoires", to prepare for the nationwide exams to go into engineering school. My parents rented a small apartment for me during that time. I was in the 13th borough (arrondissement), but my school was in the 6th. I lived there on my own for two years, having all my lunches at school. The walk was 2 km, so I sometimes cheated my way onto the bus to go avoid walking and go a bit faster. After that, I went to Telecom Paris (ParisTech nowadays), in the 13th borough, and had a room in student accommodation at the Cité Universitaire in the 14th, close to the ring road around Paris. It was a 1.5-km walk, through the nice Parc Montsouris. I was there for two years, then moved into a residence just by the school. I then went for my PhD; I guess it does not qualify as youth any more.

It's funny; I never really measured these distances (no Google Maps), so they don't seem like much today, but they seemed quite long at the time. The 2-km one in particular. There was no awareness (or at least I do not remember) of the positive impacts of walking or active transportation (the terminology is very recent).

I never tried to ride a bike at this time in Paris either (prepa was 1996–1998, then engineering school 1998–2001); not many people cycled at the time in Paris; there were no racks for parking; the bike-share system arrived in 2005.

I would take public transport to go further (films, bars), but otherwise was pretty sedentary, and stayed in students' clubs and spaces at the school for socialising. I would take the suburban train to go back to my parents' place at the weekends (50 min-1 h). Growing up in a suburb of Paris, even just a 20-min ride from Paris itself, is very different from growing up in Paris. We would go to Paris to visit my grandmother, and that's it. I started going there with my friends to go bowling, maybe when I was 14–15. I actually remember that I had a friend who had never used public transport to go to Paris the first time we went and did not know what to do with his train ticket.

GHANA (*1983)

I inhabit a part of the world where walking is a major means of mobility. Growing up in a large coastal city of over 300,000 inhabitants in the southern part of Ghana, my childhood was full of activities. The means of mobility within the most part of the city for the majority (including children and young people) was on foot. Cycling was not an integral part of the life of ordinary citizens as it was among rich people. Even at that, cycling was just for recreational purposes and not a means of transportation. Besides, cycling on the road was deemed risky by many parents and hence they would not permit their children, especially girl children, to cycle. Cycling to school was, and is still, not a common phenomenon.

Mobility for me and my peers was strictly activity-based (i.e. to school, church, or the playground). I was accustomed to accessing these places on foot. I lived seven minutes' walk from my school and thus walked to and from school five days a week. The journey from my home to church took another 12 minutes on foot and to the playground another seven minutes. I did not cycle to these locations because I had no bicycle at the time.

In the school holidays, I usually spent some time with relatives in a small farming settlement (about 500 inhabitants), which is a journey of about 105 km by car.

GREECE I (*1980)

I grew up in the 1980s in Athens, Greece. We lived at the foot of the mountain called Ymittos. School was always a 10-minute walk away. I always walked to school; with my older sister at first, later on with friends who would come and pick me up so we could walk to school together. I often walked back home with my friends. If the weather was nice we would take a longer route back, which involved some playing around, jumping off walls or talking to stray cats. Living at the foot of a mountain means a lot of walking uphill and as a child I found that quite tiresome.

My father being a mechanic of British cars, our family was always heavily motorised, so almost all other destinations were reached by car. Even visits to relatives who lived within the same district were made by car. Back in the '80s it wasn't difficult to find a parking space on the outskirts of Athens. On the rare occasions my mother would take my sister and me to the centre, we would take the bus. To be honest, at the time I found the bus rather frightening. It was loud, fumy, and dirty. I must have been between five and eight when I got on a train for the first time. My father took us to Piraeus on what was called the "electric" train, an old-fashioned kind of metro, which still exists today. That trip was considered a special experience and it was purely for leisure.

Very often we would drive to our country house in the south of Athens, about an hour's drive away. I enjoyed those rides, looking out of the window at big stores passing by, the sea, other cars and their drivers. When I think about it now, what I enjoyed most was probably being driven around without having any responsibility. One of my favourite things at the country house was riding my bicycle. It was never a means of transport, simply leisure.

Growing up meant getting more independent. My sister and I started walking to the shops or to visit friends and relatives within our district. When I was about 13, my sister had to go to the centre every day by bus. I would sometimes go with her and considered those outings as thrilling experiences. Soon we started meeting friends in town, so we would take the bus more often. When the bus drivers were on strike or when the weather was nice, we would walk to town, which took about an hour.

When I was 18 I got my driving licence and started getting around in my car. I used to love driving. But to university it was only a quiet 15-minute walk, so I always walked and enjoyed the sunshine, the neighbourhood, and nature, as the university campus is situated in the woods of Ymittos. The language schools that I went to at the time were in the city centre, and I would only go there by bus or I would walk; I'd never go by car.

Greece II (*1974)

I was born in Athens (Greece), and for most of my early life (5–23 years old) I lived in a northern suburb, Kifissia, about 17 km from the city centre.

Walking in early childhood. When I was small (5–10 years old), I used to take short-distance walks (about 20 mins in total) with my family in the neighbourhood as an entertainment activity, usually passing through a field where there were goats, and we would feed them. We would also walk towards the main places of entertainment of our area (about 20 min away), also as an entertainment activity. Still, I do not remember doing so! I was told this by my mother.

A drive to the kindergarten. My kindergarten was about 1 km away from home. My parents dropped me there by car on their way to work and picked me up on their way back in the afternoon. The kindergarten had two locations that were about 200 metres away from each other on a busy two-lane arterial road, and we would move from one location to the other on some days in a small mini-van operated by the kindergarten. I remember enjoying being transferred in it!

A drive to school. From the age of six till 11, my school was located far away from home (about a 20-min drive). My parents would drop me there by car before going to work and I would return home with a friend of mine, in her mother's or father's car.

A walk in the neighbourhood. From about the age of eight, together with several kids from the neighbourhood, I used to wander around the neighbourhood in groups from house to house, or to possible play areas: gardens, dead ends, or un-built areas/fields to ride our bikes or play football, chase, and other games.

A walk to school. When I was 11 I changed from the private school to a public school that was a 20-min walk from home. In the mornings, my parents used to drop me, my brother, and a friend who lived nearby at school by car on their way to work. At the end of the classes early in the afternoon, me, my brother (about 2.5 years younger than me), and our friend would walk back home. On days when it rained heavily, our friend's mother would pick us up by car and take us back home. My high school (age 12 till 18) was located about 20 min away from home. I would go there either by car (with my parents dropping me off on their way to work) or on foot, and return home on foot. At the age of 16 I used to make a detour on my way back from school so that I could walk together with a boy that I liked and spend more time with him!

Trip to after-school activities. Most such activities – piano lessons, English courses, etc. – were located between 20 and 35 minutes away from home on foot. Because of time restrictions in the afternoon (I had to do homework), my parents and car availability and the car-friendly mentality of my family, my parents would usually take me by car. The exception was the essay course, to which I would sometimes use my bike (10 mins by bike). I remember once on an uphill, I stepped down off the bike and rather than riding I was walking with it. A driver who was passing by commented, saying "Bikes are for riding and not for walking." I presume that after that I reduced the number of times I used it to go to my essay course.

Freedom walks. At the age of 17 I would sometimes skip school and wander around the area on my own or with friends, or go for walks in the centre of Athens (I reached it by train). I would also go by bus or train to the centre of Athens each Sunday for a chemistry course and would wander around the centre on my own for a while. These walks were really special for me. They were my freedom walks!!!

Trip to university. After school I entered the university, where I studied for five years. Courses took place from early in the morning till early or late afternoon; still, I did not attend all of them, as lecture attendance is not compulsory in Greece. There were two campuses. One was located in the centre of Athens, with good public transport connections, and the other outside the centre, with not-so-good public transport connections. I used to go to the central campus by train (25 mins) and reach the campus after a 10-min walk. I would reach the train station either by car (15 mins) or by bus and walking (35 mins). I would go to the other campus by car (parents', boyfriend's, mine) and it took about 45 mins.

Love walks. I used to meet my boyfriend at the time, D. (together from 18 and still now, with two kids), at the university and would walk a lot, either to reach destinations or just to wander around, as it gave us the chance to spend more time together. I really enjoyed these walks. I still remember walking back home one night after a rock concert in the centre of Athens. It took us about two hours; we reached home at about two in the morning and we were so tired but very happy!

INDIA (*1958)

My grandmother, who saw me growing, told me once that I started walking before I started crawling and I started running before I started walking confidently. I did not doubt her version, because everything goes fast for children here. After standing holding onto something or someone for support, I assume that I took small and exciting solo steps. This I do not remember, but I remember cruising with a wooden baby walker that has been passed down from the elder sister's children to younger and so on, in the family for ages. It was handmade in wood, with three small wheels. Some bells were also tied onto that small cart. Now I realise that it was not a very good idea to hurry a child that had just learned to stand, giving it extra speed. Although the whole family, relatives, and the neighbours cherish the moment, it's nothing but a false impression that a child is truly mobile.

When I was in pre-school or elementary school, I started interacting with my surroundings, almost always barefoot with people big and small, flowers, leaves and trees, birds, animals, fish, butterflies, and whatnot. And I loved this. I remember seeing a kid's bike in the sports stadium in the small town we lived in then, where they allow children to ride around on Sundays. Besides cycling, I liked to swing from a tree on an old car tyre or running old cycle tyres with a stick.

In high school, my father taught me how to cycle, first to monkey pedal and then normally. He had an old English BSA. That was a green bike. Since my school was opposite his workplace, he would have me sit in front and my sister at the back and cycle us back after work. At weekends, I used to borrow his cycle and visit the nearby river with my classmate and watch shoals of fish swimming and enjoying themselves. We had to travel along highways and there used to be accidents and we were always scared of crossing either on foot or on a bicycle. But accidents never bothered me in those days as they did in later years.

When I was in my second year of college, my father bought me a bicycle with a loan and my professor and my mother stood surety for me at the bank and we repaid the loan promptly. It gave me an identity and enabled me to attend our youth programmes at the local church with my peers. Also, we used to cycle to nearby towns and villages along with my friends for social work during floods and for archaeological conservation, etc. and those were very happy years, exploring my world in a whole new way.

IRAN (*1980)

I was used to walking to school since the time I started school at age six in Tehran. It is now astonishing when I think how a little child could be allowed to walk to school and back to home in childhood, given that there could be a lot of threats (e.g. traffic, being victim of misbehaviour, getting lost, etc.) on the way to school for the children without any knowledge, skill, or control over those threats. But it was the way almost everybody went to school at that time, particularly if their home was close to school. Most of the time I walked alone, although there were classmates whose homes were near to us and we could go to school together. Most of them always seemed to be light-minded crazy children, always seeking useless crazy joys along the way, and teasing others on the way to school. So my network of friends was limited to a few children.

In addition to walking some students whose homes were further away from the school came on the school bus. To be honest, I was jealous of them because the typical experiences of those guys were basically different from us, the walkers. It was because they were on the road for a longer time than we were; they were more exposed to motorised vehicles, their journey was more complicated, they saw more interesting scenes, and the students on the school bus had a private informal network, and always told stories on the way that we were not in line with. So I had never been on the school bus, but always wished to be when I was a child.

A very funny story about my education at primary school is that while our home was located only two or three minutes from the school, I was always late. I reached the school with a delay. The reason was perhaps that I was always overconfident regarding the travel time and therefore I started the school trip very late. The other funny story was that there was always some stuff I forgot to take to school. This could be a notebook, a book, a crayon, or the assignments. I am sure this was also related to overconfidence because of the short distance between my home and the school. So I always asked the staff at the school to call our home and ask my mother (who was a housewife) to bring my stuff.

Gradually, I learned to be less dependent when I got older. When I was at the high school, the school was a long way from home, so I had to take public transport to school. It was half an hour from home, so I needed to find a way to be independent. Travel on public transport gave me a good opportunity to interact with society and I learned many things.

Altogether, I would say having explored the environment on the way to school, I did learn many things on the way to school. I think despite the many developments in recent years, the children are mostly deprived of such opportunities because these days most of the pupils are carried to schools in their family's private cars. Most parents are always concerned regarding their children's journeys to school and therefore stricter policies should be in place to convince the parents to let their children walk to school. This is beneficial to the society as physically and mentally healthier children are associated with more active travel in childhood.

ISRAEL (*1947)

As a child, in the Israel of the late '40s and '50s, walking was a way of life for young and old. All the destinations in town – school, library, parks, shops, services, friends – were considered to be within walkable distance. A radius of 30–45 minutes' walking was a typical territory range covered on foot. We shared the road, often unpaved, with horses or mules pulling carts, bicycles, and motor vehicles. We took shortcuts through yards, empty lots, and connecting steps, to make walking more enjoyable or faster as much as to avoid vehicle traffic. Private cars were not common. Only medical doctors and high-ranking bureaucrats (and the very rich) enjoyed that privilege.

As young kids we played outdoors all year round. When you play outdoors you walk and run a lot. As I grew up, my after-school and leisure activities always entailed walking all over town and beyond. Parents did not chauffeur their kids in those days – they worked hard and did not own a car anyway. Public transport was not a viable option either. I know that I walked a lot because I made many visits to the shoemaker. At the age of 13 I got my own bicycle, which extended my range of mobility even more.

To travel out of town we walked to the main road to take a (crowded) bus. As kids we knew how to use the bus service, having travelled with our parents before. In an emergency or on a special occasion my parents summoned a taxi or a friend who drove a truck. This was not easy to do, as most families had no phones.

There was no public transport service on Saturdays, so we took long walks to visit family or friends who lived farther away. If you wanted to visit the beach (about 8 km away) in the summer, you joined 30–40 neighbours aboard a truck that an enterprising owner-driver turned into an informal passenger carrier for the day. The big attraction was not only the sea but the stop the truck made, on the way back, at a special ice-cream stand.

Holiday and summer vacations, with a group of teenagers from my town, were spent in a farming village or in a kibbutz. There we experienced working/walking in the fields, driving a tractor, and taking one-, two-, or three-day hikes, in the countryside or the deserts of our land.

I was a student in Jerusalem. Walking and public transport by bus were my means of transport to and in Jerusalem. The buses were noisy and crowded; people were smoking, no A/C or heating. The bus trip from Tel-Aviv to Jerusalem took three hours uphill on a winding road (now it takes 40 minutes). There was a rest stop halfway through the journey (more to cool the engines and tyres than for the passengers).

The public transport service in Jerusalem was (and still is) off from Friday afternoon to Saturday night. I spent many weekends in Jerusalem walking in its many neighbourhoods, getting to know the city pretty well.

By the early '60s, more people had started using scooters, not because walking became passé, but because public transport was terrible, cars were too expensive, and yet congestion was taxing. I too got an Italian scooter. It allowed me to rent, very cheaply, a house in the East End of Jerusalem (then near the border with Jordan) with no public transport access. This helped me to juggle better between courses and jobs, and it made it far more convenient to visit my family and friends in the Tel-Aviv area. In my early 20s the benefits seemed to outweigh the risks I took riding a scooter (no helmets yet), with cars, trucks, and buses around me going downhill on the wet road from Jerusalem towards the Mediterranean coast.

Arriving at graduate school in West Los Angeles, California in 1965 was the first time I had encountered a highly motorised city. Students drove their cars to UCLA. Bus transport was minimal. I went back to walking to everywhere I needed to go. My rental place was a 30–40-minute walk from campus. One night I was walking home at about nine. I noticed a car following me; it was a police cruiser. The car caught up with me and the policeman told me to approach him. After checking my identity, he told me it looked suspicious when a person was walking on this avenue at this hour. Did I need a ride home or to my car? "I don't have a car and I live not far away" satisfied him. I imagine that walking there today I would at least come across joggers.

JAPAN (*1952)

I was born on a small frontier farm in eastern Hokkaido. The house stood eight kilometres from a railway station, around which there were some stores and a primary school. My brother walked to school through woods with a few friends and it took two hours. On the way they had to be cautious about bears, ringing a bell to tell them that humans were approaching. In winter, they rode a horse-drawn sleigh driven by their parents to the school, as they could not walk because of the heavy snow.

When I was five years old (in 1957), we moved to the main city of Hokkaido, Sapporo, after my father could not maintain the farm because of severe weather and poverty, although my uncle's family stayed on the farm and struggled. I visited the farm every summer (1960–1963) to help my uncle mow the grass of the pasture. I travelled twelve hours to the farm from Sapporo by steam train. I remember the beautiful sunrise from the train window in the early morning. When I arrived at the small house on the farm my aunt cleaned my face, which had plenty of soot from the train. Once on that trip, my cap was blown away when I was looking outside from the open train window. But I never confessed the truth and the "lost cap mystery" was talked about many times.

It took thirty minutes to walk to primary school and I enjoyed loitering on the way, observing flowers beside the road, finding a frog in a small pool, building a dam to block the rainwater streaming along the road and breaking it again, picking an apple from a tree, etc. From when I was ten to twelve, I liked to walk home while reading a book. One day on the way, I had a bad nosebleed beside an apple orchard and it never stopped so I lay down on the road, but nobody was walking around there. However, after some time, a middle-aged woman came and she tried to stop the blood. Finally, I returned home alive thanks to her.

My first experience of a traffic accident happened when I was thirteen and was riding a bicycle (1965). My bicycle wheels were caught by thick gravel on a road, which was common at that time before asphalt. Just after I fell down with the bicycle over my leg a car was backing toward me and the driver didn't notice me in spite of my loud shouting. But at the last minute before the car drove over me I pounded hard on the boot of the car and then the car stopped at last. I was safe and that night the driver visited my home to apologise for the accident. I remember the fear even after fifty years. By the way, my grandfather was killed in a traffic accident between a bus and his motorcycle in 1950, and my younger brother was hit by a motorcycle when he was crossing a road when he was five years old (1962). The motorcycle's wheel ran over his head, but fortunately he was not seriously injured.

I used a bicycle to go to high school and it was only fifteen minutes (1968–1971). At that time, private motor vehicles were becoming common, but my family didn't own a car because nobody had a driver's licence. The subway system of Sapporo City, which used one main line through the middle of town and had rubber tyres, opened in 1971, just before the Sapporo Winter Olympics.

In my twenties (1970s), I loved to drive a car so much and I enjoyed travelling to different places. It seemed that young men who had their own cars could outcompete other boys for girls at that time. And what's more, we had fun driving with friends. I had a very basic knowledge of car mechanics so I maintained the car by myself, for example, changing a tyre, engine oil, or spark plugs. But now, I have almost no knowledge about the mechanics of cars these days except how to operate one.

JORDAN (*1970)

I was living in a small town near Amman, named Sweileh, that is located north-west of Amman. In my childhood it was not part of Amman. It was quite a small town but it was centrally located in the country and connected different parts of the country. The streets were narrow and were very friendly. The streets in the late sixties and early seventies were my second home. We used to walk to school; at that time it was not common to have a car in every home. Kids used to walk to school and parents used public transport. I used to wait by the window for my dad to arrive home to have our family lunch. Our home was a five-minute walk from the main roundabout in the town. Dad used to be very punctual; he used to finish his work at two and then take the bus to arrive at half past two. He taught me that walking is healthy; maybe we did not have the leisure to have other options, but I used to enjoy walking with my dad. I still remember how he trained me how to cross the street. My mum kept reminding us, my youngest brother and me, to watch the traffic. She used to tell us we couldn't play on the main road and she did not like the idea of cycling. My youngest brother used to sneak to rent a bike ride, a thing I did not dare to do. My first day at school was a real adventure. My eldest sister took me with her; she was eight years older and I felt I was in safe hands. Then I was supposed to do it in my own. I had to look for friends in the neighbourhood and after a few days I managed to find one. I got used to walking every day, on rainy days or sunny days. I still remember, one day it was pouring with rain, and I walked the 15-minute walk. I could have used the bus but I had spent my daily allowance on buying a sandwich and some drinks so had no money left. I arrived home soaked and my mum was shocked when she saw me. She dried me off and let me sit by the stove to warm up. In the spring, it was really a joy to walk in the town and climb the mountains and run down the valleys. Me and a group of my friends used to buy some food after the school day finished and have a picnic. There were many springs of water and we enjoyed the scenes and the colours. It used to snow quite often and when the sun hit the snow and it started to melt it was really something we waited for. Watching the tadpoles swimming in the stream was a different experience. In spring the 15-minute walk used to take 45 minutes as we had many things to do: buy ice cream and play girls' games like skipping with a rope and many others. In my teenage years, the walking experience was different. It is the time when I started to take care about how I looked and maybe try to attract attention. Our school was close to the boys' school and sometime I used to time my walking trip so that maybe I could see someone, but it was only looking and that meant a lot. At this age, I was permitted to take the bus with my friend and go to the centre of Amman on our own. At an earlier age, we were only permitted to accompany my mother or father. Now I could explore Amman on foot and climb the steps that connected the neighbourhoods and main streets and sub-districts of the city. The city was much bigger than my town. I had to watch out for the traffic. In the early seventies we had the first traffic lights in the heart of the city, just opposite the restaurant that everyone visiting the city stopped at. I enjoyed stopping at the signal and waiting for the red. Pedestrians were at fault if they crossed on red. It was an experience at that time. The centre of Amman is beautiful; we used to enjoy every minute, eating nice food, reading the magazine *Manchettes*, buying outfits and, above all, waiting in the queue for a white taxi (shared taxi).

KOREA AND CANADA (*1988)

My childhood was split between suburban neighbourhoods of Seoul, South Korea, from birth to eight years of age, and Vancouver, Canada, until adulthood.

From kindergarten, I was taught to walk to and from school independently. This was absolutely the norm in many parts of Korea. This was partly due to the fact that my family of four (my parents, sister, and myself) had to share a single vehicle. There was really not much "sharing", and it could be more accurately described as the vehicle belonging to my father. This left the rest of us to rely on public transport and active transport. During my time in Korea, it never occurred to me that I might be too young to walk without supervision.

When I was eight, my family immigrated to Vancouver, Canada. We settled down in the suburban neighbourhood of White Rock near the US–Canada border. To this day, I clearly recall my first day of school in Vancouver. Because it was my first day, my parents decided to walk my sister and me to school. I recall all four of us discussing that there must be some emergency (e.g. a vehicle crash) as there was an endless line of vehicles in front of the school. When school was over, the same traffic jam was present. We soon realised that this enormous traffic was caused by parent drivers picking up and dropping off their children at school. In the following few days, my parents encouraged my sister and me to walk to school by ourselves. But two young children walking alone was socially not looked upon fondly, despite the high level of safety and security of the neighbourhood. Adult drivers would constantly pull over and ask me if I was lost. Because of this, my parents decided to assimilate to the local mode and drive us to and from school every day. It is important to note that this distance was only 1 km. On my 16th birthday, I took my knowledge test for my driver's licence. One year later, I was able to drive without supervision. At the time these two birthdays were the best days of my life as I associated driving with freedom. From the age of eight to 18, I rarely walked for utilitarian purposes. I was chauffeured around everywhere by my parents until I was able to drive myself.

From 18 to my late 20s, I lived without a car in the urban cores of Montreal, Canada and Washington DC, US. In the first few years it was extremely challenging for me to adjust to a carless life. I actually had to learn how to cycle in traffic in my late 20s. I've only recently been able to truly appreciate the joy of active transportation. I can say with confidence now that the number one element that I consider when looking for housing is walkability. And, if and when I have children of my own, I will encourage them to walk or cycle to and from school independently.

Lithuania (*1978)

I was born in Lithuania, which, at the time, was part of the Soviet Union. My home town had about 26 thousand inhabitants. It is a one-hour walk to cross the town from one side to the other. There was some public transport that was mostly used by people to get to work or to school, from my point of view just to be on time in the morning, especially for people who were working in the morning shift in the factories. Other people either used private cars or just walked.

As I was a child, I cannot remember any instance of walking just for the purpose for walking. My parents – engineers in a factory – were busy doing full-time jobs, raising the kids, and trying to fulfil the needs of the family with the rather modest financial income that they had. Therefore, all of us worked a lot. My parents had a garden (they still have it) where we grew all our vegetables, fruits, and berries. There was no time to go walking for no purpose. If we all walked together, it was for some specific reason – to go to the grocery shop, to the garage (which was 10 min. away from our flat) to pick up the car, etc. I would say that there was no culture of leisure time walking in our country at all.

But children still had time to play. My friends and I spent the vast majority of our free time outside. We played various games and most of those were physically active games, including running, skipping, riding bicycles, hide and seek, and skiing in the winter.

Summarising my childhood walking experience, it would be fair to conclude that there was no walking, but a lot of other physical activities. Yes, I walked to school, but it was just three minutes there and three minutes back.

My walking story started in my teens. I was involved in extra-curricular activities outside the school. I went to a visual arts school which was located in the centre of town. So, together with my classmates, I went there on foot three or four times a week. It was 17 minutes' walk to school and 30 minutes or more back home. Usually, we were almost late getting to the art school from our regular school. That's why I still remember the exact time. But there were really enjoyable walks back home. With friends, having so much to talk about, just fooling around. Getting to art school and back was necessary, regardless of the season and weather, which might be really terrible in Lithuania. Both reasons for walking, I guess, were of the same importance: it was too difficult to get there by bus and it was fun to walk with friends. I cannot remember going alone even once!

Another role of walking in my adolescence was related to emotional independence from my parents and dependence on peers. In late adolescence I had a very nice group of peers to hang out with. Sometimes we stayed at someone's place, but none of our parents were extremely happy about having 8–10 teenagers in their small homes. So we just went outside and walked, and chatted, and fooled around, and nothing more. The strangest part – we always stayed in the same street. It was a one-kilometre-long straight street with a dead end at one end and a church at the other. We were doing this to and fro, walking for hours when we had time and wanted to spend it with friends. If someone who was not as close as the members of my gang in my school years came to my parents' house to look for me, my parents were sure where they could find me and the others.

PORTUGAL (*1963)

Alcobaça is a city located 92 km north of Lisbon and in the centre of Portugal. It currently has an urban area with about 10,000 inhabitants, and was elevated to the status of a city in 1995.

Alcobaça is known for its imposing Monastery of Santa Maria of Alcobaça or Real Abbey of Santa Maria of Alcobaça, which is one of the masterpieces of Portuguese architecture and history, classified by UNESCO as a World Heritage Site and considered to be one of the most important European Cistercian abbeys.

It is designated as the Land of Passion because of the story that is contained in what is considered one of Portugal's most tragic love stories: D. Pedro and D. Inês de Castro.

In the '60s Alcobaça was a village where practically everyone knew each other. My family combined baking and agriculture. My family was always one of the pillars of my life. This was quite interesting, since in a small village, my family was known and so the relations between the people were warm and gave a certain security. From an early age I got used to walking to primary school. I did it (me and my younger brother aged five years old) alone or with a group of friends.

Our afternoons were spent together, at our friends' houses and in our house, where we studied and played. Today these friendships from childhood are still sincere friendships. Walking every day was part of my mobility from home to school and from school to home, which was at least about 2 km per day. In this way I met people, talked with people, and played with friends. In parallel we did sports (from swimming to handball, among others).

A safe city with green spaces to play, with time to talk and having fun with friends. We had a healthy life in which security was inherent in each of us. There were no mobile phones but they were not necessary. We knew where we were and what we were doing.

In adolescence and until the age of 18, I continued to live in Alcobaça. The secondary school was a little farther away (3 km) but we continued to do that trip autonomously and on foot most of the time. We would go in groups, or alone if we felt we needed privacy.

From swimming to the music school and, sometimes, horseback riding, these activities filled my day-to-day life with friends and family. Summer was divided between trips to the beach by bus or by hiking (12 km) and agriculture, where, together with our school friends, we spent good and pleasant times picking fruit (apples and pears) on the grounds of my grandparents.

At the age of 18 I went to study psychology at Coimbra University (Faculty of Psychology and Educational Sciences), 100 km from Alcobaça. Coimbra, with its university, is also a UNESCO World Heritage Site, a city of alleys that enchant and dazzle, a city that stays in the memory and gets into the soul. During all my time at university time, I always walked. The long descents and ascents to the faculty were part of my daily life and of all the students of this city.

As I write these lines, I look back and I miss that time. Effectively, walking allowed for a better quality of life, more encounters with people, and the development of relationship skills. During my childhood, adolescence, and university life, I moved in these two cities. Alcobaça and Coimbra, where the most marked Portuguese love story unfolded (the story of Pedro and Inês). Two cities recognised as part of the UNESCO World Heritage.

Today, these cities are still part of my daily life.

Russia I (*1960)

A walk to kindergarten. In my childhood my grandma walked me to the kindergarten in the morning and back home in the afternoon. It was only a 5-minute walk from my home. It was convenient for all to have the kindergarten so close to home (I sometimes escaped from home and was immediately returned by my grandma).

A walk to school. When I was seven, I went to school, which I attended for 10 years. I was lucky to have it just opposite my house. It was a three-minute walk from door to door. I loved it that the school was SO close. I could easily go home for lunch and... I did not have to get up earlier.

A walk to the stadium. From the age of six to 11 I attended a figure skating school three times a week. It was a 20–25-minute walk from my home to the stadium. Sometimes I walked all the way there. Sometimes I walked to the tram stop for 10 minutes and then took a tram. It was only a five-minute ride (three stops). At the age of six and seven my grandma accompanied me, and then I walked on my own or with a friend. I did not like the journey – it seemed too long to me.

To the park. In the summertime my parents took me and my sister to the park about 5 km away from our home. A 5–7-minute walk to the trolleybus stop, then 10 minutes by trolleybus, and then we walked to the riverside, where we spent most of the day. This trip was never a burden as it was always at the weekends. We sometimes walked all the way to the park.

A trip to the dacha. When I was seven we got our country house (a "dacha" – in the Soviet Union all families with children received a plot of land in the countryside for free for summer gardening and where they could build a summer house). It was 50 km away from our home in Moscow.

Every weekend from April till October was spent at the dacha. To get there we walked to the tram stop, then 20 minutes by tram. Then a 10-minute walk to the railway station, then 45 minutes by train, then either 20 minutes by bus (always overcrowded) or we just walked. The distance from the railway station to the dacha was 6 km. The distances between various means of transport seemed long and tiring. To walk from the railway station was hard, as we always had big heavy bags with us. To go by bus was always a problem – it came seldom (one per hour) and there was always a risk that you would not be able to get on, too many people, and always a sort of a fight at the doors.

By car. My father bought a car when I was 12. From then on we went to the dacha by car. Sometimes we went to other cities in the USSR by car. Or by train. I loved to go by car when my father was free. I loved to travel with him across the country during his holidays.

Trip to the English course. From the age of 14 till 17, I attended an English course three times a week after school. To get there I walked to the trolleybus stop (5 min), then 35 minutes by trolleybus. Then another 10-minute walk. Sometimes my father would come to pick me up from the course (after his work). It was OK. I loved my English classes and the teachers and the journey there was not a burden.

Trip to the University. After school I entered the university, where I studied for five years from 9 a.m. till 3–5 p.m. six days a week. A five-minute walk to the trolleybus stop. 20 min by trolleybus to the Metro station. 20 minutes by metro with one change. And another 10-minute walk to the University. I would rather have had the university closer to my home, but it was OK and quickly became habitual.

Russia II (*1972)

When I was a little girl I lived in a small town – Voronezh (now it is a big city nearly 520 km from Moscow... That is near for Russia.)

We lived in the very heart of Voronezh... and I could freely walk to the central square. It was nothing dangerous and my parents allowed me to walk there alone. Many people were walking there in the evenings and I liked to watch them. I liked to walk there in the summer because roses were blooming and I smelled them!

There were not many opportunities to travel. But my father had a car. At weekends we drove to relax by the river and into the forest. I really liked to drive to the forest with my parents... so I loved to travel with my parents to my father's sister – my aunt – she lived in a small village outside the town.

My parents did their best to make me feel happy; they tried so hard! When my father had free time he took me with him to the park on the outskirts of the town, where we travelled by bus. I did not like buses, I always thought that they were very slow, but I really liked buying a ticket. It seemed to me that I was an adult when I bought a ticket!

In 1980, I was on a plane for the first time: my parents took me with them to Sochi (it is a Russian city, very close to the Black Sea). I saw the sea!!! Oh, how I liked it: I thought it was magical – travelling by plane. Once (!) and already so far! I really liked it: everyone got lollipops in the plane before take-off or landing; this was especially pleasant.

An important event in my life was my first "long" trip to Europe; it was 1985, and at school I was given a ticket for a trip to Lithuania (to Vilnius, Kaunas, and Trakai... then it was part of the Soviet Union) and I travelled with a group of children and our teacher by train. I remember it was an amazing trip! We drove through Moscow and stayed there for one day. I saw a very big city and liked it. There I saw the metro for the first time! Everything seemed magical to me then, because I had never seen the metro... and it was my first trip without my parents so far and by train. One year later I went to a big pioneer camp, "Artek", in Crimea by train (without my parents again). It was a wonderful place (I hope it is nice now!): a special atmosphere, many interesting and famous people, the Black Sea and, of course, new friends from different countries of the world!

When I was studying in high school I very much liked to go camping. I liked it so much because there I could relax and think nothing about school and learning. When I went camping, I could talk to my friends and I played different games, took the air, and slept in tents.

When I became a student, I had to travel to Moscow and Saint Petersburg very often: conferences, seminars, and I needed to study. And after graduating from university, I decided to leave my hometown to find work in Moscow.

After I moved to Moscow, all my childhood and youth ended and I began to work.

Rwanda (*1981)

I was born in Rwanda in 1981 into a family of five children and two parents. My dad was a vet and my mum was a teacher in a primary school. We possessed a motorcycle (a Honda XL125) that was used only by my dad to go to his workplace. My mum did not know how to drive a car or ride a motorcycle. My dad's workplace was located about two kilometres from our house and my mum's workplace was located 4.2 kilometres from our home. Walking was the primary transport mode used by my family (with the exception of my dad) for a journey shorter than 15 kilometres. We lived in a place where there was no bus service. The road network in my neighbourhood was unpaved (gravel roads) and in very bad condition (dusty in the dry season and muddy in the wet season).

Mobility in my childhood and youth:

Given the history of my country, I have described my mobility in four time periods: (1) the period before the war and genocide in 1994; (2) the period during the war and genocide; (3) the period in a refugee camp in the Democratic Republic of Congo (1994–1996); and (4) the period after 1996.

1. *The period before the war and genocide in 1994*: During these times, the main destinations of the walking trips were from home to school (Mon to Sat) and from home to church (on Sunday). My school was located 4.2 kilometres from my home. I made two walking trips every day (from home to school in the morning and from school to home in evening). Before I reached the age of seven, I used to travel with my mum to school and after this age, I started travelling with my friends. In wet seasons, these trips were unpleasant since there was no shelter (trips through the bush and farms). We used to carry our rain jackets every day in our school bags. On the other side, walking to school with your friends and peers was an enjoyable experience as we could squeeze outdoor games into our trips back home. It was also an opportunity to hang out with your peers to explore many things without parental control. On Sunday, my three sisters and my mum used to travel on foot to church. These trips were the most enjoyable for me as they were made on a different route which went through a busy business location. This was the moment when my sisters and myself expected to get something new (e.g. clothes, shoes, etc.), especially at the end of the month.

2. *The period during the war and genocide*: The normal mobility to school, church, or for business activity was limited during this period. There was no school, church services, or business activities in our neighbourhood. The capital city (Kigali) was very unsafe and when the war approached, my family left Kigali to our province of origin (63 kilometres to the west of Kigali) to stay with our grandparents. We had lost everything in our house, including the motorcycle. All trips at this time were made on foot. When the war approached again, we fled from our grandparents' village to Congo (DRC) on foot. We travelled a distance of about 250 km, each carrying a bag weighing about 15–20 kg, sometimes through flying bullets and gunfire. As it can be expected, this was the most unpleasant moment for mobility. The attached map shows the distance travelled during this time period.

3. *The period in a refugee camp in the Democratic Republic of Congo (1994–1996)*: My family spent two years and six months in a refugee camp that was located in the eastern region of Congo (DRC). The majority of trips in the camp were from our tent (home) to a water collection point (approximately a 500-m walking distance) and from our tent to a natural forest where I used to collect wood for cooking. The trip to the forest was the most painful as it took approximately 10 hours (from 5 am to 3 pm). We received food parcels from the World Food

Programme (WFP) but wood for cooking was not provided. As I was the oldest boy in my family, I had to go to the forest every week to collect wood. At that time my mum had passed away and my dad was sick. I was the only person in my family fit for the duty of collecting wood.

4. *The period after 1996*: In November 1996, a war broke out in Congo and our camp was the first to be destroyed. As in 1994, we fled from our camp to the west of Congo until we met a virgin forest that was impenetrable. We decided to go back to our country of origin and we travelled a distance of about 300 km on foot in a period of about 30 days. We were very exhausted, weak, and malnourished, with swollen feet. It took almost three months to recover from the fatigue once we settled down in my grandparents' village. After recovering from the trip back to Rwanda, I started a small business trading in local farm products. I used a bicycle to carry crops from one location to another. I used my bicycle for the majority of the trips I made. One year later, I had a chance to be admitted to a boarding school. My mobility was very limited for the period of six years I spent at the boarding school. I could travel by bicycle only during holiday times (see Figure 2.17).

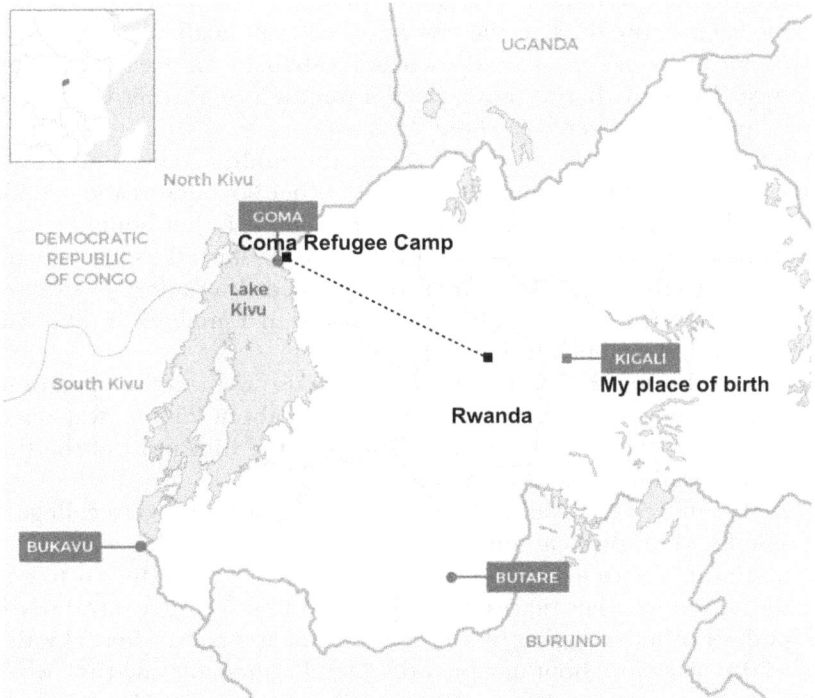

Figure 2.17 Distance travelled during the war and genocide in Rwanda.

SAUDI ARABIA (*1960)

I was born in a small town in the middle of Saudi Arabia in 1960. There were eight children in my family. I am the third after two sisters, then two brothers followed me, then one sister, and then two brothers. At that time there were no cars available to be used for transportation. All of our mobility was done on foot. The distances were not far. Normally, at that time, I got to the elementary school by walking with other children, about one km back and forth. In the afternoon and on holidays I went to visit relatives and my grandmother's house regularly every day, often many times in the day. The walking trip normally took five to 10 minutes at a maximum. Many times I also walked to the central market to buy some food or any other things required by my family. The market was one km away. I also walked to the butcher's shop almost every day to buy meat (camel meat) for the price of one Saudi riyal, then. It took five minutes to get there by walking. The reason for buying food and meat every day was that there was no refrigerator to keep things fresh. Sometimes, when the family needed to go to visit other parts of the family in other villages, we organised a car to take us to that place. The distance did not exceed 8 km. But this happened once in six months. When we arrived there, we walked all day to the farms and mountains, and to the small markets there. All this was a playground for us, and we kept on until we returned. Normally, we came back before dusk, as there was no electricity at all.

From an early age on I used to play football in an area close to my residence. Twice or three times a week, I went a little farther to play with other friends in another area about 2 km away.

When I moved to the seventh year in the middle school at another location, I continued walking to school with other boys. It was about 1.5 km each way. In my tenth year (1975) at the school, my father bought a car to be driven by me and my brothers. At that time we started using the car to go to school daily and our walking was reduced dramatically. A driver's licence was not necessary then for us as we lived in a small town. There was no traffic authority there at that time.

I continued using the car to school, but we also went to the open desert for picnics almost every day (3 km) or to sites about 25 km away once a week. During our picnics we usually walked in the hills most of the time. The average walking distance was ~5 km.

In 1980, I moved to Riyadh, the capital city, in order to go to college. By that time I had my own car and a driver's licence. My walking was reduced to a minimum, restricted to the area where I lived. I used the car to go to my college and to other places. Once a week I went to the central market in Riyadh or other shopping places by car to the car park. There, I walked around the place for about one or two hours. I remember one time when I lent my car to my cousin for a week or so. During that time I used to walk longer distances to go to bus stops to move around the city.

During my studies in Riyadh, at the weekends I left and drove to my home town, about a two hours' drive. In my home town I used to take young relatives, nephews, nieces, and others for a short picnic in the nearest piece of desert for three to four hours. We usually walked around and climbed hills just for fun. In 1983 I graduated from the university to start working. Since that time my walking – sadly – has been reduced almost to zero.

SLOVAKIA (*1980)

I will describe the period of my life when I was a child, let's say six to 10 years old. In those days we were living in a suburb of Bratislava in a prefabricated tower block building, actually quite close to the Austrian border. The best connection to the city centre was by bus; it took about 20 minutes to get there. The bus stop was right in front of the building. Buses went quite often, let's say every five minutes. In front of the building there was also a car park, usually without problems to get a parking space.

As long as I can remember, we always used to have a car. For longer trips (and family trips: all of us – my parents, sister, and me), we used the car in almost all cases. For trips within the city, on the other hand, we almost exclusively used public transport (buses, trams and occasionally trolleybuses). The only exception was a visit to my grandparents (living in another part of Bratislava) – we mostly did these visits by car.

It was also about money. I remember my parents saying that we had money for two full tanks of petrol per month. So when the petrol ran out, we had to use public transport.

From the third grade in elementary school (nine years) I started to commute to school by bus. At this stage, I changed to another school, which was in another part of the city (where my mother worked). It took about 40 minutes to get there (bus/tram) and about the same time to get back. In the morning I travelled to the school with my mother, and on the way back (afternoon) alone. So I spent quite some time on public transport during these years. I remember that during these years I wanted to be a bus driver.

For holidays, longer trips, etc. we always (as far I can remember) used the car. But, as I said, this was not an issue for trips in the city. As for shopping, we used shops that were within walking distance and did not use the car.

The last thing I want to mention is my bike. I remember that I used a bike quite often to get around the suburb – let's say up to 5 km from home. At that time a bike was a very practical means of transport (to get somewhere quickly, instead of walking). That is different from now – when it is rather a sport. I even remember bike trips to the closest Austrian village (Kittsee), which we did on bikes to buy chocolate (during the years right after the end of communism).

SOUTH AFRICA (*1963)

The good thing about growing up in Johannesburg was the weather. On the 'Highveld' we had one of the best climates in the world. Summer rainfall (late afternoons) and winters that seldom dipped below 19°C, which means that walking conditions were exceptionally good (of course, winter mornings were chilly, but they warmed up quickly). As a 'white' child, in an officially 'white' neighbourhood, walking to and from school was fairly common among my peers and I; as we got older the walking tended to be replaced with bikes, and then as after-school activities grew into the evening hours, we abandoned bikes for lifts by parents. Thinking back on the walk to and from school brings back really happy memories, especially of dawdling home in the afternoons with friends or sisters. The sidewalks took us past gardens bursting with flowers and busy with excited dogs – we got to know most of them by name over the years. In those days there was no concern about road safety, or indeed private security. We had no valuables to speak of – no mobile phones, and our watches were rudimentary at best. We carried school satchels stained with ink and stuffed full of exercise books, and really not much else apart from the occasional tennis racket or hockey stick. We certainly didn't carry any money with us. Even our bikes, when they became necessary, were fairly basic. I don't remember having a bike with gears until I was an adult, so they were certainly no magnet for thieves! Thus, walking and cycling were considered safe activities for kids in Johannesburg. Thinking back, the only other people we saw walking were domestic workers, who came in from the outer city areas to clean and garden in white-owned houses. No white adults walked anywhere (it seemed to me without much reflection) – even a short few blocks to the local shopping centre would involve a car trip. This was the seventies after all, and petrol was fairly cheap.

Walking was very much a necessary thing for children in those days, as parents were not the 'lifts on call' they became in later years. We had far more independence than the children of today, and were far more self-reliant. Walking, for me, was a means of getting from point A to point B… it always meant having a purpose. Cycling, on the other hand – now that was a fabulous and fun way of getting to know the city. My friend Susan and I would spend hours on school day afternoons cycling far and wide. We explored huge areas of Johannesburg and developed our first taste of what it would be like to be independently mobile. Cycling downhill, through parks and rose gardens, along sidewalks bumpy with tree roots and purpled with jacaranda blossoms. Fixing punctures under the hot sun, and having help along the way (we always met the kindest people this way) – these are formative memories for me, and were quite possibly some of my happiest days as a child.

THE NETHERLANDS I (*1950)

During my childhood (in the 1950s) I lived in a provincial town of about 100,000 inhabitants, with my parents and two sisters in a free-standing house in a nice and quiet district. I went to pre-school and primary school on foot. The trip was about two kilometres. At that time it was not allowed to go by bicycle; only children who lived outside the school district were allowed to go by bike.

To pre-school I was mostly taken by my mother. From first grade in primary school I walked by myself, guiding my two little sisters. Apart from one crossing, we did not encounter much car traffic. That one crossing was protected by crossing guards, consisting of one parent and the sixth-grade pupils in eye-catching vests and a ready-over sign. At that time I had neighbourhood friends to play with, next door and further down the street. We played in the street, in our garden, or the train yard that was close nearby, where wood for the coalmines was stored. We had soapbox go-carts made of old prams and wooden planks and pushed them in turn. At the weekends we often had family walks in the nearby woods, with the two dogs we had. My father got his first car in 1956, which he used for work, but, because of the high cost, very little for private trips. Those were mostly made on foot and by bike. Our first holiday away from home was in 1962. That trip was made by car.

On the corner of our street was a small shop, where we got our groceries. We walked there quite often, and we could fetch the groceries on credit or simply give the shopkeeper the grocery list, which he or his wife would deliver to us at home later.

At the age of nine I had a bike-car accident. I rode down the walkway up the street, where visibility was blocked by big oak trees. The car driver could not see me and vice versa. Luckily for me it was a VW Beetle, and not some angular car. Still, it took about two months to recover from my injuries.

From about age 10 I went independently to music school and tennis lessons by bike. Both destinations were outside our neighbourhood, but reachable mostly over bicycle paths.

THE NETHERLANDS II (*1953)

My early childhood (1950s), up to second grade in primary school, was spent in a provincial capital in the east of the Netherlands (200,000 inhabitants), where we lived in an apartment house. Then my family moved to the west, to a row-house in a satellite town (150,000 inhabitants) of the administrative capital of the country. Up to age eight I walked to school; we did not have a car at that time. Both my pre-school and primary school were quite nearby, so that was not a problem at all. For lunch we all went home.

At age eight (1960s) I got a bicycle which I used to go to school, together with a girlfriend. On the one busy street there were parent crossing guards. The bicycle was also used for independently going to ballet lessons and, later, hockey. The latter was on the other side of the town, about six kilometres away. Only when the team played outside town was I taken by one of the parents; we did not have a car before I was 14 years old.

I could also go to secondary school on foot, as it was a straightforward trip of about one kilometre, with only two busy crossings. Going by bike was not practical or allowed: there was not so much space for parking the bike.

UKRAINE (*1949)

I was born in 1949. I spent my childhood in a small town in the Ukraine. My family never had a car, and therefore I always walked to school together with my three siblings. Both primary school and high school were at a distance of about 800 metres from our house. We never went to kindergarten because my mother was a housewife and did not go to work outside the home and she took care of us children at home until we were of school age. We had a small farm and garden round our house and we worked there. We had fruit and vegetables, and we also had our own animals for meat, which reduced shopping. In our city there was a theatre, a culture hall, a stadium, and a park, and we had leisure trips there and parties. All trips there were on foot. I got my first bicycle when I was 12 years old, and that was the only vehicle in the family for the next six years. When I was 19 I began my university education in Lwow. I went there by train.

2.4.2.1   *Do these tales have something in common?*

All the stories about mobility in childhood and youth provided by colleagues from countries all over the world point in the same direction: walking was not perceived as something really negative in any of those tales. On the contrary, as children, many of them associated positive impressions with walking: being together with their mates, smelling flowers and generally enjoying nature, being impressed both by the physical and social environment, and enjoying the activity of walking itself, also in combination with the (autonomous) use of public transport. In one case, walking is sadly connected with fleeing from a war, but in all other cases – even by the colleague who fled from the genocide in Rwanda – walking was mostly something interesting and enjoyable, interwoven with many other attractive activities, fully in line with the reports collected by Chaloupka and Risser (2004) 15 years ago. There, leisure trips with parents and relatives and pets and animals play important roles. Walking is a predominant mode during childhood and youth. The first trips with different vehicles – from bicycles to cars – have left impressions; accidents have caused distress and anxiety. But when one thinks twice: what differences would one have expected? All the authors in that book came from industrial countries – with the exception of the United States, Canada, and Australia – with urban and land use patterns that have developed over many centuries, with settlements that have been made for walking since the beginning. The preconditions thus prevailing did not allow road networks to develop that would be fully oriented towards near to 100% car use. In the previous new tales, there are two reports from Canada, and the character of one of these reports is not much different, most probably because it is from rather long ago (the 1960s). In the other one, a development becomes clear: it has almost become normal to take one's children to school by car. Maybe the development in European countries is moving in the same direction? In the previous new reports, there are also some stories from colleagues from developing countries and Brazil, Russia, India, China, and South Africa (BRICS countries). In the reports from Rwanda and Ghana, but also from India, we can see an accentuated lack of the car, with more and longer walks in childhood and youth than in the other countries, while the experiences from childhood and youth in Brazil, Russia, and South Africa – all experiences of rather wealthy and white people – are not too different from those in (Western) Europe. But irrespective of where the stories stem from, we do not have the slightest difficulty in understanding the emotions expressed directly or indirectly in connection with the reported experiences. *"Walking is adventure and fun"* for all children is one of the conclusions we dare to draw from the collected materials. This is certainly a motivation to invest energy in research about soft mobility and its enhancement even in the future, not least in order to preserve for our children some very precious experiences and feelings that are, or can be, connected to walking. If one keeps in mind how many positive feelings are associated with childhood and youth mobility, that is, such types of mobility as those that include driving a car hardly at all or even not at all, then there are no obstacles to an increase in mobility from a sustainability and life quality perspective. This is a good starting point for the development of measures to increase such mobility. "Soft" mobility (walking and cycling) can increase without negative global consequences. It is usually perceived positively, if the preconditions are appropriate, and we do not depend psychologically on the car as much as we are often made believe. It is important to keep this in mind and to discuss this fact *"with feeling"*. It also seems that children are very resilient and can cope with almost all types of preconditions; in no place can one find criticism of those preconditions. This means that we can motivate children to walk and also let them walk when the preconditions for walking are poor, or in any case not very good, as is often the case at this moment, provided that one precondition is fulfilled: we need to make sure that children are safe when they are outside in the public space as walkers, where traffic safety is probably of much greater relevance than safety from the danger of criminal assaults (NZTA, 2018).

2.5   And what do adults associate with walking nowadays?

The tales about mobility in childhood presented in the previous section are recollections of grown-ups, who present their memories under the impression of their actual everyday life. It seemed interesting to compare these memories with reflections about walking by adults who live at the present time. Following the classical tradition of a qualitative research approach, to learn what walking means to people, we approached them with unstructured questions. Ten randomly selected respondents from Austria, the Czech Republic, and Slovakia answered three questions: *Why do you walk? What does it mean for you to walk? Name five words which come to your mind when walking or thinking about walking.* We received eight responses, which we coded and grouped according to the principles of qualitative data analysis. Subsequently, we summarise what we learned, including some quotations from what the respondents told us. We can see that emotions and positive feelings connected with walking are very similar nowadays to the memories recollected from childhood.

2.5.1   *Why do people walk? And what does it mean for them?*

The most frequent answers to these questions dealt with **(1) feelings of peace, relief, or happiness, curiosity, slow pace, well-being, or concentration on oneself; (2) transport – getting from A to B, low cost, flexibility, variety, being easy to manage and combine with other modes, effectiveness, independence; (3) "non-demanding" mode of transport, minimalism, perception of one's own strength; (4) activity, motion; (5) health, physical exercise, and (6) social contact.**

For each category, we summarise quotations from selected answers subsequently:

1. **Feelings of peace, relief or happiness, curiosity, slow pace, well-being, or concentration on oneself:**
    *   *"Walking also helps to slow down today's hasty life."*
    *   *"Walking helps to clear your mind; in my case it works one hundred per cent – my troubles walk away while I do my walking."*
    *   *"The main reason why I walk is just curiosity. Seeing and experiencing what lies behind the next hill, and the next, and the next. Next to curiosity comes the special impression of the world you get at walking pace. A bicycle takes your attentiveness away from the surroundings at a distance, and a car is far too fast for any good impression. Being on the move under these conditions brings relief from being tied to the everyday treadmill. The logical consequence of all that for me is well-being, a feeling of happiness. However, what promises the greatest pleasure in leaving for a good walk is the thought of coming home afterwards."*
    *   *"When I walk alone then it is in the countryside because I can find peace and quiet there and I feel good."*
    *   *"A feeling of peace of soul while walking in the countryside."*
    *   *"Noticing the power of nature."*
    *   *"The pace of walking provides a much better opportunity to get to know the areas one is passing through and living in on everyday routes, which other modes just do not offer as higher speeds require a higher level of attention towards traffic."*
    *   *"It means to walk along a street or in the countryside and notice the people and things around me, buildings, trees, flowers, everything that you cannot see while travelling on public transport or in a car, to concentrate on my*

own thoughts and feelings which spring forth from my perceptions of my surroundings. To stop thinking about your duties or problems. To enjoy the fact that I do not have to hurry anywhere, to be alert as to whether I'm on time or whether there are traffic restrictions."

- "A feeling of humbleness and gratefulness for being able to walk without pronounced difficulties."

2. **Transport – getting from A to B, low cost, flexibility, variety, being easy to manage and combine with other modes, effectiveness, independence:**

- "Movement, transfer from place A to place B."
- "Walking in the dense urban area I live in is not only one of the most efficient ways of moving (cycling would be even more efficient), but I also associate it with not being dependent on a certain infrastructure (roads, trains, etc.) or other restrictions. Except for routes with longer distances, which require public transport, walking is not affected by interruptions, traffic jams, or other obstructions. When planned properly, basically any route can be managed by walking, especially if one starts in time."
- "Walking can easily be combined with any other mode without having to think about parking, etc."
- "Without breaking any rules, walking routes can be varied easily, yielding a more diverse experience on regular trips in both leisure time and on the way to and from work. also in bad weather or when there are time or other constraints."
- "Because sometimes it is faster to walk (in city centres)."
- "Pedestrian pavements always have been, are, and, for sure, will continue to be free."
- "Walking is not connected to schedules, a certain vehicle, or ticketing, which is why I associate it with independence and a lack of structure in an otherwise usually very structured daily routine."
- "Everyday walking trips can easily be experienced in different ways (i.e. on the one hand focusing on the surroundings, the city, and the people passing by, or on the other hand listening to audiobooks and music and just focusing on the visual perceptions), making it a very diverse experience."
- "A feeling of freedom and independence – nothing is carved in stone, no time schedule, no limit, no means of transport."

3. **"Non-demanding" mode of transport, minimalism, perception of one's own strength:**

- "It does not require any special clothes; a pair of good and comfortable shoes is sufficient."
- "You can walk anywhere. All you have to do is not to get in a car or on a tram and start walking."
- "I use my body (and soul) without the need for technical systems; I feel no borders, and stay in contact with the earth."
- "Walking does not depend on people's age."

- *"Walking symbolises one of my principles: achieving your aims with your own strength, your own muscle power. I'm grateful that I'm able to walk."*
- *"Noticing and focusing on one's own body and its limitations."*
- *"I am free to go wherever I want, feel my body, and know it is healthy, and I have a feeling of competence regarding moving around without technical help."*

4. **Activity, motion:**
   - *"Walking is motion; it is vitality and vibrancy."*
   - *"I enjoy walking and do not like waiting. If I have to wait 10 minutes for a tram I prefer to walk one stop (or the whole way)."*

5. **Health, physical exercise:**
   - *"Walking is the only form of movement; it is good for my health and I enjoy walking in the countryside and doing something for my health."*
   - *"To do physical exercise."*
   - *"Making walking my main mode of transport on most of my daily routes provides me with a low-threshold physical activity which can be experienced on a regular basis."*

6. **Social contact:**
   - *"I feel good when I walk, especially for sightseeing, for shopping, and for talking with friends (mainly female friends because while we are walking we have a lot of time to talk)."*
   - *"Walking includes stopping and looking around wherever I want, being out with the potential to socialise."*

We asked our respondents to write down the first five words which came to their mind when walking or thinking about walking. These are the associations, grouped according to their meaning:

Associations connected with:

- *Motion*: Movement (2×), transfer, motion
- *Feeling of wonder*: Carefulness, curiosity, impression, awareness, participation, experience, rhythm
- *Feeling of freedom*: Freedom (2×), independence (2×), peace, time, natural, coming home, sustainability
- *Feeling of well-being*: Relaxation (2×), well-being (2×), balance, relief, leisure
- *Environment*: Mountains, nature, environment
- *Practical issues*: Pedometer, shoes, weather
- *Personal*: Health, children

To sum up, positive feelings about walking predominate. We can see that walking is very much connected to feelings, consciousness, slowness, and focusing on one's own perception and cognition. Freedom and independence are much appreciated as qualities of walking, as are well-being and relaxation. It seems that it is "only" in second place that the practical issues, such as getting from A to B or health benefits, are stressed. When promoting walking, this should be taken into account.

2.6 The elderly and walking

In[8] accordance with many other researchers (Tacken et al., 1999; Amann et al., 2006; Bell et al., 2010) who dealt with older people and their mobility, we underline that (autonomous) mobility is very important when we get older, possibly the more important the older we get. They simply state *"keep the elderly mobile"*, thereby not only aiming at the necessity to let older people drive a car as long as possible, on the basis of the facts that show that older drivers cannot generally be blamed for being "dangerous drivers" (see Langford et al., 2006). Evans (2004) even postulates that older drivers are the safest group of drivers. However, all the publications mentioned previously also argue for the provision of preconditions that allow older citizens to be autonomously mobile without the use of a car, thereby focusing mostly on walking, as the use of a bicycle becomes more difficult with increasing age. Bell et al. (2010) show that above 80 years of age, walking is the most frequently used mode of transport. In order to be autonomously mobile, these people need to have the chance to handle all their daily errands – shopping, visiting friends and relatives, attending cultural activities (Figure 2.18), or accessing a physician or the health service – by walking. The definition of the World Health Organisation (WHO) of health is *"a state of complete physical, mental and social well-being and not merely the absence of disease*

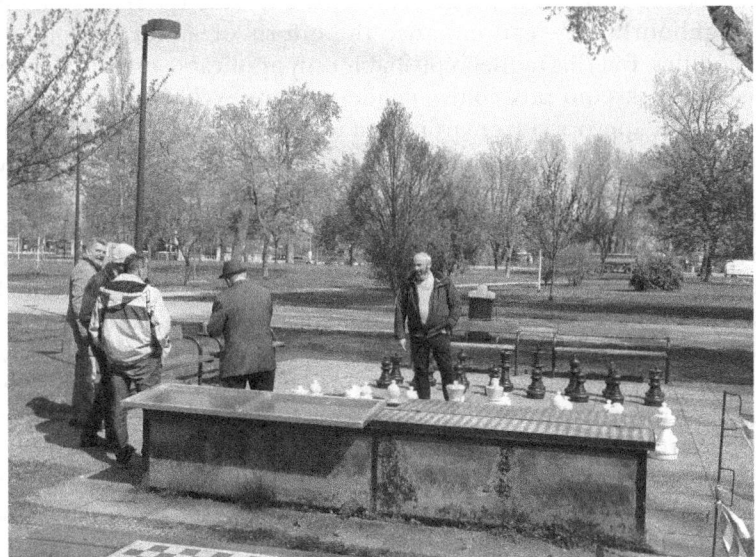

Figure 2.18 Playing chess in the park (own photograph).

or infirmity" (Benz et al., 2013), clearly supporting the idea that being able to live an autonomous (social) life is part of being healthy. A recent review noted that social participation is associated with proximity to resources and recreational facilities, public transport, neighbourhood security, and the user friendliness of the walking environment (Levasseur et al., 2015). Being able to walk, and carrying out such activity, is thus a health issue. In a less technical sense, it is, of course, a matter of quality of life. A grown-up person usually wants to be self reliant and self assured, and why should this change when we get older and when we cannot use (motorised) vehicles as drivers or riders anymore?

Walking and being able and allowed to walk are also related to health in a narrower sense. Throughout our life, it is important that we use our body, by carrying out physical exercise, by using our limbs, by dancing or – most simply – by walking. Physical exercise is necessary for children, for youngsters, and for grown-ups of all ages, but especially so for older people. The slogan *"use it or lose it"* becomes more relevant as we get older. Muscles are reduced in strength or lose all their strength if they are not trained continuously, and the same is valid for the brain and nerves. We have to think, to communicate, to socialise, to move. We have to use our bodies. Walking (outdoors) means that we use our bodies; it obviously enhances thinking, as we have learned already in the beginning of this book, and it allows us to socialise and to communicate, or at least to be among people. However, when discussing ways to make the use of public space easy for older people, one paradoxical remark should be made with reference to Lawton and Namehow's (1973) ecological model of aging: up to a certain degree, challenges in the public space – the author refers to challenges in the neighbourhood – can enhance the efforts of senior persons to train their abilities. But this model is probably only applicable under the condition that severe risks and prohibitive challenges are excluded. This means that providing an appropriate environment for older walkers that also considers Lawton and Namehow's model needs sophisticated discussion. What does a challenging environment that at the same time considers comfort, safety, aesthetics, and usability look like? One way is, of course, to make those areas where one moves about – or has to move about – as easy, comfortable, and safe as possible, so that everybody can use them without any difficulties, including those who do not want to be challenged, but at the same time provide opportunities to train and to exercise for those who like to be physically (more) active and to look after their fitness more regularly. Mayrhofer et al. (2010) carried out a study that, among other things, dealt with what are called "exercise or calisthenics parks", which can be found in many different countries in Europe, Asia, South America, Canada or the United States. They are equipped with training devices that can easily be used by everybody but are especially appropriate for older people. When passing by on walks, people can interrupt their trip and have a go on those devices, and people may start to do such exercises on a daily basis. See Figure 2.19.

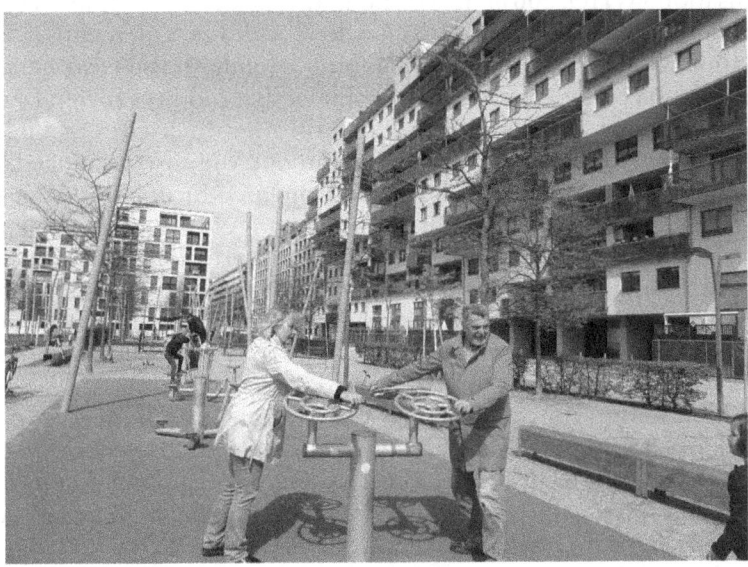

Figure 2.19 Exercise park in Vienna (own photograph).

In the discussion concerning our ageing society, the concepts of getting older and having impairments are often mixed in an illegitimate way. Not everybody who gets old is also impaired. The fact is rather that the older people get, the higher the probability is that some impairments will develop, such as physical, sensory, or cognitive ones. All these types of impairments are usually not prohibitive for walking as long as they are mild in character, but the easier the public space is to handle for walkers, the greater the possibility that people with more severe impairments will move about autonomously. Of course, there are limits on how far such adaptation of the public space can go, but this should not stop societies from investing money and creativity in the development of features of the public space that allow as many people as possible to be mobile and carry out their daily activities as self-reliant and independent people. Rosenkvist et al. (2010) and Risser et al. (2015) discussed the problems of people with mild impairments in connection with their outdoor mobility with a focus on the use of public transport, including the walks to and from public transport stops and stations, and pointed out measures that could help to improve the preconditions for mobility for these persons. There is a connection to traffic safety, again, as often roads have to be crossed on the way to the means of public transport, and in many cases, those crossings are (perceived as) dangerous and function as a barrier.

There is a truism among mobility researchers that *"having people remain in their homes and communities for as long as possible also avoids the costly option of institutional care"*, as Wiles et al. (2012) put it, citing the World Health

Organisation (WHO, 2007). It is difficult to calculate exactly and compare the costs for an infrastructure that allows as large a percentage of the population as possible to be autonomously mobile to the costs generated by a public space that is prohibitive for many that requires societal support for more and more people who cannot look after themselves to a lesser or larger degree. However, as Wiles et al. point out, the costs produced by the latter situation seem to be relevant, and from an ethical point of view, it is obvious that an environment that allows as many citizens as possible to live a worthwhile life is to be preferred to a society where more and more people need institutional help because they cannot move about appropriately in the public space. From this perspective, to provide preconditions for walking that suffice for as many groups and types as possible of citizens of all ages seems to be just the perfect way to go.

But how about the comfort of the traffic environment for older pedestrians? It is very difficult to find parameters that reflect comfort and even more difficult to find research data. Oxley et al. (1995) approached this aspect by measuring waiting times at kerbs, thereby comparing younger and older pedestrians (see Table 2.5).

It is obvious that crossing roads is a real barrier for older walkers that may considerably reduce the comfort perceived by older people when they are outside as walkers.

When discussing walking in connection with the situation of older people, we have to come back to the safety issue. One can summarise some of the safety problems of this group as follows (Tomasch et al., 2016):

- There are significantly increased shares of pedestrians who are killed and severely injured in the age groups above 65 years, compared to younger road user groups (in the year 2011, it was 46% of those killed and seriously injured);
- During the months of November, December, and January, pedestrians older than 65 years constitute 42% of all fatalities in traffic;
- 70% of all accidents occur in the daylight hours, even if the share of accidents during times of artificial lighting and darkness is increased in the months of November, December, and January;
- 66% of all victims are female.

Table 2.5 Waiting times at kerbs (Oxley et al., 1995)

(In seconds)	Approaching the kerb	At the kerb	Crossing (to the centre of the road)	Total
Younger pedestrians (<50 years)	3.1	9.2	4.8	17.1
Older pedestrians (>60 years)	3.9	24.3	6.2	34.4

The last point leads us to the next section, where one can see that women walk (much) more than males, among other things. The high portion of women involved in accidents may be explained by a difference in exposure.

2.7 Women versus men as walkers

From different studies – and concerning many of us also from personal experience – we know that women, to a large degree, have a different mobility pattern from men. Despite all the efforts to achieve gender equality, which, in some regions of the world are more intense and in others less so, women still perform more duties for the household, that is, the supply of food, bringing and fetching children, taking care of the clothes of the family members, and taking care of older relatives who need help. Data from Vienna (Figure 2.20) indicates that women's modal split, in spite of their mobility patterns being more complex, is more environmentally friendly than men's. We do not have comparable data from EU or other countries, but we can expect that in developed countries, the mode shares and type of trips among men and women do not differ significantly from the data presented here. Among other things, this is due to the different types of trips of the genders. Women, on average, cover fewer kilometres per day but make more short trips, of which a larger proportion is carried out on foot or by bicycle, as reflected in Figure 2.20 subsequently.

The different tasks that are carried out by the genders lead to this difference. Figure 2.21 (Damyanovic, 2010) represents one example of how these differences can be imagined. In this figure, bringing children to kindergarten or primary school, which is done more and more by car,

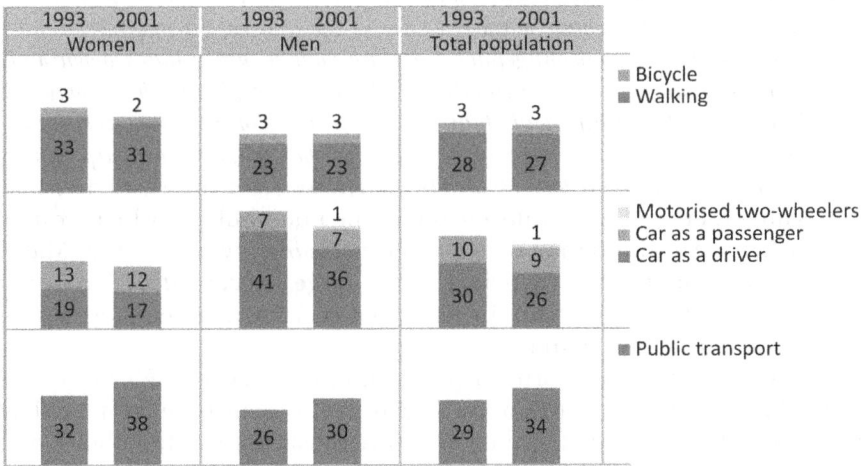

Figure 2.20 Modal split between women and men in Vienna in 1993 and 2001 (VCÖ, 2009).

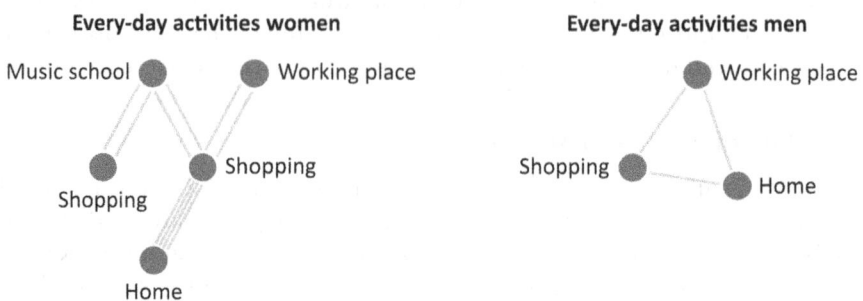

Figure 2.21 Daily mobility of women and men (Damyanovic, 2005).

is not included but rather is imagined as being done on the way to work. Concerning this latter case, Knoll and Szalai (2008) indicate that if children are brought by car, then it will more often be by men, and if they are brought by bicycle or on foot, it will rather be by women. This is far from being representative for the whole world, but there are many common-sense reasons to assume that some truth lies therein (see also the World Development Report, 2012).

Maffii et al. (2016) came to similar conclusions concerning the "gender gap" in mobility, as they call it, when looking at the EU 27 (the EU, still including the United Kingdom but without Croatia). Subsequently, Figure 2.22, produced by these authors, shows some interesting results in a perfectly understandable manner.

Maffii et al. (2016) summarise what lies behind the differences in female and male mobility patterns as follows: *"Lower employment rates, part-time roles and low-wage positions are the main factors which determine a sensible difference between genders in the labour market, in social life and in transport behaviour. Furthermore, even at retirement gender needs are notable, given that women make up the predominant part of the elderly population. The picture that emerges is one where women travel differently than men in relation to transport modes used, distance travelled, the daily number of trips and their pattern, and, not surprisingly, they also travel for different purposes."* The purposes refer mostly to activities concerning taking care of children and of the household, in which women are much more involved than men – *"escort, shopping, visits, leisure"*, as Maffii puts it. The time for these activities is to a large degree *"stolen"* from the time they spend working for an income, that is, women are employed part-time much more often than men.

The larger portion of shorter trips allows more walking, which does not mean that preparedness to walk is greater in women then in men. The previous authors state that women are more sensitive to sustainability, and specifically to ecological issues, than men are. The fact is, however, that in European countries, women use a car considerably less, they use public transport more often than men, and astonishingly, they use a bicycle slightly

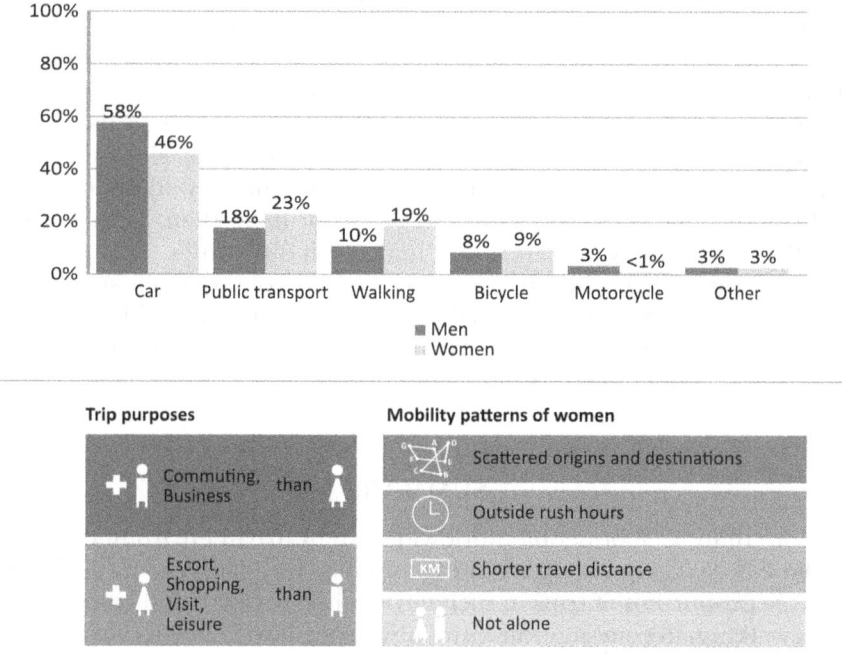

Figure 2.22 Some differences in mobility between women and men (Maffii et al., 2016).

more than men, and in any case not less than men do. But, most importantly, the proportion of walking in their mobility pattern is approximately double that of men.

Thus, to conclude, women walk much more than men. Whether this is captive walking, because, for example, there is only one car in the family and this is used by the man, walking for practical reasons (because for very short trips, walking might be more convenient than using the car), or because they consider walking agreeable, especially together with the children, does not really matter concerning the implication that the needs of women have to be considered when public space and traffic organisation are being designed. This does not mean that the social role of women, as in many cases it still is today, will be perpetuated forever. But when men take on their share of household duties more and more, they will have similar needs on short trips for shopping, for bringing the children to kindergarten, for fetching them from football or the gym in the afternoon, for having a walk with old relatives, or other duties. Until now, infrastructure planners worldwide have been men who "had a myopic focus on cars and other motorised vehicles", as stated in the World Development Report (Uteng, 2012) and who have been planning mainly for men and their outdoor activities and needs. Interestingly – or maybe one should say as a matter of fact – regions with more gender inequality have a greater difference in mobility difficulty between women and men, as a Canadian study showed (Mechakra-Tahiri et al., 2012). Good walking facilities could therefore be seen as an expression of a society's greater or lesser attitude to gender equality. A good walking infrastructure with smooth surfaces for allowing children's tricycles to ride over without falling, low kerbs of boardwalks, safe crossings, walking paths that are broad enough to walk on side by side, and many other features, such as public toilets, that make walking easy, safe, and comfortable will also be advantageous for men, then, as they will be for all other groups who walk, albeit many with difficulties. This includes a reconsideration regarding zoning and area plans of the public space where these different gender and age needs have to be taken into consideration – not to prolong these differences but to make the interim period before there is more social gender equality more comfortable.

SUMMARY

More than 50% of people worldwide live in urban environments; in the EU, 80% are expected to live in cities by 2050. Theoretically, a large proportion of trips in such environments can/could be covered by walking, in combination with public transport. The fact that today 15%–20% of all car trips in the EU are shorter than 1 km gives an impression of the potential there is for walking to replace car trips.

Walking is the most sustainable mode. It is economically sound, generating only low costs for both the individual and society. Providing infrastructure for walking is cheap. At the same time, there is usually a considerable return on investments for pedestrian-friendly infrastructure as a result of the boosting of the local economy on the micro level. Walking has positive social effects, providing cohesion among citizens and making outdoor environments safer: where there are (many) walkers outside, the risk of being harassed or robbed is reduced. Significantly, walking is, of course, the most environmentally friendly way to move about. In addition to all this, walking is healthy, boosting one's fitness and reducing the risk of different types of cancer and of osteoporosis, depression, dementia, and other illnesses.

Concerning safety, there are certain problems. Overall, accident numbers are decreasing, in any case in the OECD countries, but pedestrian accidents do not fully follow this trend, and in many cases, they are even increasing. This shows that much has to be done to improve the conditions for walking in this respect. It is especially interesting to see that pedestrian falls are not treated as traffic accidents, in spite of indications that they cause more economic damage than accidents involving pedestrians and other road users. Of course, walkers are most often killed in accidents with motor vehicles.

The portion of walks under agreeable conditions is not increasing worldwide; on the contrary. A very negative aspect of this development is that children walk or cycle to school autonomously less and less. Parents often integrate bringing their children to kindergarten or school into their own trip to work or to other places they want/have to access. Thus, children do not get motion in this very simple and efficient way, nor do they learn to cope with the traffic environment in an effective and safe way. Moreover, children are more often killed as car passengers than as walkers or cyclists, which might be an exposure effect. We do not have figures from which it is possible to conclude whether being brought to school by car is safer than walking or cycling, but what can be said is that being brought by car certainly does not fully solve safety problems.

When discussing adjustments of the traffic environment to the needs of certain segments of the total population, we also have to focus on senior citizens and on women. In the first case, it can be said that the older we get, the more we have to rely on walking. Above the age of 80, more than three-quarters of trips are made on foot. Concerning women, it is important to note that women move about in a somewhat more environmentally friendly manner within the frame of a daily mobility pattern that is usually more complex than that of males, including larger portions of walks. Thus, planners should take thorough care of the needs of both seniors and women.

As far as the general population – reflected by the average grown-up? – is concerned, there is no generally valid data. A tentative and highly qualitative survey that we conducted in Austria, the Czech Republic and Slovakia indicated that a possible perspective of "average grown-ups" on walking could be that walking gives feelings of peace and well-being, including a more intimate relationship with the immediate environment; it allows one to get from A to B flexibly and at low cost, also because it is easy to combine with other modes; in this sense, it is effective and provides independence; walking is elegantly minimalist and does not require any/much material effort, while at the same time providing a feeling of one's own physicality; it boosts health, combined with the big advantage that positive fitness effects are felt immediately and not only as an abstract notion; and, last but not least, it enhances social contact(s).

Notes

1. www.realestate.com.au/advice/how-does-internet-connectivity-affect-home-prices/
2. http://theconversation.com/life-in-the-pedestrian-fast-lane-is-no-life-at-all-lets-slow-our-cities-down-instead-50254
3. http://buildabetterburb.org/six-reasons-resurgence-car-free-shopping-streets/

4. https://www.vcoe.at/news/details/einkaeufe-fuss-fahrrad
5. https://www.scinexx.de/news/technik/autofahrer-atmen-mehr-feinstaub-ein/
6. https://www.umweltbundesamt.de/indikator-belastung-der-bevoelkerung-durch#textpart-1
7. https://www.everydayhealth.com/fitness-pictures/reasons-to-walk-your-way-to-health.aspx#walk-to-reduce-stroke-risk
8. In the frame of the SIZE project (Amann et al., 2006), in the context of a workshop, one representative of a senior citizens' association complained very emotionally about the word "elderly": "Why do you use this stupid word? Simply say older people or older citizens, instead." Here we use the word again because we cannot think of any label for this group that fits nicely. But we are aware of the fact that some people possibly do not like it.

3   Human behaviour and its change

This chapter describes in detail what lies behind human behaviour – why it is not enough to only 'know' something to change the behaviour and that it takes more than just having the correct information (or from the point of view of decision-makers, 'to deliver' the correct information). Concrete examples from readers' everyday lives are used in order to show how to build habits and to maintain them. We discuss all the (perceived) difficulties which prevent people from walking and suggest how to eliminate them. The difficulties associated with walking (it is time-consuming, it relies on your own energy, the walker becomes tired, not too great distances can be covered, the walker is exposed to weather conditions, etc.) are explained, and suggestions for planners and decision-makers as to how to deal with these issues provided.

In terms of psychology, road user behaviour is a (visible) consequence of the action of multiple factors, which can be divided into those that affect the road user from the inside and those that exert an effect from the outside. It is of course possible – and necessary – to target the factors that influence behaviour from the inside, but to achieve sustainable changes may involve long-term efforts and intensive psychological interventions, such as campaigning, education, and training. Additionally, the relevant interventions are targeted at the road user population as a whole or at specific groups of road users, rather than at individuals.

3.1   What influences human behaviour

In this section, we describe core psychological theories which deal with human behaviour and are relevant for the traffic domain.

3.1.1   *Dissonance theory*

The basic concepts of the cognitive dissonance theory (Festinger, 1957) involve cognitive elements or cognitions (our perceptions and thinking; sensations, thoughts, beliefs, opinions, and attitudes) and the relations among them. According to Festinger, cognitive elements can be independent of each other (isolated) or mutually related. Generally speaking, two types of relations – consonant and dissonant – have been described.

Cognitive dissonance refers to a feeling of mental discomfort experienced by a person with several conflicting or totally contradictory cognitions. The conflict between a decision and a perception generates inner tension. The relation is totally consonant if the elements are in full accord. The intensity of the dissonance, that is, the degree of uncomfortable tension, is expressed by the following index:

Dissonance intensity = n(dissonant relation)/N(dissonant + consonant relation)

In addition to the effect of dissonant relations, the subjective importance of the cognitions involved plays a major role. In more important cases, dissonance is felt with greater intensity and discomfort than in those of less importance.

There are two ways of reducing dissonance. The first strategy involves changing the cognitive elements to the effect that the previously dissonant relations become consonant ones. The other strategy involves the acceptance of new cognitive elements (e.g. arguments) so that the existing and new elements can enter into consonant relations, which reduces the percentage of dissonant relationships and, accordingly, the intensity of the dissonance. A combination of both alternatives is often encountered.

It is essential to note that the changes made do not necessarily relate to reality, and, indeed, they often do not. They are usually rationalisations, that is, subjective justifications of our own beliefs and the behaviours we engage in.

It is natural that people have (to some degree) conflicting cognitions (attitudes, beliefs, etc.) and that we tend to reduce these conflicts. In fact, a dissonant 'stage' is a prerequisite for change – it reminds us that there is something we need to think of or solve. The most frequent ways of solving such conflicts are to add, eliminate, or change some cognitions. It is important to note that this works both ways: we can change our behaviour on the basis of our attitudes and also, on the basis of our behaviour, we can change our attitudes. To support wished-for behaviour, in our case, support for walking or a mode shift from car use to active transport modes, we can follow both ways. We can 'add' new attitudes (e.g. by a media campaign) or, using incentives, support behaviour directly and hope for an influence on attitudes. The crucial aspect of success is that all our actions have to be consonant; for example, if we communicate the benefits of walking, it has to be possible to experience these benefits in reality.

3.1.2 Reactance theory

The theory of reactance, introduced by Jack W. Brehm in 1966, proposes that every restriction on behavioural freedom and choice, or an individual's freedom to select when and how to conduct their behaviour, is primarily felt as unpleasant. It is generally found attractive and desirable to choose from multiple options. The restriction of the freedom of choice results in the loss of these behavioural and decisional alternatives and is very likely to produce what Brehm described as a state of reactance. The concept of reactance refers to a motive, or a tendency to resist the potential restriction of the individual's freedom of behaviour and choice which also seeks to reestablish the original range of alternatives (i.e. to provoke inner resistance). It manifests itself in verbal expressions, in alternatives having their values raised or being devalued to scale up the original preferences, in attractiveness being enhanced (restrictions often make things really interesting), and in attitudes towards social objects or events being changed ('subjective reactance effects') – for example, one person finds another unlikable and tension arises. This motivation is expressly manifested as resistance to the restricting forces, which takes the form of oppositional behaviour, overt resentment, and active defiance.

Reactance processes often take place on a push-pull basis. A person being made to engage in certain behaviour would react negatively and show resistance for the reasons mentioned previously. Individuals with few opportunities to oppose coercion may resort to passive resistance – by participating in activity without immediate involvement in it, for example. It should be noted that behavioural alternatives that are imposed are ridiculed or classified as not appealing enough. Without accompanying communication, coercion may lead to a situation in which even alternatives which an individual finds positive are ridiculed or denied (this is where Festinger's aforementioned theory of dissonance also comes into play). However, in the event that a person repeatedly experiences no control, or almost no control, over an event which they find personally important or relevant, at a certain point of this experience, such a person will no longer be motivated to regain their freedom of behaviour and will succumb instead to showing reactance.

When promoting walking, we have to make sure that the way we communicate walking does not support reactive behaviour. This means that people should never have a feeling that they are being 'pushed' or 'forced' to walk. According to the reactance theory, we should offer and 'remind' people of the advantages of walking and support a change in their attitudes and behaviours but retain the possibility of also using other modes of transport, including a car.

In reality, nowadays the situation is rather the other way around. As car use is very dominant, people are rather forced to use cars, or not to walk, because of, for example, a lack of infrastructure for walking, which – according to the theory – should create a reactance against car use. We can hypothesise that this principle is one of the bottom-up movements for clearer and car-free city centres.

3.1.3   *Attribution theory*

Attributions play an important role in human behaviour. They are opinions and beliefs about the causes of events and circumstances. Why do we generally seek explanations for events and fail to satisfy ourselves with merely taking notice of them? In other words, what is the function (or purpose) of this explanatory activity which goes beyond the events being merely noticed, and what is the function of attributions as outcomes of this activity? The mere cognitive registration of events and interpersonal processes would result in a stream of events that would pass us by without us understanding them. The events will not make sense without our explanations and ensuing attributions. This is of particular importance in the interpersonal domain. When somebody pushes us on a tram and we interpret such behaviour as the person's intention to hurt us, we feel it as an act of aggression. If, however, we turn such a push into an assumption that the person stumbled and bumped against us unintentionally, we will not view this event as an act of aggression, particularly if the person apologises for it.

The way in which we classify (attribute) the push has its implications: if we explain the push on a tram as somebody else's intention to hurt us, we may be concerned that it will not stop there. Thus, in order to protect ourselves (control the situation), we take action: we try to talk to the person (it might have been a misunderstanding, after all), seek help from other passengers, or get off the tram at the next stop. When it becomes clear that the push was inadvertent, there will be no problems (e.g. no uncomfortable feelings such as fear).

Attributions, then, make it possible to understand, predict, and control events. Nevertheless, our attributions may not be consistent with reality. Misattribution of behaviour which was not malevolent may lead to escalation for no objective reason. Thus, in theory, attributions make it possible for us to come to reasonable terms with our environment, but we must constantly judge whether our attributions are accurate (Meyer, 2003).

This theory explains why it is so important to provide citizens with as much information as possible and information that is as accurate as possible in order to produce correct attributions. In other words, if we want to boost walking, we need people to attribute walking as attractive, comfortable, healthy, and costless. An example of a different attribution connected to walking can be: 'I walk because I have no time to do sports, and walking is clever because it provides all the exercise I need simply by walking on my way to work and back home' or 'I walk because I'm not afraid of doing something new and which is not (yet) mainstream, and I'm proud to do something for the environment and myself'.

3.1.4 Theory of planned behaviour

The key term in the theory of planned behaviour (Ajzen, 1991) is *attitude*. An attitude refers to the experience-based willingness of an individual to react to a person, social group, object, situation, or notion in a certain manner. This may be reflected in assumptions, beliefs, feelings, or explicit behaviours. Examples of attitudes include sympathy, antipathy, and prejudices.

Attitudes reflect either conscious or non-reflected judgements – but also simplifying concepts. They help us orient ourselves in the environment, deal with it, and find, or define, our place in it. In principle, it is assumed that a human being finds it comforting when attitudes towards various objects are in a relationship of mutual harmony (i.e. consonant; see the dissonance theory). The theory of planned behaviour explores the question of the extent to which the existing (known) attitude may be used to assess or predict future behaviour. This would be practical, as we would not need to investigate actual behaviour (which is generally very complicated, if not impossible), but the actual behaviour could be predicted by means of questionnaires, for example. This theory proposes that behaviour can best be predicted by an apparent behavioural *intention*. We could thus assume that a citizen who expresses interest in walking or cycling as an urban transport mode (e.g. in a mobility patterns survey) will also behave in this way in the future. However, such conclusions should only be reached after the following aspects are considered:

- The person's attitude towards such behaviour;
- Their perception of the subjective norm (expectations of what their significant others would think of the planned behaviour or what these individuals consider appropriate);
- Their perception of behavioural control (how easy it is to realise the intention).

Ajzen's model thus also explains the role of significant others and relevant groups. For example, when awareness-raising campaigns succeed in convincing '*significant others*' about certain behaviour, there will be a great chance of generating a '*snowball effect*', as such an attitude will be reflected in others' intentions and behaviour.

This theory gives us a solid basis when forecasting future mode choice behaviour on the basis of surveys, questionnaires, interviews, or other relevant empirical data. A nice example of how to use this theory in practice can be preparation and implementation of a media campaign to support walking. The aim of this campaign can be to make more people walk more. According to this theory, we can assume that the wished-for behaviour will take place if people's attitudes towards walking are positive (the campaign must aim at a change, or rather to add a new attitude towards walking), the perception of subjective norms must be consonant with behaviour (e.g. we can use peer groups as role models in the campaign), and the perception of behavioural control must be high (e.g. in the campaign, we should highlight that the preconditions for walking in the selected area are good and that it is easy to start walking – one does not need any equipment).

3.1.5   Rosenstiel's model of behaviour

Rosenstiel's (2003) model of behaviour explains the behaviour of an individual as being influenced by personal and situational variables. Situational variables include '*empowerment and obligation*' and '*situational enabling*'. Personal variables include '*individual desire*' and '*individual skills*'.

As illustrated in Figure 3.1, the variables interact with the behaviour and with each other. It is quite possible that the behaviour that is performed is in contradiction of one of the four domains. For example, individual desire may contradict the actual behaviour, as the person's desire appears impossible to realise at the moment, or the person may be influenced by others. Sometimes, when crossing a road as a pedestrian, we may behave differently when other people are also present than when we are alone. In the latter case, we may well cross the road at a red light (if the situation allows it), but when other road users (e.g. children) are there, we are more likely to wait until the green light comes up (social control). We will now provide a more detailed explanation of how to facilitate the understanding of the variables.

3.1.5.1   Situational variables

Empowerment and obligation: This variable implies that people always adjust their behaviour to societal norms and rules. The behaviour a person engages in reflects their individual system of values. Such an individual

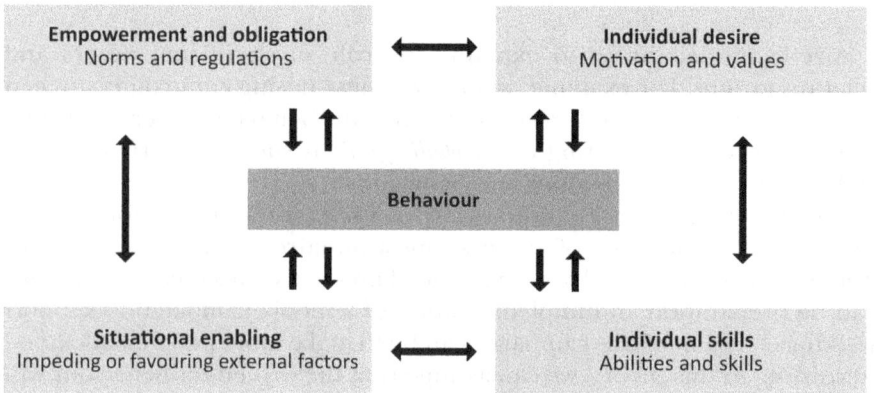

Figure 3.1 Behaviour and its conditions (Rosenstiel, 2003).

system of values develops according to the attitudes and values which are tolerated and considered desirable in social society. A pedestrian crossing the road against a red signal can serve as an example. If this behaviour is accepted, and it is a social norm and is often seen on the streets, people will tend to internalise this behaviour and perform it in the future.

Situational enabling: This variable refers to impeding or facilitating external factors influencing individual behaviour. An individual has no control over these external factors. In traffic, this domain includes the development of infrastructure, for example. If the infrastructure is not satisfactory (e.g. missing infrastructure for pedestrians), a person cannot perform the desired behaviour despite the existence of resources (e.g. physical strength = individual factor; see subsequently) and the person's determination. At present, this aspect is being addressed in relation to pedestrians and cyclists in an effort to meet the criteria for barrier-free movement in public spaces. The other example might be air pollution, which, in some cases (e.g. Beijing), is so bad that for health reasons it is not possible to walk or spend time outside near streets.

3.1.5.2   Personal variables

Individual desire: This variable comprises a person's attitudes, needs, and behavioural intentions. To a great degree, the development of these factors is shaped by the person's individual system of values. The individual system of values is linked to the given societal value system and is strongly influenced by the social environment. 'Traffic socialisation', in which youngsters observe grown-ups (especially parents) and create their system of values on the basis of this, can serve as an example.

Individual skills: This variable refers to a person's abilities and skills. A person must be fit to engage in certain behaviour. In general, this relies on the following aspects:

- Physical condition – is the person in good physical health, and can he or she participate in the traffic system as a pedestrian? Or is he or she physically disadvantaged, and does he or she need additional assistance or aids?
- Mental condition – is the person mentally capable of participating in the traffic system as a pedestrian? For example, understanding the traffic rules, possessing the ability to anticipate the behaviour of others and to perceive social norms, and so on?
- Last but not least, experience and learned abilities and skills are important. Past experience with walking at concrete locations – to know how to plan a route so as to be comfortable, how to overcome barriers or to bypass them, unsafe places, and so on – can serve as an example.

This theory can be used in practical work as a kind of checklist, when, for example, designing new pedestrian areas, covering these areas:

- Are citizens used to walking in such an area? Is it a social norm, or is it, so to say, common to walk here?
- Do all the situational factors (e.g. barrier-free, accessible, air and noise pollution, crime) support walking?
- Does a communication campaign count on influencing citizens' attitudes and needs?
- Do the majority of the citizens have the necessary individual skills (physical, mental, social)? How can we tackle minority groups with special needs?

3.1.6   Social comparison processes

In his theory of social comparison processes, Festinger (1950, 1954) assumes that individuals are driven to evaluate and compare their opinions and abilities by comparing them with those of others. This is especially true when there is not any objective fact to which people could compare their opinions or abilities (e.g. how good a lover am I?). Specifically, people will seek others who are close to their own opinions and abilities for comparison because accurate comparisons are difficult when others are too divergent from oneself. By comparing themselves with those others, people build their self-concept. According to Leon Festinger, social comparison processes belong among the main reasons people seek the company of others.

New situations involving several people may give rise to uncertainty if efforts to determine or discuss a unified opinion fail. Personal uncertainty of opinion persists until an opinion is at least subjectively confirmed or refuted. While physical realities are relatively simple to describe, it may be a challenging task as far as social realities are concerned. Opinions pertaining to this area (e.g. attitudes to social norms) are difficult to verify empirically and rationally.

If opinions are not defined and communicated, uncertainty about the reactions arises, as a range of behavioural alternatives is on offer. A difference of opinion within a group also generates uncertainty that is experienced as aversive, that is, causing discomfort (see cognitive dissonance).

The concept of social comparison processes is not limited to opinions only; it can have a broader scope of application. It covers cognitive contents in general and visible behaviours.

In promoting walking, the potential for the use of this theory may lie in the building of the (self-)image of pedestrians – as proud, modern, and clever citizens. Those who walk (often) in the city and prefer active traffic modes over car use are (still) often labelled as 'weird'. Also, as nowadays the norm is still to have a car and use it on a daily basis, the self-concept of the 'city walker' is not established. What is the identity of city walkers?

What do they share? When trying to promote walking, we should also focus on the establishment of, and support for, a community of walkers which would boost the social life of pedestrians. A smartphone application which would record distances walked, number of walks, and so on, and sharing this information with others in the community, with the possibility of a comparison, of setting 'challenges' and the like, can serve as a nice example. This approach is very well known in the domain of public health and sports, for example, mobile phone applications for sports such as *Endomondo* or *Runtastic*.

3.1.7 Model of ecological behaviour

A model devised by Fietkau and Kessel (1981) explores the ways of facilitating ecological behaviour and reducing non-ecological behaviour. It posits five major factors. In addition to relevant environmental *knowledge* and its impact on environmental *attitudes and values, opportunities to act* pro-environmentally, *incentives* for pro-environmental behaviour, and the *perceived consequences* of behaviour play a salient role (Figure 3.2).

Environmental knowledge is understood as a factor of indirect action which is realised by means of a person's attitudes and values. If a behavioural change is initiated, general awareness must also be accompanied by the knowledge of the measures to be taken in order to perform the desired behaviour.

This model can be used in the practical work of enhancing walking and other active and pro-environmentally oriented traffic modes. It summarises the relevant factors which have to be tackled and which have to act in the same direction in order to support the wished-for behaviour. We have to

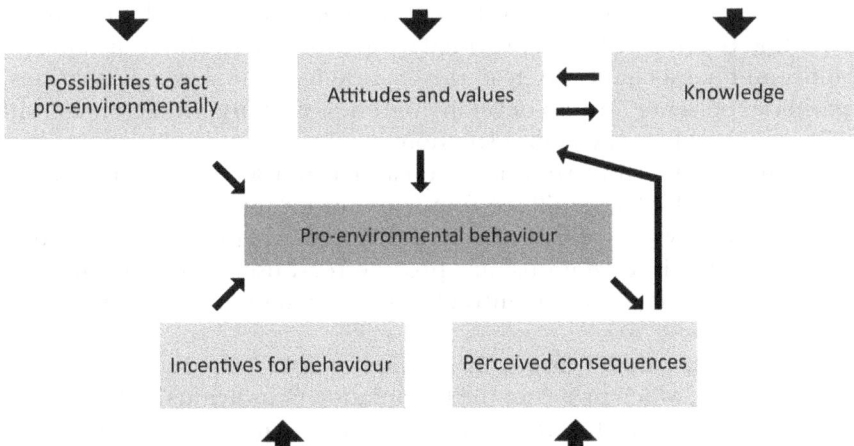

Figure 3.2 Model of ecological behaviour (Fietkau & Kessel, 1981).

make sure that citizens have relevant information about walking and its (positive) impact on the environment. Furthermore, we have to support pro-environmental attitudes and values, for example, by media campaigns, school education, or campaigns in the workplace. Opportunities to act pro-environmentally would refer to good infrastructure for walking, low crime, and connectivity to public transport. Incentives for wished-for behaviour in this case might be a free ticket for public transport for those who do not own a car (and park in the city) or benefits offered by employers, such as, for example, a day off for those who walk to work and back. Perceived consequences of pro-environmental behaviour refer to the fact that the acceptance and performance of pro-environmental behaviour provide positive feedback on attitudes and values and thus support future behaviour.

3.2   How to influence human behaviour in traffic

The model presented subsequently, suggested by the authors of this book, describes possible ways of influencing people's behaviour in traffic (Šucha, 2019). It is based on the assumption that human behaviour results from people's efforts to satisfy their needs. Behaviour is thus shaped by individual needs and preferences, that is, motives. Motives – and thus behaviour – may vary according to internal factors, such as individual personality structure, values, and norms, or to situational external factors, such as the quality of the infrastructure, aesthetics, accessibility, and so on.

The most common interventions to influence people's behaviour in traffic at the level of human-specific factors are education and socialisation. The rationale for these interventions is to educate road users (provide them with information) and improve their insight, awareness, and sense of responsibility. Interventions are delivered at the individual level, either universally or selectively.

The expectancy of the effectiveness of such interventions is based on the assumption that if a person is provided with information about sustainable mobility and has a chance to 'test' this knowledge in real-world situations, to gather experience, and to develop awareness and insight, he or she will opt for sustainable mode choice solutions.

Situation-specific interventions are carried out at the societal rather than the individual level. Their implementation and effectiveness are the responsibility of society, not of individuals. Figuratively speaking, situation-specific interventions may provide road users with a framework within which they can subsequently choose their (more or less sustainable) behaviour.

In general, the model draws on the *diamond model* by Ralf Risser (see Chapter 2.1.2.1), which proposes the formulation of individual categories in terms of situation-specific factors. The model was empirically tested using qualitative analysis of ten interviews with experts in traffic psychology, the criteria for the selection of experts being at least 10 years of work experience in the area of human factors in traffic, with relevant publication activities in the field. The objective of the interviews was to collect data used to uphold, modify, or reject the model. Given the nature of the problem under scrutiny, the semistructured interview method was employed, and the following areas and questions were looked into:

1. What do you think does influence people's behaviour in traffic?
2. How do you think we can influence people's behaviour in traffic?
3. What measures do you think are the most effective/suitable ones for ensuring people's behaviour in traffic (including both drivers and other road users, such as pedestrians)?
4. Do you find this model useful/suitable for describing people's behaviour in traffic, or factors which influence their behaviour? Why is it so? Why not?
5. What new aspects do you think this model brings in?
6. What use do you think we can make of this model in road use practice?

The majority of the experts who were interviewed agreed that people's behaviour in traffic is conditioned by a range of factors and that a comprehensive approach is needed to change or influence road users' behaviour. Such a multifaceted approach is also believed to help in achieving the sustainability of situation-specific interventions (see Figure 3.3), which the experts seemed to emphasise.

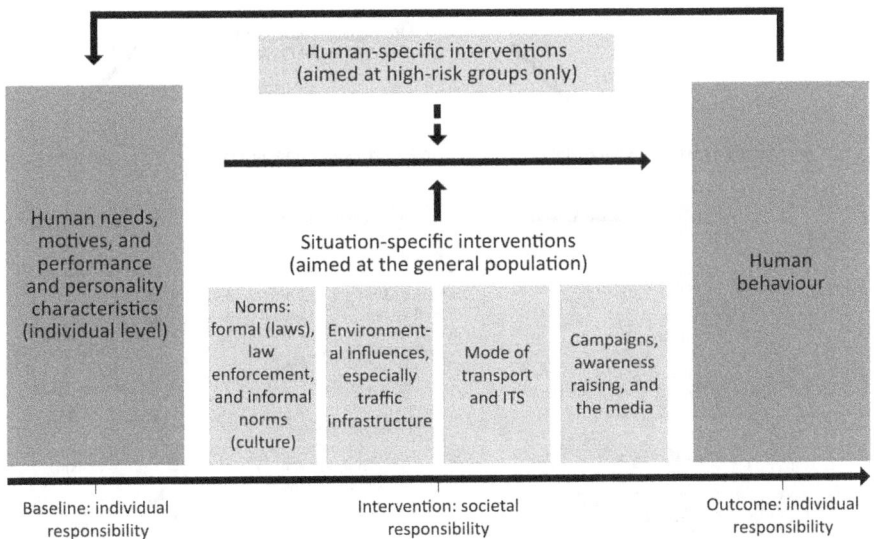

Figure 3.3 Model of influencing road users' behaviour following adjustments reflecting comments provided by experts (Šucha, 2019).

The model (and the results of the analysis of the experts' feedback) suggests that factors which have an impact on road users' behaviour can be divided into *individual* and *situational* or *social ones.*

The model, as revised in response to the feedback collected from the interviews with experts, is presented subsequently (Figure 3.3).

3.3   What keeps people from walking and how can we support walking?

Alfonzo (2005) suggests a transdisciplinary, multilevel, theoretical model that can help to explain how individual, group, regional, and environmental factors affect physical activity behaviours. His model offers a social-ecological concept for how both urban and non-urban factors may interact to support walking (Figure 3.4).

The model posits that individual, group, regional, and physical environmental variables affect an individual's choice to walk at different points in his or her decision-making process and that some factors are more prominent in the decision-making process than others. Alfonzo (2005) argues that a hierarchy of walking needs exists. These needs are 'organised into a hierarchy of prepotency'. The same hierarchical structure can be applied to the needs that people consider when deciding to walk. According to the model, there are five levels of needs that are considered within the decision-making process. These needs progress from the most basic need, feasibility (related to personal limits), to higher-order needs (related to

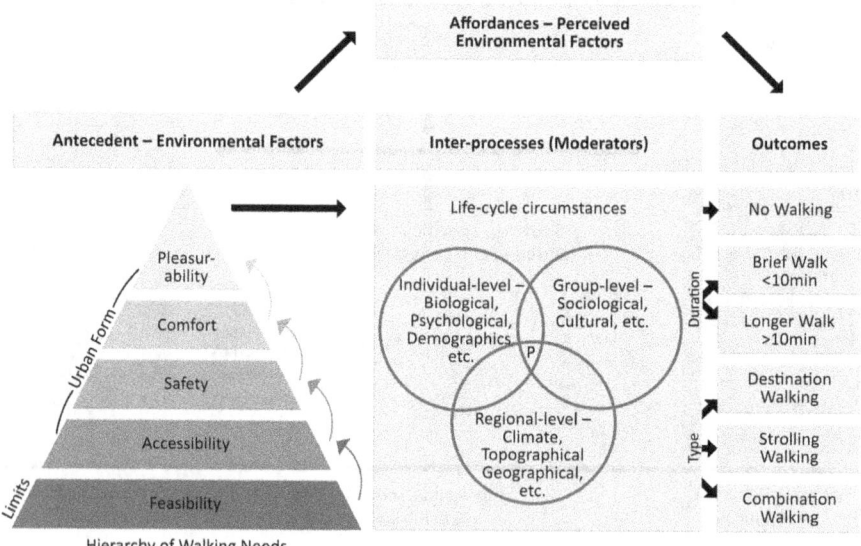

Figure 3.4 The hierarchy of walking needs (Alfonzo, 2005).

urban form), which include accessibility, safety, comfort, and pleasurability, in that order. Within this hierarchical structure, an individual would not typically consider a higher-order need in his or her decision to walk if a more basic need was not already satisfied (Alfonso, 2005). This is reminiscent of Maslow's hierarchy of needs (see Chapter 1.1).

Later on, Mehta (2008) elaborated on the model further and added three more levels (Figure 3.5).

Usefulness is the ability for the environment to satisfy the individual's basic day-to-day needs for shopping, eating, entertainment, and so on, and this ability or lack thereof affects walking behaviour. The *sensory pleasure* derived through a sensory experience of the street depends on various stimuli perceived from the environment – from the lights, sounds, smells, touches, colours, shapes, patterns, textures, and so on. *Sense of belonging* refers to a community place that helps shape community attitudes and to establish the community's identity, become significant to the neighbours, and achieve a social value and meaning. The characteristics of land use and the physical and social environment are all important to provide a useful, safe, comfortable, pleasurable, and meaningful setting for people to walk in urban public spaces (Mehta, 2008).

These models lend themselves well to use in the daily work of decision-makers and urban planners when designing urban areas with the intention of enhancing walking. They are practical and easy to understand and can be used as a kind of checklist with this logic: prerequisites (environmental factors) – moderators (individual, group, regional) – outcomes (duration

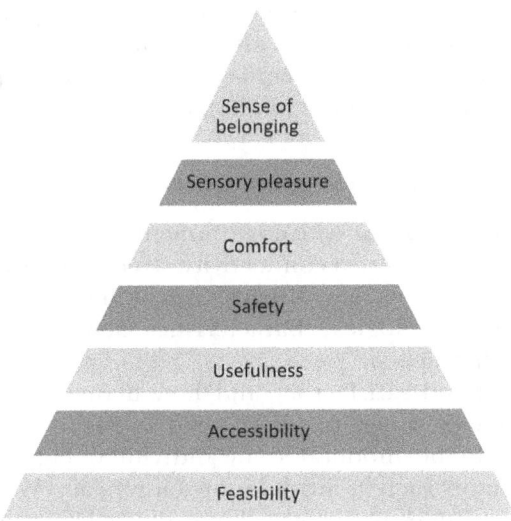

Figure 3.5 Hierarchy of walking needs on the neighbourhood high street (Mehta, 2008).

and time of walking). The prerequisites, organised in a hierarchical manner, describe where to start with changes in the environmental factors, for example, infrastructure changes or planning according to the pedestrians' needs. *Feasibility*, which refers to the personal ability to walk, is an exception – in this respect, special attention has to be paid to groups of citizens with special needs, with the aim being to make it feasible for everyone to walk or to move on the pavement with some aid (e.g. a wheelchair or crutches). 'Hierarchical' means that lower levels have to be tackled before upper levels become important. Urban planners should check that the planned public space or an existing one which should be revitalised is accessible, useful, or logical (e.g. regarding connectivity), safe, comfortable, and aesthetic, and if it has its *genius loci*.

The moderators, the most prominent and important factors from the psychological point of view, show us that prerequisites are perceived in a very different manner by different citizens. This means that, for example, for some groups of citizens, safety is much more important than comfort or aesthetics. Furthermore, the social norms and shared beliefs (culture) of the community (place, district, city) differ and influence the outcome (walking behaviour). Importantly, regional moderators such as the topography (is this place hilly or flat?) have to be taken into account. To consider all the relevant moderators, a psychological and sociological approach has to be implemented, as described in other chapters of this book. The needs and preferences of different groups of citizens have to be identified, and the prerequisites have to be adapted accordingly.

The outcomes are reflected by the walking activity (how many people walk, and how much?), the types of walks (for pleasure, for what purpose), or the time spent walking (preference for short or long walks). Outcomes should be measured and evaluated all the time with the aim being to give feedback with respect to the prerequisites, how these are perceived by the citizens, and what the role of the moderators is.

3.3.1   Psychological and environmental factors

Walking is known to correlate with environmental factors such as population density, type of land use, street connectivity, street design, aesthetics, traffic safety, and violence. As we have already seen, walking is also influenced to a large degree by psychological characteristics such as attitude, preference, intention, and self-efficacy.

What is considered satisfactory and how many levels (in the model described previously) need to be satisfied to make individuals engage in walking should be moderated by individual factors, for example, psychological factors such as attitudes or self-efficacy. When a person has less favourable attitudes towards walking (e.g. is less motivated to walk), more levels within the hierarchy would need to be satisfactory to make him or her decide to walk.

However, our understanding of how the interactions between psychological and environmental characteristics influence walking remains limited. As suggested by the hierarchy of walking needs (Alfonzo, 2005), environmental characteristics are not necessarily considered simultaneously, and the decision may resemble a tree structure; that is, some conditions need to be satisfied before other conditions are considered, depending on a person's psychological characteristics. As an example, we can show the role of habits in behaviour. A strong habit allows a weak relationship between attitude and behaviour (behaviour is driven by habit, not so much by attitudes; positive attitudes are not needed, so to say). On the other hand, when the habit is weak, the relationship between attitudes and behaviour needs to be strong in order for the behaviour to be performed.

Two interaction mechanisms have been proposed (Beenackers et al., 2013). In a *competitive mechanism*, the environment is more important to walking among those who have less positive attitudes towards walking. In contrast to this, in a *synergetic mechanism*, the environment is more important to walking among those who have more positive attitudes towards walking. To put it in other words, positive attitudes towards walking can be seen as a supportive factor which causes people to be willing to walk even though the environmental prerequisites are not fully adequate (e.g. aesthetics, connectivity), while, if a person does not possess a positive attitude towards walking, it takes much more 'work' on the prerequisites in order to achieve the wished-for behaviour.

Yang and Diez-Roux (2017) proposes a framework that integrates both mechanisms and includes the role of habits. The basic assumption of this framework is that people with very positive or very negative attitudes towards walking may walk or not walk, regardless of the environment. Furthermore, in citizens with strong habits, the relationship between attitude and behaviour may be weak, while when the habit is weak, the attitude-behaviour relationship is strong (Yang & Diez-Roux, 2017).

The practical value of this theory lies in the identification of those groups of citizens which are the most 'prone' to change their mode choice towards active modes, especially walking. On the basis of this model, one can basically see three groups of citizens with specific attitudes towards walking: those with very positive attitudes, those with moderate attitudes, and those with very negative attitudes. The role of the environment is of the greatest importance for the middle group, with moderate attitudes, because the first group would walk anyway and the third group would not walk in any case. In daily practical work, one can use this model to prioritise those citizens whom we will primarily address with supporting measures for walking, as this is the group for which there is the highest chance of a mode shift. One should start with this one. As for the very-positive-attitudes group, one should make sure not to 'lose' some of them, for example because the walking infrastructure deteriorates. As for the very-negative-attitudes group, adequate measures, such as media campaigns, should be designed

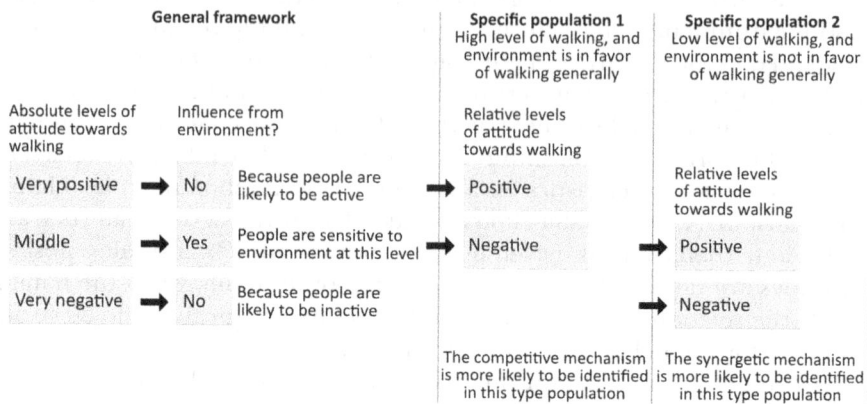

Figure 3.6 A general framework of the interactions between attitudes towards walking and the neighbourhood environment (Yang & Diez-Roux, 2017).

to push them from the pre-contemplation to the contemplation phase, according to Prochazka and DiClemente's stages of change model (1982).

The moderator (according to Alfonzo, 2005, and Mehta, 2008) in this model is the habits. As shown, when habits are weak, the potential of attitudes to shape behaviour is higher. Thus, when discussing the groups of citizens which are most susceptible to a mode shift, those groups with weak habits in either direction are the most promising ones to address. For instance, decision-makers should aim measures supporting walking at groups which have (so far) weak habits concerning mode choice, such as, for example, those who have recently moved to the city and have not yet had time to develop habits (Figure 3.6).

3.4   Interventions to support walking

The nature of walking behaviour must be considered carefully, because different types of walking (e.g. strolling, recreational walking, walking for a purpose) may be influenced by different motivational processes. In order to promote walking effectively, there is a need to identify the determinants of these different kinds of walking behaviour. The most commonly cited motives for walking are for recreation, to reach a destination (transport), and to maintain good health (Gobster, 2005). Among all types of physical activities, both structured and unstructured, research findings have shown that recreational walking which promotes relaxed walking behaviour generates the greatest gains overall for the health of a population (Patterson et al., 2017). Reducing sedentary activity is a major public health challenge requiring action around health behaviours and the environmental and social determinants of those behaviours. The promotion of walking as a physical activity that most individuals can engage in, either as a means of transport or as a leisure activity, offers considerable potential for raising the population's health level. As also mentioned previously, the main arguments are as follows:

- Walking can easily be integrated into people's daily routines.
- It is the most effective strategy for the promotion of physical activity in sedentary populations.
- It is suitable for most people in a community.
- It has been reported to be the most common physical activity, especially for those who are concerned about their health.
- It is an accessible form of activity and is suitable for all socio-demographic groups.

All these arguments should be used in practical work to promote walking, as the general population is obviously not conscious of these facts. Despite the multiple purposes and benefits generated by walking activity, walking rates still remain low in most countries (Hall et al., 2018). This suggests that there is an urgent need to persuade people to engage (more) in regular walking in order to gain its maximum benefits.

Although interventions at an individual level (e.g. education) can promote walking, research studies have shown that a single-level approach will only have a short-term impact on behavioural change (Hall et al., 2018). As also stressed in other chapters of this book, a holistic approach is needed. Therefore, in order to sustain a longer impact on the population, walking intervention strategies have to consider all factors, as shown in the Alonzo model previously: individual, group, regional, and physical environmental variables.

The challenge for policy makers is to identify walking intervention strategies that reduce barriers, as well as to increase people's motivation to walk regularly. Subsequently we describe examples of interventions which can be used to enhance walking, according to the Alfonzo model (2005), on the regional, the group, and the individual level.

3.4.1 *Interventions on the regional level*

Environmental changes aimed at encouraging walking or cycling may promote activity and improve health, but evidence suggests small or inconsistent effects in practice. Panter et al. (2019) conducted a systematic review on this topic and identified three common resources that interventions provide to promote walking and cycling: (1) improving the accessibility and connectivity of an area or route, (2) improving safety from traffic (segregation from motor vehicles) and personal attacks (perceptions of crime), and (3) improving the experience of walking and cycling (areas that are more aesthetically pleasing). Almost all the studies identified improving accessibility or connectivity to destinations as the main intervention function (e.g. *'to make it easier for pedestrians and cyclists to reach destinations in the local area'*) (Ogilvie, 2008). This empirical evidence is in line with the theoretical models presented previously (Alfonso, 2005; Yang & Diez-Roux, 2017).

3.4.2   Interventions on the group level: Lay-led group programmes

There are a variety of models of community-based walking group programmes, both professional and lay led, and these range from primary prevention to those targeted at individuals with existing health conditions. Hanson and Jones (2015), in their systematic review and meta-analysis of outdoor walking group programmes, found evidence of positive health effects, including reductions in blood pressure and body mass index and increased physical functioning scores.

3.4.3   Interventions on the individual level: Life-changing experiences

Long-distance walking (LDW) is an increasingly popular and diverse activity, known to attract participants from a wide range of age groups, including mid-life adults. As Solnit (2001) implies, walking can reduce the perceived pace of life and create opportunities for contemplation and reflection. Long-distance walking was found to facilitate moments of insight through which issues were seen more clearly or placed in a new context and therefore contributed to significant personal change. Long-distance walking may offer important experiential opportunities for those in mid-life who are searching for, or at least receptive to, significant personal change (Saunders et al., 2017).

3.5   Communication models and theories

Subsequently, we will present some selected psychological theories on communication. Communication is crucial both 'in' walking (between pedestrians and other road users or between cars or infrastructure and pedestrians) and 'about' walking (e.g. promoting walking). The first one is especially important for the safety and comfort of pedestrians, the latter for the promotion and enhancement of walking.

3.5.1   Communication model according to Shannon and Weaver

A classical communication model is that designed by Claude E. Shannon and Warren Weaver. While originally developed as part of the theories of mathematics and informatics, it is still widely cited (Shannon & Weaver, 1949). The model consists of six elements – *information source, transmitter, receiver, information sink, information channel,* and *noise source* – which determine whether communication can take place in line with the original intention and content. Shannon and Weaver assume that the transmitter uses various signals to convey a piece of information to the receiver. In communication via telephone, for example, the message is converted by the transmitter into a signal (*code*) which then travels through the channel (*line*) to the receiver, where it is decoded again. For a message to reach the destination in order, the transmission must be free of noise. However, sources of noise, such as line noise in the given example, mean that this is not always possible.

In verbal communication, possible sources of noise include sound distortion (on the telephone) or signals which are attached inadvertently during the transmission (e.g. facial expressions, tone of voice, etc.). In spoken language, the information source is the brain and the transmitter is the vocal cords, which produce variable sound pressure (signal), which is transmitted through the air (channel).

In addition to the previous aspects, emotions play an important role in the exchange of information: the expectations one has regarding other people, stress, anger, or fear may significantly affect the quality of the information exchange and may thus also act as sources of noise in the communication process.

The main message of this theory for practice is that '*what someone says is not the same as someone else hears*'. This is true for person-to-person communication (mostly verbal) but also for communication between people and infrastructure or vehicles. A pedestrian countdown signal on a pedestrian crossing can serve as an example. Pedestrian countdown timers show the amount of time left to cross the road before the red man appears. The message which road designers are communicating is that this allows pedestrians to decide if they have enough time to cross the road. But do we know how this message is 'decoded' by pedestrians? From empirical evidence, we can see that there is considerable variation in the way that people react to such signals.

3.5.2   *Schulz von Thun's model*

Another theory of interpersonal communication was formulated by Friedemann Schulz von Thun. It features a communication square, also known as the '*four-ears model*' or '*four-sides model*'. This model proposes that what we say has a fourfold effect. Whether we want it to or not, every statement we utter conveys four messages at the same time (Schulz von Thun, 2001):

- **Factual information** – what we inform about
- **Self-revelation** – what we reveal about ourselves
- **Relationship** – what we think about, and how we relate to, the receiver
- **Appeal** – what we want to make the receiver do

In figurative terms, Schulz von Thun interlinked the four sides of the square with the '*four beaks*' of the sender, whose messages hit the '*four ears*' of the receiver. Both the sender and the receiver are responsible for the quality of communication, and comprehensible communication is the ideal rather than the rule.

It is essential that information be sent and received in the correct sense on all four levels. On the factual level of the communication, matter-of-fact statements such as data and facts, that is, the content of the utterance, come to the fore.

- Content is relevant or irrelevant: is the subject matter of the message to the point or not?
- Information is sufficient or insufficient: is the matter-of-fact information enough, or do other aspects need to be taken into consideration?

On the **factual level**, the sender's task is to communicate the subject matter clearly and understandably. According to the criteria, the receiver may respond on the '*factual ear*' level. Whether consciously or unintentionally, every statement contains **information about the sender** – his or her feelings, values, unique qualities, or needs. This may occur either explicitly (*self-expression*) or implicitly. Implicitly or explicitly, intentionally or unintentionally, the sender reveals information about himself or herself by means of the '*self-revealing beak*', while the receiver intercepts such information with his or her '*self-revealing ear*': What is he or she like? What mood is he or she in? How does he or she feel? What message is he or she trying to get across?

On the **relationship level**, we indicate what attitude we hold towards the other and what we think of him or her. Both the self-disclosing information and information about the relationship are communicated by way of formulation, intonation, mimicry, and gestures. The sender transmits such information implicitly or explicitly. Depending on the information received by the '*relationship ear*', the receiver feels accepted or rejected, ignored or valued, respected or humiliated, and so on.

Influence on the receiver is exerted on **the appeal level**. Generally, when a person has something to say, he or she wants to make a difference. Such a person expresses his or her wishes, appeals, advice, or instructions. Appeals are communicated openly or covertly. Using his or her '*appeal ear*', the receiver asks himself or herself: What is it that I should (not) do, think, or feel now?

This model extends *Shannon and Weaver's* model and states that the four levels on both sides of the communication process have to be matched correctly for the communication to be successful. In practical work, this model can be used in media campaigns promoting walking. The core of each communication campaign is a message which should be delivered. Using this theory, we can make sure that our message will be delivered to the audience (potential walkers) in the way we intend. On the factual information side we formulate **what** we want to communicate, for example, 'there is a new facility for pedestrians in the vicinity'. On the self-revelation level, we communicate what we **think and feel** about the factual information, for example, we can communicate that, newly, the mayor and other city officials are using this facility and walking to their offices. On the relationship level, we communicate **how we relate to our audience**, for example, if the campaign is smart and 'fresh', we communicate that we think that our audience is also smart and fresh. On the appeal level, we communicate **what the wished-for behaviour is,** for example, 'walk more'.

3.5.3 *Transtheoretical model*

The transtheoretical model (TTM) proposes that, in relation to specific subject areas associated with their behaviour, people find themselves in different states of awareness (Prochaska & DiClemente, 1982). This involves various stages of willingness to do something about possibly problematic behaviours that are linked to the subject areas in question. The term 'problematic' may refer to the fact that a certain type of behaviour may be harmful to us, to society, or to both. For example, a lack of physical activity may cause damage to our health. When a physician raises a suggestion of walking more as an issue of physical activity, however, he or she may encounter a range of reactions, from a person's complete denial of the fact that a shortage of physical activity is harmful to a description of the specific strategies he or she has already adopted in order to walk more or to perform other physical activities. Additionally, when we want to make people pursue certain social goals, we need to be prepared for their diverse attitudes to specific subject areas.

The TTM is thus a motivational stage-based model which has been used in a number of areas, for example, public health issues such as smoking cessation or nutrition (obesity prevention). However, it holds universally that strategies aimed at producing a change in a person's behaviour must take account of the attitudinal state of the person being addressed. The TTM also includes a stage of relapse and seeks to prevent it. The model describes the stages of change as follows:

- Precontemplation: a person does not plan to change certain behaviour or may be totally unaware that the problem exists at the moment
- Contemplation: a person is considering a change in a behaviour but has no specific plan as to how to achieve it
- Preparation: a person decides to try to achieve a change in a behaviour and takes the first steps in preparation for it
- Action: a person seeks to realise his or her intention and engage in a desired behaviour or refrain from an undesired behaviour

- Maintenance: a person seeks to sustain the change in their behaviour; precautions must be taken to prevent relapse
- Change adopted: the desired behaviour has developed into a habit; no efforts to resume the previous behaviour are experienced.

The model suggests that a change in behaviour, such as that concerning physical activity, for example, achieved through active mobility such as walking or cycling, involves a learning process which may take place in several rounds before a sustained change is accomplished. This process may be conceived of as a spiral: a certain starting point is left in an effort at change. When a change is successfully brought about – which often takes much effort and several attempts – a person finds himself or herself on a higher level of the spiral. As previously mentioned, external measures (to support the change) must then be adjusted to the given state of awareness (insight).

This approach has been successfully used in the public health domain, for example, in connection with the reduction of smoking. We believe that it can also be used successfully in other areas, such as within the frame of attempts to shift mode choice from car use to active modes. As described previously, the most important point is to detect the stage of awareness (e.g. interviews with target groups or surveys) and to apply interventions accordingly. For example, if our target group is in the precontemplation stage, it means that they do not perceive that there is a problem or do not realise that there are alternatives to their behaviour. For this target group, an appropriate intervention would be to cause a dissonance (see also dissonance theory). For example, facts can be presented that show how beneficial walking is both for the individual and for society. This will cause a dissonance, because this information is in conflict with their actual attitudes and behaviour. To put it in other words, we should make this group of citizens aware that there is another, more beneficial alternative for them and raise their interest in this fact by creating an intrapersonal conflict. Once we have directed their attention towards active traffic modes, we can offer appropriate alternatives (concrete plans or steps for how to go on). For the groups of citizens in the maintenance stage, we should make sure that we do not lose them, for example, because of negative experiences with walking. In other words, we have to make sure that interventions are also targeted at those who already walk, with the aim being to make them walk more, to make their walks more comfortable, and to prevent their deterioration.

3.5.4 *Elaboration likelihood model*

The *elaboration likelihood model* (ELM) describes the effects of persuasive messages depending on the way such messages are processed (Petty & Cacioppo, 1986). The model proposes two pathways of processing, central and peripheral; see Figure 3.7. A *persuasive message* is aimed at persuading somebody about something.

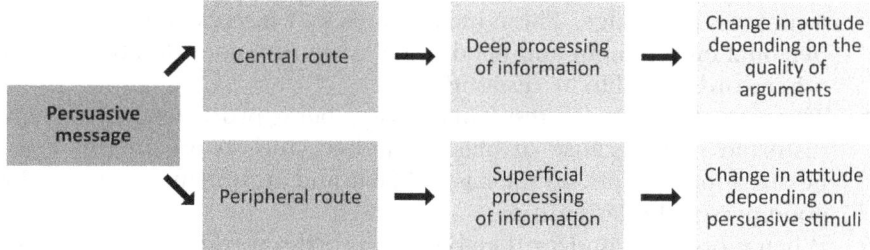

Figure 3.7 Elaboration likelihood model (Petty & Cacioppo, 1986).

With the *central route*, a new message is compared with the existing knowledge and considered, as, for example, it may be personally relevant or more information may be needed. Connection with the subject matter and willingness to deal with it already exist; the addressee of the message already possesses relevant motivation and is capable of receiving the information. Information processed in such a manner results in a stable change in attitude. Information communicated via this route can, or should, even show a high level of elaboration (minute accurateness, completeness, and dialectic quality).

With the *peripheral route*, attitudes tend to be shaped by factors which are independent of the content of the message. The change in attitude is brought about by persuasive stimuli rather than the quality of the arguments; for example, when information is presented as favoured and valued by 'everybody' or when a person communicating the information looks good, is likable, and gives an air of authority. The peripheral route may work well with people who lack motivation or have poor skills of receiving certain information. This learning process applies to children, in particular, but is also effective in adults, especially in relation to topics which are of no particular importance for them.

The ELM involves several propositions concerning information processing and behavioural change.

1. People are motivated to adopt conforming attitudes. This corresponds with the theory of social comparison processes, which holds that an individual seeks to compare his or her own opinions with those of others (Festinger, 1954). Differences of opinion are perceived as unpleasant (dissonance); a human being strives for conformity of opinions.
2. The intensity of people processing certain information relevant to their attitudes and the way they do so depend on their abilities and motivation (see the transtheoretical model previously). These two agents are further influenced by individual and situation-specific factors. The degree and direction of the change in attitude are influenced by a number of variables, such as the content of communication and the signs of the communicator or context of the communication – these need to be taken into account in the communication process.

3. There are variables that influence motivation and/or a person's ability to process a message. These include a lack of interest and absence of personal engagement and need to be taken into consideration, or, in other words, need to be responded to.
4. There are variables that result in messages being processed in a strongly distorted way, because of bias, prejudice, and so on. In this case, persuasion may work on the basis of facts and arguments supported by good personal relationships.
5. When motivation and/or the ability to process arguments are limited, peripheral information stimuli come to play an important role. While the intensity or accuracy of the way information is processed increases (in terms of the transtheoretical model, when a person advances to a higher level of the spiral), the peripheral information stimuli become relatively insignificant influencing factors.

Changes in attitudes produced by good processing of arguments or information, that is, via the central route, are more stable in time, predict better behavioural prognoses, and show greater resistance to counterarguments in comparison to changes in attitude which result from mere responses.

In practice, this model can be used in connection with the transtheoretical model in order to approach as wide an audience as possible in an appropriate way, for example, in campaigning or promoting walking in any other way. On the basis of qualitative data, for example, interviews with citizens, one can define to which stages our audience refers (e.g. precontemplation, contemplation...), and then one can define which communication route (central or peripheral) one should use in one's campaigning. In fact, both routes have to be used, so that one can reach citizens in all stages of change, but the important aim is how to mix and find a 'best ratio' between the central and the peripheral route. For example, if one uses too much information via the central route, but one's audience is still in the precontemplation stage, one will miss the goal. Vice versa, too much information distributed via the peripheral route for an audience in the preparation stage will be discarded and, in the worst case, be considered annoying.

3.6   Institutional framework for practitioners

In order to identify strategies that may be most effective at increasing walking, practitioners need a greater understanding of the underlying motives that make people select different travel modes. For this reason, we provide the five-step operational theory of routine mode choice decisions (Figure 3.8), proposed by Schneider (2013). Walking could be promoted through each of the five steps: awareness and availability (e.g. carry out campaigns), basic safety and security (e.g. introduce pedestrian facility improvements and increase education and enforcement efforts), convenience and costs (e.g.

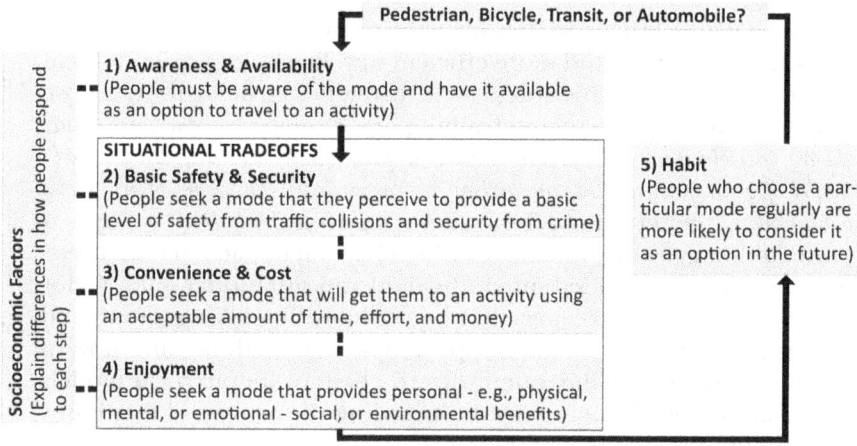

Figure 3.8 Proposed theory of routine mode choice decisions (Schneider, 2013).

instigate mixed land use and introduce limited, more expensive automobile parking), enjoyment (e.g. plant trees along streets and increase awareness of the benefits of non-motorised transportation), and habit (e.g. target information about sustainable transportation options to people making key life changes) (Schneider, 2013).

Strategies to increase walking include the development of pedestrian infrastructure, land use planning, and individual and social marketing. Larger mode shifts require a clearer understanding of the barriers to choosing walking for different types of citizens in different communities (Schneider, 2013). Operational theories such as the theory of routine mode choice decisions are useful because they can provide concise, understandable frameworks to summarise previous research for practical application.

This model of Schneider's is a very practical one that puts several theories together (also mentioned previously) in order to form one strategy for enhancing sustainable transport modes. This model leads us to the next chapter, in which we have combined different theories in order to form and suggest one holistic approach for achieving mode change, in our case, to the advantage of walking.

SUMMARY

Road user behaviour is a consequence of the action of multiple factors which can be divided into those that affect the road user from the inside (individual factors) and those that exert an effect from the outside (situational factors). It is more promising to address those factors that affect the road user from the outside. These can be shaped in an easier, quicker, and more efficient way. Psychology offers a great variety of theories which deal with influencing behaviour. Those most relevant for enhancing walking are *dissonance theory, reactance theory, attribution theory, the theory of planned behaviour, Rosenstiel's model of behaviour, social comparison processes,* and *the model of ecological behaviour.* A general model on *how to influence behaviour in traffic* is presented, suggesting that factors which have an impact on road users' behaviour can be divided into individual and situational ones. As for the traffic domain and especially when enhancing walking, situational factors are prominent. What keeps people from walking and how to support walking are illustrated with the help of hierarchical models and a hierarchy of walking needs, including the aspects of feasibility, accessibility, usability, safety, comfort, sensory pleasure, and a sense of belonging. To promote walking effectively, there is a need to identify the determinants of walking behaviour; different types of walking are influenced by different motivational processes. The challenge for policy makers is to identify walking intervention strategies that reduce barriers, as well as to increase people's motivation to walk regularly. Communication is crucial in promoting and enhancing walking. Selected communication theories are presented, namely the *communication model according to Shannon and Weaver, Schulz von Thun's model, the transtheoretical model,* and *the elaboration likelihood model.* The institutional framework for practitioners puts several theories together to form one strategy for enhancing sustainable transport modes which can be used appropriately and easily in practice.

4 How to support walking

This chapter is aimed primarily at decision-makers and politicians. It also addresses other readers, as one of the most important activities to promote walking is community-based initiatives. We present arguments to promote walking and describe them in a general context with examples. The principles of campaigning and social marketing are shown, with a focus on enhancing walking.

How can walking be supported? The starting point for any larger change of preconditions to the advantage of walking is whether there is interest in achieving such a change on the decision-makers' side and what roles different stakeholders take on with respect to supporting walking. What efforts are made to generate quality white papers and development plans for traffic and transport, is money invested, are laws adapted to the needs of pedestrians, are public campaigns launched? This is an approach that we could call top-down.

Of course, there is another type of *starting point*, as well, which is more difficult to identify. It refers to the question of when and how processes start that result in real-life policy changes, based on developments in the awareness of the public that politicians or policy makers (have to) react to. Such a discussion would probably fill a whole book of quite a different character than this one, dealing with the questions of how societal attitudes develop and change over time and what factors contribute to such changes, how they contribute, and how much they do so. No doubt the single individual can play a role in such a process, but that role will remain limited unless more individuals join together in making efforts to give the development a certain direction. Joint activities and joint forces, however, need coordination. A single individual does not know whether others will join or oppose him or her beforehand. There needs to be some forum where it is recognisable that one will not stand alone if one tries something unusual. Because, of course, it is unusual to walk to work if nobody else does so, and if many people walk a maximum of 500 metres to work, then it is unusual to walk 1½ kilometres (which will still only take 20 minutes at most). But if people from the public media become aware of such an activity and find it an interesting idea that should be promoted, and if they write about this idea in an attractive way, then it also becomes visible to other persons who may have been thinking of walking to their job but decided not to do so, maybe out of fear that this might appear ridiculous. More generally speaking, any person and any institution that can make himself/herself/itself heard in public has the opportunity and the power to attribute (more) importance to any activity that citizens might carry out. This is what we could call a bottom-up approach.

4.1   Pedestrian-friendly: Yes or no?

Psychology is the science of behaviour and its understanding and control. We have written that before. However, at this point it is important to point out that psychology can help to 'control' – or better to say 'change' – the behaviour of a single individual, that is, to direct such behaviour in a wished-for way, only if there is a chance to address individuals, of course. Such 'addressing' would, of course, be an impossible mission if every citizen had to be addressed individually by a psychologist or any other person who knows how to apply psychological tools. There need to be ways to address as many people as possible simultaneously and to convince or persuade them to change their behaviour. If anybody makes the criticism that we are talking of interfering in people's private lives or of manipulation here, the answer would be: any psychological measure aims at changing the behaviour of different groups of people: patients, customers, consumers, voters, pupils, or employees. Within the frame of analyses of human behaviour, in order to understand it, researchers have to be as disinterested as possible, with the goal being to achieve results that are not biased. But when we start to implement measures, then it has been decided that a certain direction should be taken. If this direction is not shared by the individual whom we address, efforts to convince, to shape, to persuade, to motivate, or the like become necessary.

Interestingly, hardly anybody objects to their daily manipulation by advertising, which has the goal of convincing people to buy goods or services. In order to address people with the goal of convincing them of the quality of certain products, a lot of money is spent. As Figure 4.1 subsequently shows, the car industry is a giant spender in this respect.

If one looks at the car industry's expenditures on advertising, one can easily agree that to invest money with the goal being to change people's behaviour and make them walk (more) is nothing unusual or worthy of condemnation. This is even less so if one looks at the contents of many car advertisements: beautifully styled cars alone on the road (no congestion mess) or in some beautiful and healthy wild countryside (when SUVs are

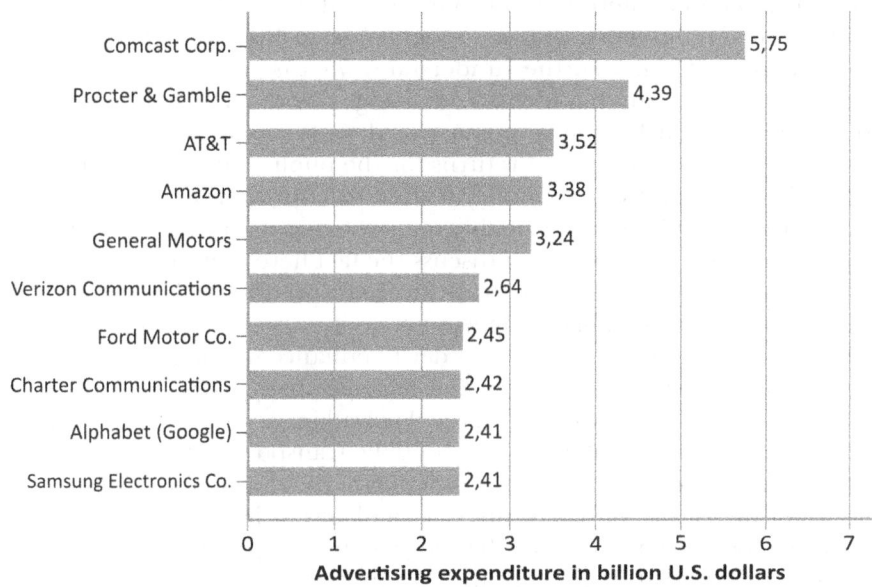

Figure 4.1 Money spent on advertising in the United States (largest advertisers in the United States, 2018).

being sold), providing either total freedom for the individual or an idyllic shelter for the family. This is very nicely described in the research done on explicit and implicit messages in the car manufacturers' advertisements. Generally, the explicit content is prosocially oriented (safety, time with family, positive attitudes), but, on the other hand, the implicit message is very different, aiming at individualism, being seen, domination of others, and aggression (Donovan et al., 2011). The reality is very different from what is presented there – nothing unusual where advertising is concerned. But in times of global warming, when one wants car use not to increase much more, one may easily conclude that much more money should be spent to market freedom, family cohesion, and environmental protection in connection with walking.

The difference from the car industry, however, is that there is hardly any strong business case for any private investor in connection with walking. The shoe industry does, of course, make money, but that is not very closely connected with the goal of promoting walking. Everybody buys shoes, even those who hate walking – shoes are rather a matter of fashion than of functionality. To make people walk (more) is not part of the interests of any branch of industry, with the possible exception of producers of hiking equipment, which, among others, sell shoes for mountaineering, but, again, this is rather a matter of sports than of everyday city walking. The one group of people with the chance to address many people simultaneously and who should be interested in promoting walking is the representatives of our states; politicians, that is, policy makers. But do they recognise the value of walking? Can they understand what is gained by enhancing walking? And also, can they identify advantages for themselves if they stand up for walkers and for improvements in the preconditions for walking? Can they point their fingers at returns for the public budgets if somebody makes the criticism that tax money is used to improve the infrastructure to the advantage of walkers, who, in contrast to car drivers, do not pay any transport-related tax? We do not discuss the fact here that, by paying their transport-related taxes, car drivers are far from covering all the costs of that they receive from the public budgets.

Anyway, what should be done in order to enhance walking? Do we know enough to produce preconditions that make as many individuals from as many different groups as possible agree that walking is an option, both from door to door and in combination with public transport, for a given doable distance to be covered? The fact is that we know roughly what is relevant and important for pedestrians. But when we look at the literature, we have to realise that pedestrians are a very heterogeneous group (indeed, it is unsure whether one can call them a group at all from a sociological perspective) with many different and partly contradicting needs in terms of detail. Furthermore, their needs vary over time and space. Surveys with similar questions and procedures lead to different results with respect to needs and their satisfaction, not grossly so, but still quite substantially concerning certain details. What does that mean in practice? It means that if the authorities are prepared to get active with the goal of supporting walking, they can do so at any time, because there is enough know-how concerning things that all agree upon: give pedestrians more space, see to it that walking networks are complete and without gaps, make crossings safe by reducing road width and introducing refuge islands where these are currently lacking, control motor vehicle drivers' behaviour when turning left or right and thereby crossing the pedestrians' path, give pedestrians enough time to cross the road (adapt to a speed of 1 m/sec), reduce waiting times for pedestrians in order to avoid crossings with red lights, reduce car speeds wherever there are (many) pedestrians on the road (where the definition of 'many' is difficult; thus, technically speaking, introducing a 30 km/h limit in whole cities would be the technically easiest way to go – but, of course, politically [still] difficult at this moment), and on a more general level that would permeate all the elements connected to walking: take all possible types of measures to attribute effectiveness, efficiency, and attractiveness to walking, thus freeing the image of walkers from that of being second-class road users.

Here, we want to refer to a graph produced by Methorst et al. (2010), citing Fleming (1999; Figure 4.1). Fleming's arguments reflect how decision-makers in any society appear with respect to any certain field of public interest. Walking in the public space is such a field, as virtually every member of society is a walker to a minor or major degree (with the exception of a few persons who cannot walk, either since birth or later, who have to use a wheelchair or who have to be transported).

4.2   The role of policy makers

It is necessary to pay attention to what changes are required (and why) with regard to the institutional framework which is tasked with improving the conditions for pedestrians, that is leadership, knowledge and professional skills, strategic policies, resources, and cooperation and partnerships. Politicians need to buy into the idea that walking is important and implement measures that make cities walkable in order to have the public walk more. But politicians will not work towards this unless the public buys into it. In other words, to implement measures supporting walking needs both approaches: bottom-up (initiative[s] from the public) and top-down (initiative[s] by policy makers).

In order to assess the chances of a positive development of the preconditions for walking, it is, of course, relevant what position the policy makers in any city, region, or country take. What value do they attribute to walking? Do they understand the positive effects that the enhancement of walking would have? How do they assess those positive effects compared to the comfort that a policy of business as usual – that does not provoke any opposition and does not require much effort – provides? Are they personally involved? Do they walk and enjoy it?

Figure 4.2 describes different levels of maturity that decision-makers and stakeholders can adopt in these respects.

According to the arguments of Methorst (and Fleming), the *pathological* state would mean that politicians and policy makers care less about the quality of pedestrians' situation than about the personal disadvantages they would suffer if they were 'caught' and sued for neglecting their official duties. They do not feel any need to become active with regard to the goal of improving the preconditions for walkers and do not have to fear the media, because at this stage of maturity of politicians and policy makers, public opinion will probably not be very interested in walking issues. Thus the risk of being caught and sued is low.

At the *reactive* level, problems are solved that appear to raise enough interest that there could be negative consequences for the decision-makers if they do not react. In other words, the importance of walking is admitted, but in practice no pro-active measures are taken. Outside signals by citizens and the media that indicate something could be wrong are reacted to but without any (good) scientific basis and without enthusiasm. Pedestrian problems are not considered important and, for example, no efforts are made to understand these problems, for instance, by taking steps to acquire appropriate knowledge about pedestrian problems in the given traffic and transport system. Research and activities aimed at learning from other countries are not supported.

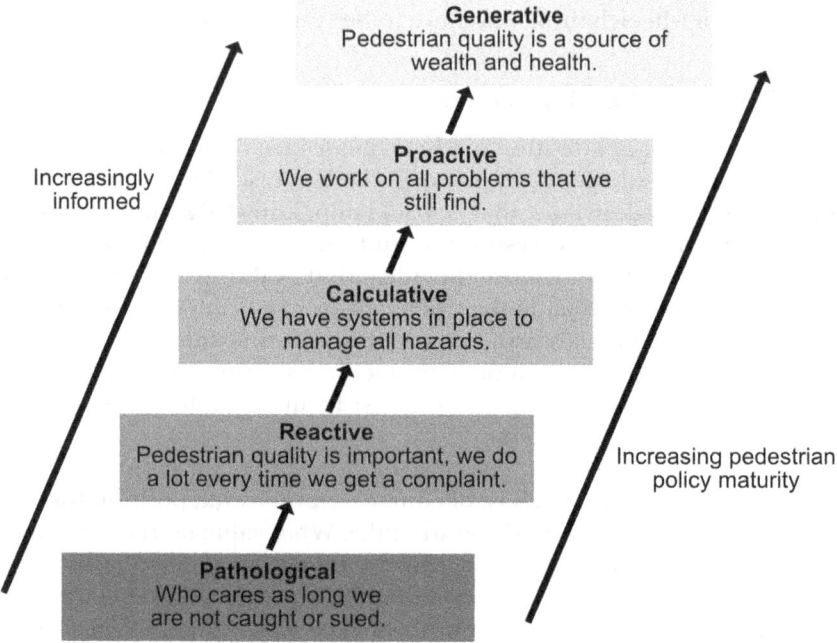

Figure 4.2 Status of society concerning awareness of problems and preparedness to act (Methorst, 2010).

The *calculative* stakeholder is rigid in the sense that he/she has systems in place to solve problems. He 'knows what works'. Staff, management, and stakeholders are informed about, and involved in, tackling short- and medium-term issues more or less ad hoc, and they know how to carry out the necessary activities to keep things going. Learning, searching for new and probably better solutions, and taking long-term effects into account are not (yet) part of this type of policy. To evaluate interventions does not belong among the routines, and more thorough assessment only takes place when unexpected problems arise. The problem at this stage is that calculative systems are self-assured; they have good solutions at hand and are not interested in improving – although there maybe is some notion that improvements could be possible.

The *proactive* organisation does everything right. It knows how to tackle problems ad hoc but also what measures to take in order to further develop and improve the preconditions for walking. Everyone in the organisation is motivated and actively involved in achieving the goals set by ambitious plans and schedules. There is not only knowledge but also the belief that it is worthwhile to support pedestrian quality, not least for economic reasons. The people involved *'know their figures'* but at the same time strive to be continuously at the state-of-the-art level, both concerning policy rationales and the management and maintenance aspects that are so important in practice. Monitoring and evaluation have become routine and are carried out in the knowledge that they do not cost money but save money. Public relations work is carried out routinely and professionally.

An illuminating comment concerning the generative organisation would be to say that in such an organisation, walking would be treated in a similar way to how the car is treated in most societies nowadays: quality deficits are detected immediately because the level of awareness is optimal. Everything that is done is accompanied by the question of whether this is good for walkers and whether *'the walking public will be satisfied'*. In psychological terms, the understanding that every solution in the public space needs to fit pedestrian quality needs would be internalised by everybody in the organisation, both decision-makers and executors. Both daily business and activities with a medium- and long-term perspective, including research and education, are steered by intrinsic motivation to support walking from all angles.

Starting from the assumption that there is no society on the national, regional, or municipal level that has achieved the highest stage and that there are very few societies on the proactive level, most of those few probably on the municipal level, the question arises of what can be done to make public organisations strive for higher stages and also to reach them. This brings us back to the discussion previously: interest in becoming active and motivation to do so arise in individuals. Individuals communicate and forums may pop up where people realise that there is support for certain ideas. If individuals with the power to move things – media people, decision-makers, or opinion leaders – support or even join such interest *'movements'*, the importance of a certain topic may be raised to a higher level. Facts about the importance of walking and its positive effects in many different areas change from *'known by some'* to *'considered relevant by many'*. If the advantages of walking are experienced and felt by a sufficient number of people and are no longer a matter of *'the literature says'*, a society could develop in which walking is treated in a similar way to how the car is treated today. We need to reach a *'critical mass'* to start the change. Who would oppose such a development? Of course, those who lose shares of the market, that is, the car industry and everything that is connected to the production of cars, to the construction and maintenance of infrastructure for cars, to the use of cars in practice with all its implications, such as insurance issues, the part of the health sector that earns money from car accidents, the petrol industry, and so on. Some call all these groups the car lobby and related lobbies.

How can we estimate the chances of a change in a wished-for direction, that is, to the advantage of walking? The decisions as to which politicians steer democratic countries are taken by voters. Voters do not mainly have traffic in mind when they vote, maybe not even as a side issue. Whether a politician is for or against walking certainly does not play a predominant role in voting decisions. But in today's situation, many voters will probably be against (too many or too harsh) measures to reduce car traffic. However, there is a chance that reducing car traffic could become an issue for more people once the relationship between climate change and car use is acknowledged by enough people. It seems to us that this goal should be reached before the effects of climate change have grown to catastrophic dimensions that nobody can deny that they see any longer. The big cities in China are a good example of this scenario. Can you imagine if politicians in European countries had to explain to their voters that during some days they should stay at home, because the air is too polluted for them to walk outside? Thus, hope lies, among other things, in the work of psychologists and social scientists who should apply tools to promote facts and figures in such a way that the relationships between facts concerning climate change and the citizens' own daily practice become clear and that bottom-up movements develop and get stronger, supported by many citizens. Of course, a lucky strike is always possible, if a committed politician with charisma gets interested in the topic of walking, succeeds in convincing enough citizens that the topic is not only important but vital, and sees to it that steps are taken to make a village, a city, a region, or a country a *'place for walkers'*. Until then, we (i.e. researchers) need to think of ways to influence society from the perspective of us scientists working in positions without the power of deciding and implementing. Not least, we need to convince sponsors to pay for research that allows us to provide facts, arguments, and methods to address the public. Then, from an optimistic perspective, as the result of a bottom-up process and without having to hope for a top-down development initiated by wise politicians, enough pressure on the politicians could build up to make them support walking in a similar way to how they support car traffic today. To sum up, both approaches are needed (bottom-up and top-down). But as far as the current stage of our societies (reactive or calculative) is concerned, the bottom-up approach seems to be the one that has more power to achieve a change.

4.3   Arguments: to push and to pull

When there is the wish to enhance sustainable transport modes with a special focus on walking in a day-to-day set of activities of the residents of any place and make walking an integral part of their daily mobility patterns, there is also a need for decisions with complex consequences and lasting effects on traffic planning, traffic management, and the design of infrastructure. The results of these decisions, that is, the resulting preconditions for walking, need to meet the exigencies of people who walk or who would be prepared to walk under certain conditions. In the EU project WALCYNG (Hydén et al., 1997), the following quality dimensions relevant for the subjective well-being of road users and mode choice were summarised, which were later elaborated by Bein et al. (2004); see also Amann et al. (2006):

- Safety: low risk of an accident, low risk of criminal infringements (thefts and robberies)
- Flow and progress: smooth flow, stops and goes are not appreciated, speed not as important as continuous progress without disturbances
- Comfort: agreeable for body and soul (temperature; weather protection; facilities such as buffets, toilets, benches, etc.)
- Aesthetics: do we like what we see (the surroundings), what we hear (agreeable sounds), and what we (do not) smell?
- Equity and respect: are we treated with due respect in the course of our journey (by other walkers, cyclists, car drivers, the police, etc.)?
- Social climate: what is the contact with other people/road users like (communication, considerateness, politeness, etc.)?
- Costs: perceived financial costs as well as time 'costs' (travel time is experienced as short[er] if all the previous assessments are of a positive character)

These quality dimensions encompass both objective and subjective aspects. Anyone who wants to enhance walking should consider them accurately and appropriately, thereby remembering that especially the subjective parts have to be tackled thoroughly. This means that appropriate measures to assess needs and their fulfilment have to be applied. What is an agreeable social climate, when are parents satisfied with the prevailing road safety conditions in the places where their children play or walk? And so on. The perspective of the users has to be understood; otherwise, planning measures will not work sufficiently well. Practitioners in the traffic, mobility, and city planning area have to be aware that people (or at least most of the people) will only accept measures that they experience as being, or believe to be, linked to an improvement in their own quality of life. Therefore, it is of great importance for practitioners and planners to stay in permanent contact with the residents of the city, in order to understand citizens and thus to win their cooperation.

4.3.1   Push measures and arguments

'Push' measures are measures that should push people away from a certain behaviour that they perform at the moment. Push measures could be in words, such as explaining in detail the negative consequences that a certain behaviour shown at this moment could have immediately or in the medium or long run; to list and communicate all the known disadvantages of car use both for the individual and society are examples in this respect. They could be of a regulatory character, such as making behaviour that should be *'pushed away'* more expensive or more laborious: higher taxes, road tolls, or

that one has to apply for a permit to enter certain areas with a car are such measures. Importantly, they could be of a technical/physical character, such as not providing parking spaces for cars at shopping centres; not allowing parking on the streets, combined with law enforcement and fines; not building new roads as soon as the existing ones are full; and allowing cars to enter cities only if there are at least two people in them (see, among others, Rye et al., 2015). In some cases, push measures and push arguments of the advantages of walking mostly consist of measures that, one way or another, make car use less attractive, less easy, and less effective. This is, of course, strong meat, and many people will oppose such measures, although we should make one observation here.

Deutsch (1985) suggests how measures that affect the public, or certain parts of it, should be applied. First, he considers it most important that everybody be equally affected by the measure (the principle of equality/ fairness); second, however, equality does not mean that everybody should be affected by absolutely equal measures but in such a way that everybody is treated in a proportionally equal way concerning income, contribution to, for example, environmental problems, and so (the principle of equity); third, Deutsch suggests that relevant characteristics of persons or groups should be considered, for instance, if older people with difficulties in walking should be supported when it comes to parking fees in city centres, and so on (the principle of need). How these principles should be tackled in practice is case related; that is, it seems reasonable to systematically develop implementation plans that take care of these three principles for any push measure (Gärling & Schuitema, 2007).

The variety of push measures and arguments seems to be limited. It is all about making car use less easy in a reasonable way and explaining why such measures are 'reasonable' so that the majority of the general public (both walkers and non-walkers) can agree – for example, by applying the principles of Deutsch (1985), mentioned just previously, both in words and facts.

4.3.2   Pull measures, arguments, and the diamond model

When discussing pull measures and arguments, we realise that there are many of them, in contrast to push arguments. It seems necessary to have a broader and more systematic look at what options we have to address people. Thus, we need to include the characteristics of the traffic system and its role in shaping our mobility choices and habits. An understanding of this role is a precondition for the development of both arguments and measures to achieve change. It is obvious that factors from both inside (personal factors) and outside the person (situational factors) affect behaviour. The diamond model, which was already introduced briefly in Chapter 2.1.2.1 (Figure 2.2; see also Ausserer et al. 2013) can be used as a theoretical model, as a checklist, as an integrated warning device, as a source of help in order to detect problems, and as a supportive framework when it comes to the finding of solutions. The last point will be dealt with subsequently.

4.3.2.1   *Personal characteristics (individual level)*

Over time, individuals develop attitudes, values, considerations, motives, and specific points of view which have been influenced, and will be influenced, by the various levels of the diamond; they can also be modified in the process.

The preconditions of individual behaviour are personal characteristics: attitudes, motives, emotions, cognitions, habits, performance, and so on. They are the contents or the focus of work that is dealt with in assessment, education, training, campaigning, rehabilitation, and so on (e.g. Dorn, 2012). On this level, it is not least the (rather negative) image of walking, and prejudices concerning it, which can be, and should be, dealt with by applying different measures. For instance, travel times are overestimated; walking is often considered more laborious than it actually is; the advantages of walking are not seen, not felt (of course they cannot be felt if experience lacks), or not believed in; or it seems difficult to combine modern comfort with a mode in which one has to use one's own energy. Of course, attitudes concerning walking vary greatly in the population. To identify and define different groups with different propensities for walking will be important if we are to find and apply measures that are appropriate for addressing various population groups with differing views on walking as a mode, different mobility habits, different attitudes concerning health and lifestyle, and so on.

Measures addressing the individual level are, among others, represented by education both for children and parents in connection with the children attending kindergarten and school, campaigns to raise awareness of the advantages of walking and to counteract mental barriers, activities in the workplace to influence the mode choice of the employees, recommendations by physicians to their patients to walk (more), and information to individuals and households distributed both by snail mail and email or other digital channels containing both facts (new walkways, new regulations, new findings, etc.) and arguments.

4.3.2.2   *Society*

Society comprises media and the related public discourse; moreover, family, friends, the social environment, and regular groups are also part of this structure. This establishes the way in which the role of different forms of traffic participation is viewed and discussed in all these areas. This process is also mirrored in laws and regulations and in informal norms which reflect values such as fairness and equality.

This dimension of the diamond model refers to laws and informal norms, the characteristics of the public discussion, the traffic 'culture' that becomes transparent, the media, and what people of public weight do and say in public (e.g. Rundmo, 2014). Social structures are the frame for many different types of attitudes concerning walking. Laws and informal norms reflect the value that is attributed to walking. Public discussion, displayed, reflected, and partly driven by the media, depicts the importance, or lack of importance, attributed to walking by the society, and a certain mobility 'culture' becomes transparent, not least through how politicians and decision-makers comment on walking and walking issues. Our own socialisation is influenced by these aspects; we internalise attributions to walking and discuss them in the family, in the workplace, or in the pub – if the topic is important enough at all to be a matter of discussion. The worst case is that walking is of such little importance that people do not even talk about it and most of us simply avoid it as much as possible, which is easy, at least in industrialised countries, given all the other possibilities that we have.

Influence can be wielded via the activities of all kinds of stakeholders that are in favour of walking; great help in this respect would come from politicians, decision-makers, opinion leaders, and media people who make the topic theirs and spread facts and figures that show the advantages of walking and counteract prejudices and image flaws. More specific steps to improve the image of walking would be represented by campaigns of different types addressed to the individual; they would underline the societal importance of walking, mention the advantages both for the national health budget and the health of individuals, point out the environmental effects to be achieved by more walking, and refer to the importance of walking for different groups of the population. Any individual citizen exposed to such campaigning would certainly belong to one of the groups being addressed and be of what is called a projective character: being told that walking is good for 'them', that is, for others, thus avoiding giving the citizen the feeling of being patronised. Other important activities on the societal level would be changes in the laws, thereby attributing to walking a more prominent role as a mode of travel. One very important societal measure is, of course, to open ways and allocate budgets for high-quality research in connection with walking. Careful consideration needs to be given to the role of public funding when designing preconditions for walking and how prominent the role of public funding should be when it comes to sustainability and the promotion of walking (Methorst et al., 2010).

If we agree that walking should be enhanced and that car use should be reduced, we have decided that walking is the wished-for behaviour. But if we are speaking about wished-for and non-wished-for behaviour, we have to understand that a large amount of such behaviour probably arises as a result of the shortcomings of the social system rather than of individuals. Thus, the following aspects should be considered:

- Mobility education from early childhood on should start as part of a sensible socialisation process. We have to demonstrate which educational steps are effective within the frame of a lifelong learning process.

- Quality assurance and proof of the effectiveness of mobility education in schools are needed, and if there is no mobility education, it should be introduced, because car-based mobility contributes severely to different types of sustainability problems.
- Psychological principles should be discussed in connection with infrastructure, law enforcement, social marketing, and the questioning of target groups that provides reliable and valid results. Further elaboration of psychological theories is necessary.
- Appropriate methods for awareness raising have to be based on better knowledge concerning these issues, that is, making use of psychology, social sciences, and communication sciences.
- We need to gain a better understanding of resistance to change, for instance, the resistance to making more use of one's own body by using active modes.
- Important issues such as problems related to speed and speeding are not treated with sufficient importance – the problems that car speeds cause for pedestrians, both objective and subjective, are largely ignored.
- There are important questions related to societal measures, for instance, concerning children's bodily exercise or when wanting to keep the elderly mobile.
- Implementation performed in a proper way is an utterly important issue when our research and findings should be the basis for a change in people's mobility.
- Last but not least, evaluation that makes use of empirical results is necessary in order to learn what measures provide success.

Without taking too much risk, it could be predicted that the top working areas in the future will be the two last ones from the list previously: the evaluation of measures and implementation issues.

4.3.2.3 Communication

The behaviour of individuals in public spaces depends on the actual communication history one has experienced within the frame of specific forms of participation in traffic. What was this individual experience like? How does the balance of power manifest itself in these communication processes?

To start this section, we want to underline that we adhere to Paul Watzlawick's point of view that interaction and communication are identical things. Everything that we do in the presence of other people, where we or the others are aware of each other's presence, is per se an act of communication. We usually call it interaction when reactions to the actions of one party become visible. But for psychology, behaviour – reactions to the actions of the other party – includes attitudes, thoughts, feelings, and so on that are not visible but that we all know of. For instance, if we get angry about the behaviour of another person, this does not necessarily become visible to others, for example, depending on how we have learned to cope with (strong) feelings. Paul Watzlawick says that *'one cannot not communicate'*, meaning that the presence of others always has effects on us and vice versa (Watzlawick et al., 2011). Yielding and crossing the road are interactive types of behaviour. They cause direct reactions on the part of the communication partners involved. These issues have to be dealt with within the frame of education, training, and rehabilitation, most of all of car drivers (e.g. Risser, 2010). Interpersonal communication has an immediate effect on our behaviour: having to wait in spite of having the right of way when crossing the road as a pedestrian, being passed with a narrow margin by a car, and being supported politely when waiting midblock at the kerb (where we do not have any right of way) are all actions which are interactive types of behaviour. They cause direct reactions on the part of the communication partners involved, and along with them, expectations are established of how different types of interaction do work and should work. Concerning the interaction between walkers and car drivers, a rather negative impression on the side of the pedestrians seems to prevail: ruthless behaviour on the part of car drivers, car drivers not respecting one's right of way, car drivers parking their vehicles on pedestrian paths, and so on have been criticised by walkers in a series of studies in which pedestrians could express their opinions (Amann et al., 2006; Bell et al., 2010; Ausserer et al., 2013). However, our view on how our own behaviour is perceived by others is impaired by the fact that we do not see ourselves, both in a narrow sense and in a more symbolic sense (the blind spot of communication; Luft & Ingham, 1955). To understand our own erroneous behaviour – both when alone and within the frame of communication with others – is therefore especially difficult and should be a prominent part of the content of driver education programmes, as well as of campaigns aiming at improving interaction between pedestrians and car drivers, to the advantage of walking as a mode.

If it seems unfair to anyone that we underline the training of drivers and not (so much) the training of pedestrians, we can give two reasons for this. First, fatal danger only emanates from cars to others, never from people in their role as pedestrians within the frame of traffic and mobility, and second, virtually all people are pedestrians, young and old, fit and impaired, healthy and unhealthy, sober and drunk, you name it. There are no laws that forbid people to be outside as walkers, except that in many countries, there is a defined age until which individuals (children) are not allowed to be in the public space alone without a custodian. It is very difficult to imagine any education programme that takes all these heterogeneous groups into consideration. Moreover, when it comes to children, youngsters, or very old (but healthy) people, it seems ridiculous that these groups should look after adult people driving cars instead of having things the other way round.

It is often said that cyclists are a problem for walkers when issues of interaction between road users are being discussed. The studies mentioned just previously that deal with the problems experienced by walkers show that there are some problems within the frame of those interactions but that they are far from having the same relevance. Often, problems are due to the fact that too little space is allocated for walkers and cyclists, thus 'programming' conflicts between them.

There are several ways to improve communication to the advantage of pedestrians, but the most important principle is probably that vehicle speed is low in those places where pedestrians and motor vehicles interact. It is not possible to say in absolute figures what a sufficiently low speed is. In many cities in Europe, areas with a limit of 30 km/h have been extended, and that is certainly an improvement compared to higher speed limits. A very nice example of this is the city of Paris, which has gradually spread 'zones 30' areas across the city by 2020, capping the limit at 30 km/h across central Paris, except for a designated network of major roads, on which the limit will remain at 50 km/h. Thus, limiting speeds to 30 km/h, combined with appropriate law enforcement, is certainly a step in the right direction. In addition, one can introduce infrastructure elements that reduce speeds even further where communication takes place, such as extended boardwalks that force vehicle drivers to slow down even more when they turn right (in right-hand traffic). Other measures could consist of infrastructure design elements that direct the trajectories of both vehicles and pedestrians in a way that makes sure that pedestrians and car drivers see each other and that they do so at an appropriately early stage. Even if experts agree on such principles, an experimental approach in order to develop elements that work well at different types of meeting-points is necessary.

4.3.2.4   Infrastructure

When speaking about infrastructure, it is important to know what kind of support the infrastructure offers when using different transport modes. How easy and convenient is the use of these modes? How does the infrastructure support the relations between different road users, and what are the communication processes that the infrastructure supports?

Starting from the point made previously that '*elements need to work well*', we can continue discussing infrastructure issues. If cycle paths are designed in such a way that they make journeys longer, many cyclists will move on illegally; if the red light for pedestrians is on for too long, they will cross when it is red; a road that looks like a motorway will be used like a motorway by car drivers, thus endangering VRUs (e.g. Theeuwes et al., 2012). Psychologists should get involved in urban planning much more; in parallel, we need to establish a better knowledge base concerning all of these issues in the way which will be understandable for other professionals than psychologists. Education and campaigning are not the only measures that can improve the interaction between walkers and car drivers (or walkers and cyclists). The infrastructure can influence both the mentioned interaction processes between pedestrians and car drivers but also the life of pedestrians generally in a positive way. On the one hand, this would be infrastructure that reduces car speeds, that incites car drivers to respect the right of way of pedestrians (more), that raises the awareness of car drivers concerning where to look and what to mind, and that reminds car drivers that there are unprotected road users around; on the other hand, we think of infrastructure that considers known pedestrian needs; short waiting times at intersections, green light (crossing) times that allow even slower walkers to cross without stress, mid-road refuges, minimal kerbs that suffice for vision-impaired persons to recognise road or boardwalk margins, narrowing of roads where pedestrians cross in order to shorten crossing times (and also to reduce car speeds), connective and complete walking-path networks, or planning that allows the walking distances between destinations to be minimised. When thinking of the three usability aspects – effectiveness, efficiency, and satisfaction – we also need to include aesthetics in the discussion of important infrastructure elements. Architectural and ensemble planning aspects, but also greenery and comfort elements (benches, toilets) play important roles.

Many relations between infrastructure and behaviour can easily be studied empirically; for instance, if the red light phase is too long for pedestrians, they cross the street at a red light, or if a lane is wide, the speed of motor vehicles goes up, and so on. By now there is already extensive knowledge about all this that is based on empirical research (e.g. Theeuwes et al., 2012), while there is room for improvement concerning implementation.

One important thought when walking is concerned is that you cannot take away the principal 'burdens' of walking. Walking is slow, 'driven' by one's own energy and therefore tiring, consequently only allowing limited distances to be covered, and so on. However, you can provide infrastructure that makes walking easier and more attractive, and you can give a different value to the characteristics of walking, with arguments, so that these elements which in the general discourse are seen as 'negative' – slow, tiring, susceptible to weather conditions, and so on – can be perceived as more positive or even joyful. To move slowly and to feel one's body when walking give one a chance to be present, to live 'the life of the moment', to explore and cherish mindfulness and the inner 'silence'.

In connection with what has been stated previously, infrastructure should assist road users in communicating in a safer and more agreeable way. But, of course, one most important demand, to start with, is to give pedestrians enough space. First, there should be pedestrian infrastructure everywhere where people live. Second, such infrastructure should allow pedestrians to walk comfortably, also in company with others. Facilities should allow at least two people to walk side by side. In more densely inhabited areas, this is not sufficient, however, because people will walk in both directions everywhere. Third, in order to support walking, a close-meshed network of walkways without 'holes' in it is necessary. Walkers are very distance-sensitive, and thus every measure to make journeys between different points of access as short as possible is to be recommended.

4.3.2.5 Traffic mode

With regard to the chosen mode of transport, the question arises of what advantages this mode of transport offers or whether, for instance, certain road users are forced to use a particular mode of transport without gaining any advantage from using it. Which burdens and frustrations does the use of a certain mode of transport entail? What role is assigned to certain road users? What needs can be satisfied – or not – with a certain mode of transport?

The vehicle that we use or the mode that we choose defines both opportunities and limits for our behaviour and for interaction with others and is thus a catalyst for the generation of many features of our behaviour. The '*walking vehicle*', our body, is very susceptible to physical efforts, such as long distances, steep flights of steps, and so on. These limitations of walking – the 'burdens' of walking – for instance, quite often result in the development of informal norms (if we do not want to talk of rule-breaking): people crossing roads in forbidden places in order to shorten their journeys, crossing roads against a red light when waiting times are too long, producing trails over meadows that lead directly to walkers' destinations, climbing over mid-road barriers when the bus stop is on the other side of the road and the 'legal way' following the itinerary envisaged for walkers would be too long, crossing illegally in order to avoid bridges or tunnels, and so on. Both the (more or less) illegal behaviour of single individuals and informal norms that develop as a result of many individuals indulging in such (illegal) behaviour express needs of pedestrians: of distances from A to B that are as short as possible, of interconnected and complete networks, of itineraries that do not take too much time, of waiting times that are not experienced as being too long or that are experienced as being unfair. At the same time, there are places that are considered dangerous by pedestrians, not least, or especially so, by the parents of children and youngsters. In those cases, walkers, or the people responsible for very young walkers, are susceptible to danger and try to avoid such places. Those who cannot renounce walking have to negotiate those places in spite of their objections, or they have to choose other and often longer routes, in direct opposition to their usual intentions and needs. Those who can renounce walking, on the other hand, will use another mode instead. If we want to support walking, all these aspects need to be considered by both city officials and traffic planners.

One more comment concerning the vehicle, or the mode, that refers back to the issue of communication is the following. Car drivers get very little feedback concerning their speed behaviour (or behaviour in general) and how this is perceived by the outside world: noise, vibrations, headwinds, physical effort, and personal feedback from outside have vanished stepwise. Not least, communication is impeded by shaded car windows. Especially drivers who do not have experiences with walking or cycling are 'blind' to the needs of other road users. Thus, the characteristics of cars also have to be considered when discussing mode or vehicle aspects, their effects on walking, and measures to improve the preconditions for walking.

To take appropriate care of walking as a transport mode, one has to consider the characteristics of walking: it is relatively slow, and thus the distances which can be covered are limited. Walking makes use solely of the personal energy of walkers and is tiring, which again limits the times and distances that one can walk. The elements of infrastructure mentioned previously are helpful in this respect: provide a close-meshed network, keep the routes from A to B as short as possible, avoid barriers such as flights of steps, high kerbs, or guardrails that extend for longer distances. The latter are often implemented under the pretence of improving traffic safety, but another interpretation is that they allow motor vehicles to proceed more undisturbedly without having to mind pedestrians too much, while at the same time making pedestrian routes longer.

But do measures that we take off the shelf fit? A lot of those measures that were mentioned previously are known to work well in principle. But are they detailed enough? Are the lists of measures complete? Are they up to date, that is, do new types of measures have to be envisaged as times have changed? Do they cover all groups of pedestrians according to their (different) needs and preferences? To make sure that all these questions can be answered in the affirmative, we suggest a structured approach that will be discussed subsequently.

4.4   Mode choice marketing

Mode choice marketing is a structured process of communication with target groups concerning mode choice that is based on understanding them. If we want to achieve a certain behaviour, as many individuals as possible – or in any case as many sceptical or reluctant individuals as possible – have to be convinced. One way to convince people is to make use of communication theories, the most appropriate in our eyes being the marketing model by Philip Kotler (Kotler et al., 2016). According to this model, the necessary steps are to make people interested in the type of behaviour that you want to achieve, to provide appropriate preconditions, and thereby to work on the side of the environment as well as of the individual and the interface between the two, that is, on usability.

Social marketing helps to increase voluntary compliance with new suggestions, regulations, laws, and policies that are introduced. The use of social marketing has been proven effective in many social programmes, including reducing smoking rates, increasing immunisation rates among children, increasing the physical activity of senior citizens, changing nutrition habits in the population, and many more. The concepts, theories, and design components for nutrition education and enhancing physical activity among older people have been well described, and everything suggests that mode choice can be influenced effectively and efficiently with the help of social marketing measures.

If applied appropriately, social marketing can help to influence the mode choice of the target population in such a way that the outcomes will provide for better sustainability. To this end, it is a precondition to identify the reasons people resist change, to uncover affordable benefits which the audience cares about, and to create strategies to display those benefits in compelling and cost-effective ways.

Marketing, including social marketing (also addressed as non-profit marketing) is characterised by the five Ps (Product, Price, Promotion, Place, and People), displayed in Figure 4.3 subsequently.

The development of informative and persuasive communication (P = Promotion) ensures that the product (programme) is provided in an appropriate manner. This includes formulating the objectives of

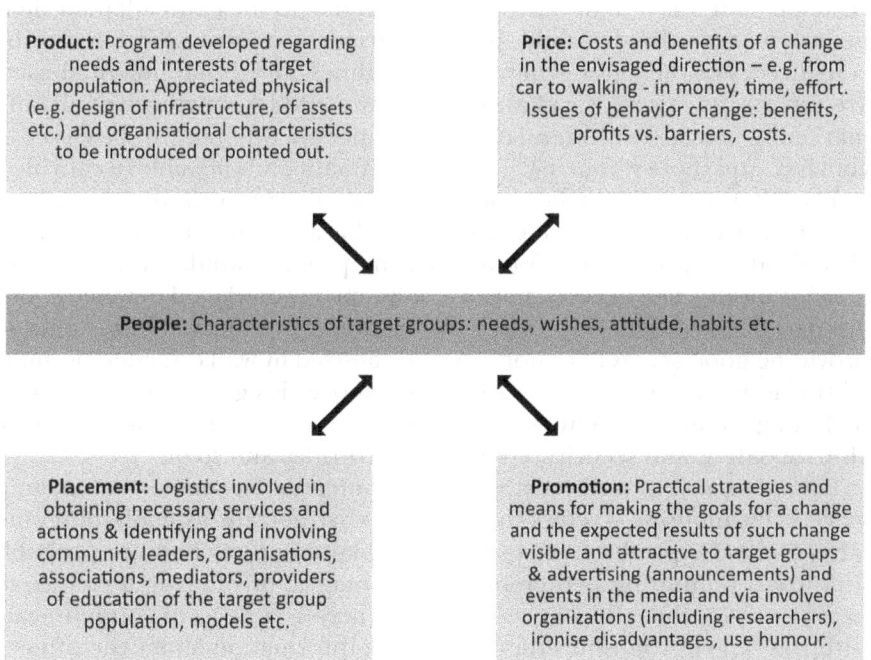

Figure 4.3 Application of marketing mix strategy to mode choice modification (Kotler et al., 2016, modified by authors).

mode-change efforts, addressing the appropriate persons and institutions in an appropriate and efficient way (P = Placement), discussing the necessary efforts (P = Price) in juxtaposition to the advantages, and tracking both exigencies *a priori* and responses to the programme (P = People) in order to adapt both offers (P = Product) and arguments (P = Promotion) to the users' needs and expectations. It takes into account what the audience wants, needs, and expects, that is, their satisfaction or dissatisfactions. This means that social marketing has to consider the social context of the behaviour, the available resources (human and financial), the organisations involved (competitor analysis, coalition-building), and the attitudes and habits of the target audience (P = People): socio-demographic and psychological characteristics, perceived benefits and barriers (P = Price), mass media usage, important others, membership in community organisations, road user associations, and the like.

In other words, marketing is about making people interested in something to such a degree that they 'buy' this 'thing'. Social marketing or non-profit marketing mostly deals with 'selling' or 'buying' ideas. Mode choice marketing with the goal of achieving more sustainable mobility habits in the population wants to sell the idea of making use of certain modes, of changing to another, more sustainable, mode. The 'customers' are the people addressed in the marketing process. The 'users' or active customers are those who have already adopted an idea and adapted their behaviour accordingly, while 'potential users' are those who need to be convinced. For the latter group, it is sometimes added that potential users are those where there is a chance that they could be convinced at all, and marketing activities differentiate between people whom it will be easier to convince and those whom it will be more difficult or impossible to convince.

The 5 Ps previously can be grouped and labelled in a different way, where the first key element is the *product* and its characteristics, analogous to the (P = Product) previously. In our case, the product would be the idea of 'change mode'. The necessary efforts to adopt any marketed new behaviour are part of the aspect (P = Price). For instance, product measures refer to providing good access to important goals desired by walkers; good usability of traffic infrastructure by walkers; attractive design of infrastructure, including greenery, architecture, and design elements; a friendly social climate, safety, and security; connective networks, and so on.

Communication towards customers and potential customers – analogous to (P = Promotion) – refers to measures that pertain to explaining and advertising the product, for example, explaining facts that are probably unknown, reminding people of the advantages, or offering a chance to experience the benefits of the product. There is a need to communicate with the target groups in order to provide information about the offers – networks, city plans and guiding infrastructure, a combination of walkways with the public transport network, interesting design elements. There is a need to apply professional advertising to mitigate mental barriers to walking and find arguments and take other necessary steps to give the product *'walking'* a good image. Any manufacturer would do that as a part of both its advertising and public relations work. However, there is also a need to explain failures and problems connected to walking. Any person who tries out walking as a result of good communication measures delays and gets taken by surprise by the fact that walking trips take longer than expected or by other unexpected negative aspects could be lost as a customer for ever ('I tried it out and it was awful – I'll try never again') – as is very well known from a marketing specialist: *'Your customers will give you only one chance to try your product'*. Thus, communication also encompasses the aspect of (P = Price) as far as explaining the downsides of the idea being marketed and putting them in perspective is concerned. The costs and benefits of a change in the envisaged direction – for example, from car use to walking – are discussed in terms of money, time, or effort: benefits and profits versus barriers and costs.

Incentive measures encompass offers to potential customers to try out something – in our case, that would be the wished-for behaviour – without effort, in situations where the use of the product provides direct (contingent) positive enforcement. The nature of incentives in psychological terms is that one provides extrinsic motivation and hopes that this will produce intrinsic motivation: *'Try it, find it OK, and stick to it'*. Incentive measures would also belong to (P = Promotion).

What are the incentives that influence mode choice on different levels? This question can only be answered on the basis of a better understanding of the incentives that would work effectively and efficiently for different groups: road users, decision-makers/politicians, industry managers, employers generally. Incentives can be provided on a national level (subsidies, tax refunds or tax reductions, etc.), on a regional, and on a local level (free or reduced tickets for public transport that make people walk more than today because of the somewhat longer walking trips to the public transport stops). To find new and effective types and combinations of incentives that should be applied more often is the task and the goal of sound marketing work.

Distribution – analogous to (P = Placement) refers to efforts to place both physical elements and references connected to the product – *walking* – in such a way that as many people as possible have the chance to become aware of them (e.g. a broadcast about walking) and to experience them (e.g. an attractive walk network recently implemented in the city). In other words, place and distribute your offers, your communication, your arguments, your advertisements, and your incentives in such a way that you reach an optimum number of your potential customers.

Last but not least, before all these steps are taken, information measures need to be implemented (see also Figure 4.6). One wants to find out what the interests of the potential customers and users are (P = People). Information work in the sense of the marketing model is constituted by finding ways to understand the needs and interests of customers and potential customers in order to be able to adjust all other measures appropriately. What features of the product do they appreciate and what should be changed, what arguments are accepted and effective within the frame of communication measures, and what incentives are considered interesting and motivating? In order to find these things out, one needs to *inform* oneself about the characteristics of the respective target group: how it is segmented, about the needs and resistances of different subgroups (e.g. users and potential users), about the values they support, about the conditions for cooperation and for compliance. Concerning potential customers, this means:

• Estimating who and what percentage of the total population could be won over as walkers: one needs to identify those people and groups that can be defined as *'depending on car use'* in connection with their trip to work or with the character of their work, which would refer to jobs where the use of one's own car is necessary, for example, salesmen. Among other things, the distance between home and the workplace is a relevant parameter;

• Concerning both practising walkers and potential walkers, one needs to analyse the existing preconditions for walking and to compare their needs with the given situation. What is found within the frame of this process is important material to be used in connection with the development and the refinement of product, communication, and incentive measures.

One may expect potential walkers to make comments which are only partly based on experience but more on hearsay and prejudice or on skewed experiences resulting from the restricted radius of practice. Thus, potential walkers, people who are to be convinced that they could walk (more), need to be met by appropriate communication and incentive measures; prejudices that reflect wrong information about facts and that generate a negative image of walking need to be counteracted, and people need to be provided opportunities to try out walking (more).

Feedback from practising walkers is certainly more relevant as far as the actual preconditions in practice are concerned. Negative criticism from this side will probably make improvements of the product characteristics necessary, but practising walkers will also be able to point out what works well and thus could be implemented more generally in the network, in other places, or in other cities and towns. In marketing language, we could term them our *'walking ambassadors'*.

Concerning the preconditions for walking and efforts to market walking, very much also depends on employers, authorities, politicians, and decision-makers. Their attitude concerning walking and its promotion and support is crucial and thus needs to be assessed in order to be able to approach those groups in an appropriate way, not least within the frame of lobbying (Chapter 4.5.1).

Successful social marketing, in our case, would result in increased numbers of walkers and in improved satisfaction expressed by practising walkers. It is important to note, though, that marketing procedures will only be successful if carried out in a holistic way (see also Figure 4.4). If, on the one hand, one has a wonderful product that is not communicated or distributed well, a suboptimal number of people will know about it and adhere to it. If, on the other hand, one announces one's product in a highly professional and effective way so that many people try it out, but they then find that in practice things do not work out as well as communicated – or in other words, that the product is rubbish – (many) customers will be lost for ever. *'I have tried it and I was really disappointed. I will not do it again'.*

4.4.1 Appropriate information measures

For information work to provide good results, two paths have to merge, in our opinion. (1) The compilation of all the measures that are known and proven to be effective with respect to making walking more attractive, thus motivating more people to walk more, in principle has (2) to be matched with new situations, new populations, and new contexts. To make sure that measures that were applied earlier also work under such new preconditions, the principles of marketing may be applied: inform yourself about the new

Information (People): Learn about user preconditions to fulfil needs & to avoid barriers. You need to learn as much as possible of existing and potential customers of the product and systematically collect information about customer's attitudes and motives (needs, interests, moral concepts...).

Product: Define what is to be marketed and propose precise objectives. Pinpoint the precise behavioural change which you want to achieve, e.g. to increase the share on walking trips to work by 5%. Provide easily useable and attractive products embedded in an agreeable context. The product has to be designed in accordance with the customer's needs and wishes while compromises have to be found between the work of experts and the wishes of the customer.

Communication (Promotion): Address your (potential) customers with arguments that meet acceptance and do not forget the downsides (Price). Information, instructions, PR measures, advertising, etc. have to be provided in a way that they will attract the addressed persons' interest and that will appeal to them.

Incentives (Promotion): Provide opportunities to test the product and to experience it as convenient and giving. These measures help to provide direct (contingent) reinforcement for the customer if they "use the product" (in our case: if they behave in a wished-for way = if they walk).

Distribution (Placement): Place products, communication and incentives efficiently so as to achieve high probability that citizens become well aware of them.

Holistic approach: A combination of all the mentioned steps is necessary for a successful marketing process.

Figure 4.4 Overview of the marketing steps (Kotler et al., 2016, modified by authors).

target groups and their attitudes, motives, and habits and fine-tune the product, communication, incentives, and distribution accordingly. While interacting with the target group in this way, new approaches and new measures might pop up that could open up new ways to motivate people to modify their mode choice in a wished-for way. Many improvements for pedestrians have been developed and implemented by engineers (many of whom had earlier been involved in developing a traffic system tailor-made for cars). In particular, changes in the infrastructure came from the engineering departments, while communication measures were either missing or carried out on the basis of common sense rather than on psychological or sociological know-how. The result was often that the measures did not have the wished-for effects. Measures of a technical character – concerning infrastructure and mode in the diamond – often missed the goal, as well, because the perspective of the users was not considered sufficiently. In psychological terms, the behaviour of the people who were addressed was not understood sufficiently well. From this perspective, the marketing model is the most appropriate approach for the development of effective measures because it calls for a systematic communication process with the target populations.

4.4.2   *The mixed-measures approach*

For this communication process, the American researchers Creswell and Plano Clark (2018) have suggested combining qualitative and quantitative ways of questioning people. Qualitative ways of asking people are individual interviews (narrative, semi-structured, rapid, etc.) or focus-group interviews, all types of dialogues with people where it is possible to ask for the '*why*' of certain attitudes, motives, habits, and behaviours; questions, for example, about why one does not like to walk have to be answered in the person's own words. Explanations can be longer and differentiated and help to understand the person's motives. The qualitative part of the questioning thus helps to find many different explanations that could play a role in connection with any issue relevant for the populations being addressed. If one wants to find out what could lie behind the pleasure that certain people perceive in connection with walking or behind the reluctance to walk of others, a qualitative approach is the way of choice. Or, to keep it simple – if we want to find out why people choose a certain type of behaviour, what their motivations for this behaviour are, if we want to research what cannot be observed, we need to use qualitative methods. Qualitative questioning is usually carried out following the principle of saturation, meaning that the researcher or the psychologist realises after some time that no new explanations are being given, that everything that could be relevant has been mentioned. The question of how many persons are asked thus depends on when the point of saturation is reached. At that point, the researcher has a list in his hands with as many possible explanations for a certain behaviour (attitudes, motives, habits) as possible in this case. In connection with qualitative questioning, representativeness is not an issue. The goal is to collect explanations that play a role for the people who are interviewed and that could play a role for the total population.

To find out what role the explanation plays for the total population, a quantitative and representative approach is needed and has to be added. To this end, what has been learned within the frame of the qualitative procedures is transformed into an instrument that can be answered by ticking or by scaling pre-formulated answers to questions. The sample of people that is questioned in this way needs to be representative, as said. This means that a statistically relevant part of those persons whose position we want to understand needs to be questioned. For instance, the statement that group A is put off by motor vehicle noise more than group B has to be based on a thorough procedure concerning the sampling of people that should be asked.

To structure the answers received within the frame of a qualitative dialogue with the population, different methods can be chosen. Here, we want to suggest making use of the usability principle according to ISO/IEC 9126-4 Metrics (Usability Metrics – A Guide To Quantify The Usability Of Any System, 2015), which specifies that the concept of usability reflects '*the extent to which a product can be used by specified users to achieve specified goals with effectiveness, efficiency and satisfaction in a specified context of use*'. The effectiveness of any product, service, or idea refers to the necessity that it clearly serves to reach defined and relevant goals. Efficiency reflects the easiness and economic viability connected to adopting any new behaviour or buying any new product; no exaggerated investments should be needed. Satisfaction points to the necessity that the wished-for behaviour should be comfortable and feel good.

To sum up: The qualitative steps have the task of detecting phenomena related to any topic that might be relevant for any defined population from the perspective of members of this population. The quantitative ones should measure the distribution of these detected phenomena in the defined population. Without this combination, formulating the questions for a standardised questionnaire that should be applied in order to achieve representative quantitative results is a risky endeavour, with some probability that the questions will be irrelevant to the target group and that the questionnaire will miss important issues.

So generally, both for analysis and development of measures, we have to work in the areas outlined in the diamond model, being aware of the interdependencies among them. Thus, when we make efforts to identify attitudes and behavioural problems and to influence behaviour in a desirable sense, we have to be aware that the effects that we introduce on the individual level, addressed to the individual, are only a small part of a large 'orchestra' of effects that all contribute to the shaping of mode choice behaviour.

4.4.3 Marketing steps together with the diamond model

Subsequently, we will give an example of how one could use the diamond model and the marketing model in combination with the goal of reaching good coverage of all the possible steps that could be taken in order to make (more) people walk (more).

4.4.3.1 Individual

Product: Provide information about all the options that could be relevant to the individual: goals that can be reached, available networks, shops, cultural sites and facilities, and so on. Provide a full list of all the advantages for the individual that walking is known to have: fitness, health (lowering the probability of many diseases), pleasure and a good mood (endorphins), knowledge of connection to the environment, relaxation or stimulation of the brain (see also product measures associated with the walking mode further subsequently; Hansen, 2019).

Communication: Discuss and challenge arguments against walking, for example, walking is slow – this is not true for short distances; in the city you often can take short cuts; walking is tiring – if you do it regularly, you will find that it is not that tiring, because you will be in better shape, sometimes you will want to be a bit more tired physically, which makes you sleep better and feel more relaxed, and using your body is always an advantage; as a walker you are exposed to (bad) weather – 'there is no bad weather, there are only bad clothes' (as Norwegians say); the weather is not as bad as we usually think (the number of rainy days is lower than most of us would suppose); walking is unsafe – that is correct, as a pedestrian you are more exposed and endangered by car drivers, but should that remain as it is? The more pedestrians there are out on the road, the safer any pedestrian is (what is called the 'safety in numbers' phenomenon); as a walker you are exposed to criminal acts – compared to road safety problems, endangerment by criminality is a minor problem, but of course it troubles us more, and here too the statement is valid that the more people you have out on the road, the safer you are (and we do not mean people that are sitting in a car but people that are visible as people).

Incentives: Incentive measures are always addressed to the individual by providing a direct advantage to the person being addressed. Usually, these are measures related to ease of use and reduced costs provided in connection with infrastructure and mode-related measures, and they can be nicely combined with communication measures; for example, announcing a new walking area in the city with hints about new shops that provide special offers during the first two weeks to those who come by walking from more than 1 km away (testified to, e.g., by their mobile phone), such as special prices, and so on. Another example of an incentive: employees who live more than 500 m away from their work and who do not come by car get a reward or a day off each three months. Of course, it is difficult to make such incentives look fair for all those who live nearer or have other disadvantages. Creativity and knowledge of good practice are required.

Rewards or tokens within the frame of incentive measures could include free public transport tickets; bonuses for fashionable sports shoe shops; equipment such as reflectors, pedestrian GPS, pulse-meters, or step-counters; reduced entrance fees for museums, theatres, and so on; more days off at the company (more holidays); a km-tax refund for distances walked; physical condition checks for free; and many others.

Distribution: Provide the product, communication, and incentive measures listed previously in as efficient a way as possible. Figure out how many people as possible can be reached in an effective way without investing inappropriate amounts of resources by distributing different types of measures accordingly.

Costs: The cost issue is closely related to incentive measures; many incentives are characterised by the fact that one gets something cheaper or for free. The hope, in psychological terms, is that extrinsic motivation (low or zero costs) will turn into intrinsic motivation (*'I tried it out and it works nicely, so I will buy or do it again'*). Of course, the costs have to be calculated in such a way that in the end, the benefits for society from more people walking more are bigger than the expenditures invested in the incentives.

4.4.3.2 Communication

Product: Describe well-functioning communication between pedestrians and other road users and ensure walkers know about their rights in those interactions, for instance, where the right of way is an issue, thereby not forgetting that they are the weaker party in those processes. Another aspect that should be pointed out is how well communication between pedestrians functions; where there are many pedestrians, and only pedestrians, there is usually no interaction problem and processes run smoothly. Walking and being among other people is experienced positively by many, and this can be shown with, for example, pictures, videos, or animations.

Of course, many products that help in the marketing of walking lie on the infrastructure side. The aspects of interaction between pedestrians and other types of road users that have already been mentioned often have a problematic character. There are many infrastructure measures that (could) help to mitigate or solve these types of problems, such as, for example, elevated crossings or humps before pedestrian crossings that reduce vehicle speeds.

Communication: Here again it can be seen that demonstrating well-functioning cohabitation between pedestrians, as a *'product'*, is not easy to differentiate from a communication process to market walking. A difference may be seen in the sense that marketing communication makes use of arguments to make things more visible or to make fun of erroneous assumptions (e.g. the prejudice that pedestrian zones are full of thieves). In communication activities addressed to all road user groups, the relaxing effect of taking *'stupid things that others do'* more easy (and the fact that we tend to overlook the stupid things that we ourselves do – think of the blind spot of communication discussed by Luft and Ingham, 1955) should be stressed. This is, of course, an approach that can be of great advantage in many other areas of life as well.

Incentives: All the incentive measures mentioned in connection with the other areas of the diamond model have the potential to improve communication between walkers and other types of road users.

Distribution: Provide the product, communication, and incentive measures listed previously in as efficient a way as possible. Figure out how as many interaction spots and processes as possible can be reached in an effective way without investing inappropriate amounts of resources by distributing different types of measures accordingly.

Costs: The cost issues to be addressed in connection with the area of interaction are similar or equal to those referring to the individual aspects displayed in the diamond model.

4.4.3.3   Society

Product: Implement laws that support walking efficiently and that strengthen its position in relation to motorised traffic but search for alliances with other sustainable modes; allocate budgets for research into walking and the possibilities it offers. Opinion leaders, decision-makers, and politicians should walk themselves and be visible as walkers in a credible way (a photo of a walking opinion leader when everybody knows that he/she in reality only travels in a car driven by a chauffeur is not credible and has a deleterious impact on the 'product' walking). There is also a nice connection to infrastructure: an infrastructure that supports walking is the clearest indicator that walking is taken seriously and thus is something good and important. Compile the advantages of walking for society in figures – savings in health costs as a result of the physical exercise of the population, reduced costs for the protection of the environment, less public money paid for compensating for damage done by car transport as a result of the potential transfer from car use to walking.

Communication: Communicate all the previously mentioned product characteristics appropriately. Discuss and challenge arguments against walking; *'walking infrastructure is expensive'* – infrastructure for car use costs very much more; *'the accidents of pedestrians cost society a lot of money'* – but the reduction of health costs clearly outweighs those costs; *'you cannot motivate people to walk and thereby expose them to the risk of accidents'* – the more pedestrians there are on the road, the better the per capita safety of pedestrians, and the more one walks, the more experienced one becomes and thus the safer one is (which is especially valid for children).

Incentives: Possible incentives provided to the individual by society include tax refunds or reductions if it is proven that healthy modes are used on the way to work (at the moment, the opposite is the case in many countries; there is refunding related to the number of kilometres people '*have to*' drive to their job by car); companies or employers can be rewarded by the state if they encourage their employees to move to and from work in a way that requires a certain amount of walking. Usually, walkways are longer for people who walk to public transport stops than for those who just walk to their parked cars – thus, the use of public transport could also be supported with the help of incentives such as reduced ticket prices and so on. Otherwise, incentive measures for walking are measures such as reducing municipal tax for activities to enhance walking, considering companies in the transport master plan, mentioning walking-friendly companies in the journals of the municipality for free, providing lower ground prices for walking-friendly companies that see to it that fewer employees arrive by car, and giving certification to the most walking-friendly companies and activities alike.

Distribution: Provide the product, communication, and incentive measures listed previously in as efficient a way as possible. Figure out how many public institutions on the national, regional, and municipal level can be involved in research and the implementation of results and how as many employers as possible can be reached in an effective way without investing inappropriate amounts of resources. Develop strategies for how to address the public within the frame of communication measures in an efficient way.

Costs: A relation between public costs – or savings on public costs – and costs for the individual, that is, individual cost reductions, needs to be established, for instance, by showing that cost reductions resulting from increased walking can release budgets for other important purposes (while it is a matter of public discussion to define what an important purpose is).

4.4.3.4   Infrastructure

Product: The infrastructure is a '*product*' element in itself according to the marketing model. Are there walking facilities? Are walkways well equipped and broad enough, and are there seating facilities and toilets? Are pavements kept free from obstacles, and is there enough space for people to walk side by side? Is there protection from rain, for instance, at bus stops? Is it seen to that walking distances are kept as short as possible, and is there a consistent and complete walking network where people live? How are crossings designed? There are plenty of handbooks and guidelines that display and summarise how infrastructure that supports walking should be designed; for instance, see Morar and Bertolini (2013). One can add that many traffic engineers and traffic planners probably know how to provide good infrastructure for walkers, but decisions to implement such infrastructure are very often not taken. A good example is waiting and crossing times at traffic lights. Almost all over the world, traffic lights make pedestrians wait much longer than car drivers, while at the same time crossing times are too short. These, according to what many experts demand, should allow a low walking speed (e.g. 1 m/sec or 3.6 km/h). But in reality, this is hardly ever the case, which produces stress, especially for older people, people walking with small children, or impaired people.

Clearly, weather aspects need to be borne in mind when infrastructure is planned and implemented. In many regions of the world, it may be pleasant to walk for most of the year, but what about walking in Siberian cities, Scandinavia, Canada, or the Northern United States in the winter, when minus 20°C is common day after day and temperatures dip to minus 30 and even minus 40 at night? Or in southern climates when the temperature in the shade exceeds +40°C and clouds rarely block the sun? It is necessary to create shaded spots in hot climates and wind-protected walking facilities in cold climates (Givoni, 1998; Mander et al., 2006), causing expenditures that are not easily made 'just for pedestrians'.

Communication: Provide information regularly about new walkways and about new decisions taken by the city that concern pedestrians (such as: *'the municipality has decided that all new pavements shall be 3.5 metres wide, without exceptions to this rule'*). Show comfortable walking facilities in a convincing way, for instance, by producing animated demonstrations of new solutions. Work with testimonials – from opinion leaders, decision-makers, and influencers – who walk the new infrastructure and explain what advantages these new elements provide. We would say that such a type of communication is the least covered part of any marketing of walking.

Incentives: The use of new infrastructure, *'trying out'* new infrastructure, can easily be motivated by organising festivities where new infrastructure has been implemented. According to the size of the new product, this can be everything from single persons distributing stickers and other tokens up to fairs or festivities at those sites.

Distribution: It is almost self-explanatory that good infrastructure should be implemented everywhere people walk. Of course, more resources will be invested in places where there are many pedestrians, but less densely walked areas should not be neglected. Often, the assessment that *'nobody ever walks there'* comes together with poor quality of the preconditions that keeps people from *'ever'* walking there. In any case, *'holes'* in the walking network can have a deterrent effect.

Costs: It is clear that good walking infrastructure is not for free. But we state that those costs are peanuts compared to the costs for the construction and maintenance of the infrastructure that is needed for motorised traffic (Gössling et al., 2019). This needs to be communicated to the public.

4.4.3.5   Traffic mode

Product: In the sense of non-profit or social marketing, the idea of walking has to be presented as a '*product*'. Thereby, the characteristics of walking need to be described, with all its advantages and disadvantages. In the end, if our view of things is correct, a positive balance of results will be shown. What is done by walking and what can be done by walking is described, is made visible, as is how omnipresent walking is and that it is automatised to such a degree that we do not even realise how much we walk. We need to be reminded of this in some way. In other words, it is a SWOT presentation of walking that we envisage when we want to see the idea of walking presented as a '*product*' – its **S**trengths, its **W**eaknesses, its **O**pportunities, and its **T**hreats. More '*materialistic*' products include bags, shoes, clothes, and other outfit items that give walkers an attractive look, where attractive can be stylish, functional and practical, easy-going and comfortable, or creative. When talking about usability, we have to remember that usability equals effectiveness, efficiency, and fun. We should make these things clear and thereby strengthen the image of walking.

Communication: When an idea is presented as one important product aspect, it is rather difficult to discriminate between such product aspects and communication measures. However, the focus on communication would reflect professional ways of presenting the idea of walking and its characteristics and of assets associated with, or connected to, walking. Communication would also include irony ('*there is no bad weather…*'), absurd humour ('*silly walks*'and that '*one can do better than that*'), and exaggeration and cartoon-like presentation of both the advantages and disadvantages of walking. In other words, the SWOT elements should be played with in an intelligent and surprising way.

Incentives: Incentive measures concerning the idea of walking are similar to, or the same as, those mentioned in connection with the individual check previously; one needs to provide reinforcement for people who come to certain places by walking on certain occasions or select winners of prizes from those people who came by walking to work, to some event, or to a shop. With respect to assets associated with walking, the most simple incentive measures are prizes offered at tombola events, in competitions, in bingo halls, or for winning a quiz.

Distribution: Again, good distribution is about presenting the idea of walking and the assets associated with walking as efficiently and comprehensively as possible and trying to reach as many people as possible.

Costs: The societal costs of walking are very low compared to the societal costs of motorised transport. Similarly, the costs of walking for individuals – for personal stamina and motivation and for the equipment needed for walking – are very low compared to the costs of car use: the German ADAC (an automobile association in Germany) calculated costs of between €540 and €670 per month for a middle-class car, that is, €6480–€8040 per year (ADAC, 2019). How would you compare this to virtually everything that you need for walking, even if you are the greatest snob?

4.4.4　*How are changes to be communicated to citizens?*

Whenever any measures '*against*' car traffic are envisaged, there is loud protest, in municipalities, in cities, in whole countries, or on the whole continent – currently, unified taxes on combustibles are being discussed in the EU. We write the word 'against' in quotation marks, as any measure to reduce car traffic is considered a hostile act by some stakeholders (especially car manufacturers) and some parts of the population. These parties are powerful in influencing debates in this direction. Any evidence-based discussion of how to turn mobility into a sustainable direction thus becomes more difficult. Measures that support and enhance walking almost as a rule bring some disadvantages to car drivers: the reduction of space for cars when space for pedestrians increases; inhibitions on the '*freedom*' of choice of speed, which is not total freedom but the perceived freedom to break speed rules within certain '*accepted*' margins; the questioning of the '*right not to be bothered by too-low speed limits*'; disturbance by law enforcement measures, frequently labelled rip-off activities, and so on.

Anyone who wants to interrupt this automatism (suggestion of measures automatically leads to loud protests) should know, however, that '*loud*' does not necessarily mean '*representative*'. For instance, the Sartre studies (Cauzard, 2004) showed that more than half of European car drivers are in favour of speed reduction measures, including law enforcement by the police. Table 4.1 shows the positions of car-driving citizens in 23 European countries concerning speed-limiting devices, black boxes, and electronic identification. The majority of the people who were interviewed were in favour of implementing speed-limiting devices and black boxes in cars, and almost half of the population that was addressed would even accept electronic identification in their vehicle. We consider this example relevant because it deals with one of the most difficult areas – speeds and speed enforcement – where politicians tend to say '*citizens will never accept such measures*' without any empirical evidence that would support such a worry. In our eyes, this indicates that there would be even more support for other measures of a less sensitive character. Still, experience tells us that there is (most) often loud protest even in connection with the implementation of measures that should be easier to handle. But, as said, those loud ones are, as a rule, quite powerful (or at least, they simulate power), and they obviously succeed in intimidating decision-makers.

Our suggestion to decision-makers is twofold. First, collect empirical evidence concerning the attitude of concerned citizens with respect to envisaged or planned measures. Second, compile all the known facts associated with the envisaged or planned measure and treat them according to the marketing model: present them in an appropriate, highly visible way to as many concerned citizens as possible, provide incentives to make people come to presentations of the plans by means of animations and models, distribute animated clips via social media, and embed everything in professionally produced frames of arguments.

Table 4.1 Support for speed management measures in the vehicle:
either 'very' or 'fairly' much in favour (Cauzard, 2004)

	Speed-limiting devices %	Black box %	Electronic identification %
Austria	54	47	26
Belgium	62	58	49
Denmark	40	47	45
Finland	64	64	49
France	70	67	54
Germany	54	50	31
Greece	77	67	50
Ireland	81	77	69
Italy	70	72	51
Netherlands	41	52	38
Portugal	73	79	53
Spain	63	57	44
Sweden	44	54	31
United Kingdom	68	75	70
Average	*62*	*62*	*47*
Croatia	63	64	50
Cyprus	78	70	54
Czech Republic	45	53	48
Estonia	47	56	64
Hungary	50	55	58
Poland	57	76	75
Slovakia	75	55	66
Slovenia	64	61	50
Switzerland	46	45	30

If decision-makers walk that way firmly and also maintain their position against very loud protest – from which we know as said before that it absolutely need not be representative – there is an important side effect related to '*society*' (check in the diamond model): citizens then understand that the topic – in our case to do something to promote walking – is important and is given importance and that the promises of politicians to advocate a sustainable development of transport and liveable cities are not just lip service.

To be prepared for such cases, research that summarises what is known concerning different measures to enhance walking is recommended, thereby maybe following the scheme displayed by Methorst et al. (2010), showing the great advantages both for the individual and for society that can be harvested from all efforts to support walking. Convincing arguments that the losses for those who are against measures to support walking because those measures may mean disadvantages for themselves have to be included in this process.

However, it is important to think of marketing procedures in a holistic way, as already underlined earlier. Results in practice to be used by the citizens should work nicely, in line with how they were communicated. Otherwise there will be a kind of a boomerang effect: '*They promised wonderful things and now look what happened – never again will I…!*'

4.5   Campaigning

When one discusses communication in connection with marketing activities, it is only a small step to coming to think of the concept of campaigning. One could say that these two things are the same, except that when we talk of campaigning, we usually think of a set of measures carried out as an isolated activity, not within the frame of an orchestrated and holistic process. As soon as it becomes part of such a process, campaigning can be seen as communication in the sense of the marketing model. However, this is a play on labels and not really relevant. To know how to carry out a good campaign means that you know how to carry out communication measures well.

What is the aim of campaigning?

- It can make the advantages of a change of behaviour visible, for instance – an easy and '*primitive*' example – that walking is the cheapest transport mode and you save money if you do not use a car.
- It points out needs one does not think of as long as no deficits are perceived, for example, to feel fit and healthy; you do not perceive any problem when you are young, but you will come to feel negative consequences at a later point in time. For example, if you only move about in your car, you will have problems with your back and your neck.

One thing is clear: if the preconditions are not good enough, then they have to be improved. But let us assume that in spite of not being optimal, the preconditions are not so bad that one has to use the car for a 500m trip. Why, then, do people still use the car for such short distances? The reason might be laziness or erroneous assumptions concerning facts and feelings: for instance, people might have biased assumptions concerning facts like the weather statistics: they have the feeling that '*it rains so often*', but, for instance, in Hamburg, which is usually seen as a very rainy city, in 2007 only 850 hours of rain, night hours included, were measured, out of the 8760 hours in the year in total. Biased feelings or expectations could be another reason: walking is boring, it is time-consuming, and it is exhausting. To be honest, if a trip of 10 minutes is exhausting, you should definitely do some exercise!

Campaigning should support a more sober view on preconditions, present facts, and let testimonials express different views on preconditions – as one can always look at things from different angles. It is also necessary to discuss the difficulties of walking, but with a bit of irony, not least in order to neutralise exaggerated expectations in this respect.

When you look at campaigning in its function to make people change non-wished-for behaviour into a different, wished-for one, then campaigning should try to achieve what is reflected in Figure 4.5 subsequently. This figure displays speeding as non-wished-for behaviour and not to speed as the wished-for one. You could replace speeding and not speeding by walking and formulate the disadvantages and advantages slightly differently from the graph of Delhomme et al. (2009): insert the perceived disadvantages of walking on the left and the perceived benefits on the right, and it should turn out that the benefits weigh more.

One could summarise the envisaged result of a targeted campaign to enhance walking as follows:

$$M_{walking} > M_{avoid\ walking}$$

meaning that the motives for walking should be, or should become, stronger than the motives for avoiding walking because of campaigning activities.

Campaigning includes the use of print media (newspapers, magazines, direct mail, etc.); broadcasting media (radio, television); display media (billboards, signs, posters); online media (the internet, social media); and (interactive) events such as press conferences, shows, and much more – basically speaking, all the types of media that we know. But experts will also

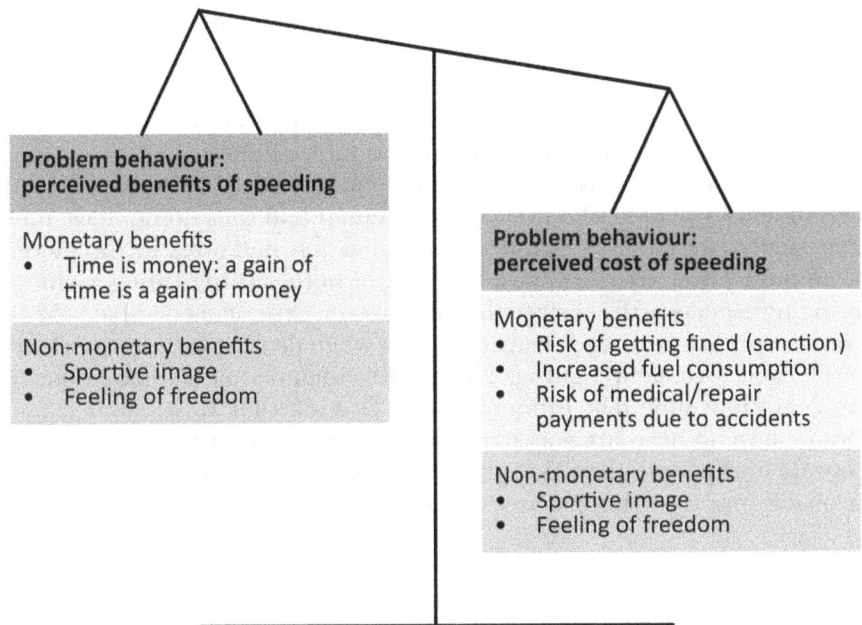

Figure 4.5 The 'motivation balance' (Delhomme et al., 2009).

have their eyes open for emerging new ways to address target groups and target people in an effective and efficient way.

Specially designed environments, pilot areas, or model districts can reinforce the message of any campaign, for example: environments which animate people to walk, where life can be filmed and shown, thus demonstrating the advantages of walking in reality and hearing 'real' people speak about them.

At this point, we want to underline the fact that how people perceive any preconditions is important. Experts may consider these preconditions excellent, experience may tell us that the situation is perfect, but walkers and those who need to be convinced that they should walk (more) might still find a fly in the ointment. This is what brings us back to the information measures discussed in connection with the marketing approach. Assessment of the usability of any measure must rely on the perspective of the addressees, and any new measure to be implemented has to undergo appraisal by the addressees. Bein et al. (2004) divided objective parameters into: Presentation – the prevailing image of, and respect for, walking in any society; Environment – the impact that walking has on energy consumption, air quality, noise, and so on; Economy – the costs that walking causes for both the individual and for society compared to the benefits; and Policy – infrastructure and budgets provided for walkers. There are certainly many other ways to structure objective parameters, for instance, according to the diamond model. However, the important message of Figure 4.6 is that the individual relevance of all preconditions and measures is always filtered by their subjective assessment.

Figure 4.6 illustrates how objective preconditions translate into subjective ones by listing the parameters that are relevant for individuals: security or perceived safety; the social climate that is experienced; comfort, aesthetics, perceived costs, spontaneous mobility,[1] and perceived accessibility are of great importance (Hakamies-Blomqvist & Jutila, 1996).

As we know that the assessment of preconditions can be flawed, especially assessment by people who do not walk (much) and thus do not have much experience, we need to include communication measures in the picture. Communication activities have the goal of both putting things right and bringing aspects to the surface that maybe even experienced walkers are not conscious of, as we already learned earlier when dealing with the marketing model and with campaigning. The way in which people perceive objective preconditions should be influenced in such a way that $M_{walking} > M_{avoid\ walking}$. But we have to be aware – as stated previously – that if we convince people to walk and people then find the preconditions in practice lousy, we will probably lose those people as walkers 'forever'.

4.5.1   Lobbying

Pedestrians have weak representation compared with car drivers; there are no strong private pressure groups, nor do they appear to be strongly

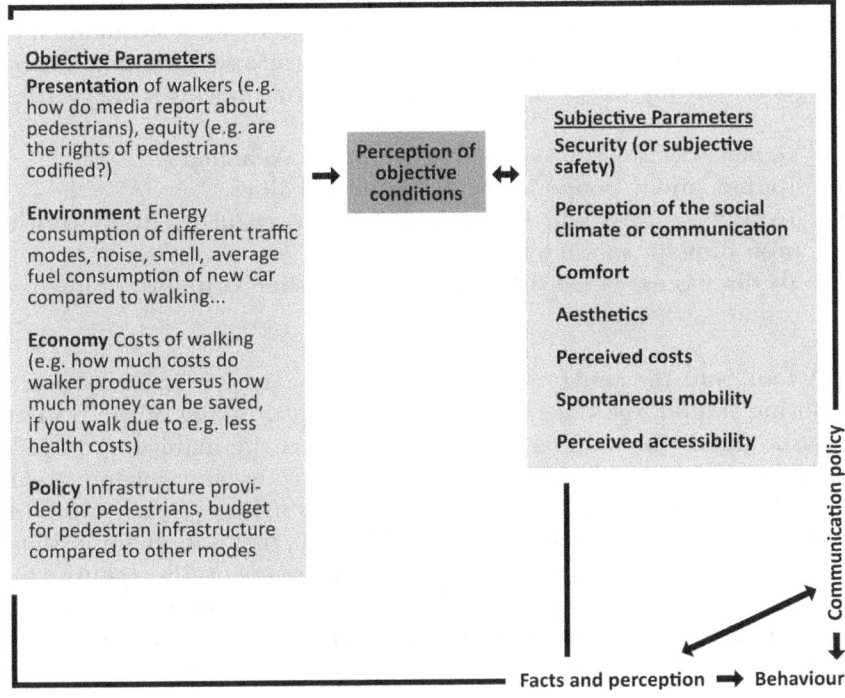

Figure 4.6 Preconditions and their perception (Bein et al., 2004).

supported by public institutions. Departments that are responsible for pedestrians do exist in many cities. But if we take the example of Vienna, this department is 'without teeth' – it has no money and no official power, only a consulting function. However, those institutions where there are at least workplaces connected to the topic of walking could work on their lobbying competencies and thus contribute to achieving improvements for walkers. In fact, all people and groups who want to support and enhance walking should deal with lobbying, thereby making use of the literature in the realm of psychology and the social sciences (e.g. Baumgartner et al., 2009).

Seen from the perspective of an advocate for walkers who wants to promote the implementation of measures to the advantage of walkers, one needs to address structural issues related to industry, nongovernmental organisations (NGOs), transport experts, authorities, politicians, and decision-makers. In order to encourage those people to work for the enhancement of walking not to give up too early, one needs to assist them in preparing for the problems they are going to meet, how these problems usually develop, and how the problems can be overcome. To be prepared for the difficulties to be expected when working for walking means in the best case that one is inoculated against (immune to) those difficulties (Banas & Rains, 2010).

We do not want to go into detail about how to do good lobbying; this has to be done with the help of professionals. They have to be acquainted with the theoretical background, practical experience, and know-how as a basis for good lobbying work. In any case, parts of any lobbying strategy are:

- To meet decision-makers and influential stakeholders,
- To find, and to cooperate with, (potential) allies,
- To provide facts and figures and forward them in an appropriate, professionally sound way,
- To discuss expected difficulties and possible counter-arguments or counter-strategies.

A look into the budgets that, for example, the car industry uses for lobbying should not make us pessimistic when thinking of the restricted sums available for walking issues. For instance, the main work of NGOs which deal with issues that concern pedestrians and related areas is some kind of lobbying anyway. The point is to strive to do this work in as professionally sound a way as possible. We think that it is not impossible to find good specialists from the '*second row*' who are not overly expensive to do this job. On the other hand, experience tells us that this work is often done by amateurs who work wholeheartedly for the common goal – to enhance and support walking – but lack the necessary background.

SUMMARY

In order to support walking, the population needs to be addressed. Steps to support walking may result from a top-down or a bottom-up process. Such a process needs to start from a decision to change the behaviour of citizens. When we start to implement measures, then it has been decided that a certain direction should be taken. If this direction is not shared by the individuals whom we address, efforts become necessary to convince, to shape, to persuade, to motivate, or the like. A bottom-up process would be likely to start on the initiative of interested individuals, most easily so if steered by economic interests. However, at first glance, there is no strong business case connected to walking. Thus, it is up to governmental institutions to take steps within the frame of a top-down process to start with.

In expert circles, it is quite clear what should be done in order to support or enhance walking. The question is what status decision-makers have achieved concerning awareness of any necessity to support walking. If there is sufficient awareness, they will accept recommendations from experts concerning different push and pull measures that 'push' people away from car use and pull them towards walking where this is reasonable. Lists of such measures can be compiled with the help of social marketing measures according to the diamond model: product improvements, communication measures, incentives and placement and pricing measures addressing the individual, envisaging improvements to communication between pedestrians and other road users and to the infrastructure, aiming at adapting societal preconditions, and considering the needs inherent to the walking mode.

A precondition for successful marketing, though, is to thoroughly analyse the needs and interests of the citizens being addressed on any occasion and at any place where measures to support walking should be taken. There we discuss the application of a mixed-measures approach: identify the possible needs and interests of defined populations as thoroughly as possible (qualitative) and measure the distribution of the identified needs and interests in the same population (quantitative).

Convincing people to adopt a certain type of mobility behaviour – or also just to continue performing such behaviour – means that for the individual, the advantages of the wished-for behaviour should outweigh the advantages of the behaviour that should be changed, while the disadvantages of this behaviour should outweigh the disadvantages of the wished-for one. The motivation balance presented in the EU project CAST is taken as a model for this approach. To achieve such a goal is the task of campaigns, and lobbying plays an important role in connection with the attempt to gather as many allies as possible within the frame of these attempts.

Note

1. Spontaneous mobility refers to how freely one can move by walking from any point without taking (too many) precautions – without (too much) strategic thinking and planning.

5 Success stories

In this chapter, good examples from different cities and countries around the world are presented. We focus on both concrete measures which were implemented and steps that were taken and also on the process: how the change was introduced to the general public, which needs (and whose) were considered, and how the public accepted the change.

This chapter is divided into two subchapters. The first one deals with general considerations and recommendations for successful projects. In this subchapter, we include good practices and recommendations on a more general level which were only implemented in some respect, or at least discussed. We consider them an indicator of the state of awareness of relevant decision-makers. In this sense, cases where a municipality asked for the advice of experts for how to enhance walking were also taken as good examples.

In the second subchapter, we include examples of success stories where measures were implemented. We tried to find cases where evaluation is available, though this is not the case for all the examples that are presented. Success stories in this respect are scarce. Unfortunately, while talk is universal, action is much harder to find. In many cases, measures which have a potential to enhance walking (or cycling) were implemented, but because evaluation is lacking, we do not actually know if it really is a success story. Thus, we also include cases where measures based on solid empirical evidence have been taken and where one has good reason to expect the wished-for impact.

5.1 General considerations and recommendations for successful projects

5.1.1 Measures

To start with, here are some general recommendations: to create an environment which supports walking, where walking is comfortable and pleasant, and where fewer or no accidents happen between motor vehicles and pedestrians, measures can be taken at different levels. On the level of infrastructure, measures can be taken to limit exposure between pedestrians and motorised traffic. This can be done by separating different modes of transport. When this is not sensible or not possible, the option of speed reduction must be considered. Better visibility must be ensured, not only at the infrastructure level but also from the point of view of the road user. Education and awareness play an important role. Pedestrians need to know that they are not that visible, and driving lessons need to pay extra attention to vulnerable road users. Measures can also be taken at the level of vehicle technology; there are systems which can regulate speed and also help to avoid accidents. When an accident is unavoidable, the consequences need to be limited. Of course, the measures that are taken must be supported by clear and understandable regulations (Pelssers, 2019).

5.1.1.1   Examples from Vienna

A study conducted in Vienna in 2009 by Karin Ausserer and her colleagues, 'Bef(w)usst unterwegs', meaning 'consciously underway on your feet', had the aim of determining the factors which make walking a pleasant, safe, and attractive mode of transport.

The authors found that, in line with what is known from earlier literature, citizens consider walking healthy, reliable, environment-friendly, flexible, communicative, and safe. On the other hand, pedestrians stated that they frequently feel unsafe because of inappropriate car speeds, motor vehicles ignoring the right of way, and motor vehicles running red lights. Furthermore, pedestrians complained about lacking smoothness and easiness (traffic light regulations to the disadvantage of pedestrians), missing infrastructure (e.g. detours being necessary), shared infrastructure for pedestrians and cyclists, the recklessness of car drivers (car drivers parking on pavements, among other things), and problems with an unattractive environment.

The authors also analysed why many car drivers in Vienna do not like to walk. The main reasons were too much car traffic (paradoxically), missing or inadequate infrastructure, the slowness of walking, difficulties with transporting things, and exposure to traffic-related risks and criminality.

On the basis of their findings, the following recommendations were formulated: reduce waiting times at traffic lights; use the weakest (children, old people, etc.) as indicators for the ease and safety of the use of the public space as walkers; introduce constructional measures such as speed humps and elevated intersection plateaux; broaden pavements considerably and consistently; introduce strict enforcement concerning speeding, running red lights, and turning manoeuvres at intersections; introduce higher penalties for speeding and illegal parking, among other things; and, last but not least, shift the burden of proof in the event of an accident onto the driver.

Chaloupka and Risser (2016) conducted another survey in Vienna that was related to walking and pedestrians' needs. Their findings showed that setting slow speed limits (30 km/h) is essential for pedestrian safety. It is also of great importance to enforce these limits rigorously. Setting limits without enforcement has detrimental effects: motor vehicle drivers learn that limits have no significance and one does not need to obey them. Furthermore, the treatment of all road users has to be fair and equal, which is not the case in most cities nowadays, including Vienna. Traffic is mostly organised in a way that favours car traffic, while a smooth flow of pedestrians is not considered. For example: pedestrians have long waiting times; there are often unnecessarily long walking distances because of infrastructure characteristics; walkers often face unclear (e.g. lacking signage), laborious (tunnels, bridges), and dangerous situations; to avoid time losses is usually an explicit goal only as far as car drivers are concerned; (too) little space is dedicated to pedestrians, while most of the road space is allocated to car traffic, where in the year 2019 100 cars transported 116 persons (https://www.vcoe.at/news/details/vcoe-jede-5-autofahrt-in-oesterreich-ist-kuerzer-als-zweieinhalb-kilometer).

In order to promote walking, dealing with safety issues is not enough. More is needed to make walking attractive. This includes aesthetic aspects and comfort. The infrastructure for walking should be 'usable'. This means that it should be effective; one should be able to reach one's everyday goals. It should be efficient; it should be possible to reach one's goals easily, without much effort, and safely. Not least, it should be satisfying; it should be a pleasure to walk. The infrastructure has to be 'user friendly' for pedestrians. Such pedestrian-friendly infrastructure should include areas where people can sit and relax (also without having to buy food or drinks), appealing street furniture, and a well-accessible and safe network of routes. Toilets are most important but are regularly 'forgotten'. If cars are allowed, they should go slowly and this should be enforced rigorously. Finally, anyone who wants to enhance walking should consider that the perspective of the users has to be understood. Otherwise, planning measures will not work sufficiently well. Practitioners in traffic, mobility, and city planning should be aware that people will only accept measures linked to an increase in their own quality of life. It is of great importance to stay in permanent contact with the residents of the city in order to understand citizens and thus to win their cooperation.

5.1.1.2 Germany and the Netherlands

The Netherlands and Germany have long recognised the importance of pedestrians' and cyclists' safety. Over the past two decades, these countries have implemented a wide range of measures to improve safety that mostly also have a positive effect on the comfort of walkers: better facilities for walking and cycling: auto-free pedestrian zones; clearly marked crossings; pavements on both sides of all streets; pedestrian and bicycle traffic lights;

modifications to intersections, bicycle streets, bike lanes, and bike paths; urban design sensitive to the needs of non-motorists, such as pedestrian zones; zebra crossings (sometimes raised and extra-wide) with highly visible striping, usually with special overhead illumination and sometimes with flashing yellow lights to alert motorists; pedestrian-activated crossing signals, both at intersections and at mid-block crossings; pedestrian refuge islands for crossing wide streets; and wide, well-lit pavements, often furnished with benches for resting. Other measures are traffic calming measures in residential neighbourhoods, such as speed limits of 30 km/h or even lower, physical barriers such as raised intersections and crossings, roundabouts, road narrowings, zigzag routes and curves, speed bumps, and artificial dead-ends created by mid-block street closures. Restrictions on motor vehicle use in cities are another recommended measure and one that is being implemented more and more often. Traffic education of children in order to teach them to protect themselves has high priority. Rigorous traffic education of car drivers with a heavy emphasis on and special attention to avoiding collisions with pedestrians and cyclists is becoming the rule, combined with strict enforcement of traffic regulations protecting pedestrians and cyclists. Even in cases where an accident results from the illegal behaviour of pedestrians, the motorist is almost always found to be at least partly at fault. When an accident involves children or the elderly, the motorist is usually found to be entirely at fault. In collisions between pedestrians or cyclists and motorised vehicles in the Netherlands, the insurance company responsible for the motorised vehicle automatically pays the damages, regardless of guilt (Pucher & Dijkstra, 2000).

5.1.1.3   New Zealand

The New Zealand Government Policy Statement on Land Transport 18/19–27/28 (The Pedestrian Experience, 2018) stresses that, most importantly, there is a disparity between the many available design guidelines for accessible pedestrian environments and the real-world physical barriers still faced by pedestrians. Thus, the question of pedestrian experience is an important one, as it can help to shape the streets in a way that will encourage more people to enjoy them as pedestrians.

A study in Auckland found that there were many positive perceptions concerning walking in Auckland. But many factors were deemed to be unpleasant for walking. There were safety problems for pedestrians, especially children, and many women felt unsafe when walking at night. They pointed out the risk of being involved in an accident and the risk of falling victim to a criminal offence, violence, or threats. Important shortcomings connected to walking are the limits to the distances that can be covered, the time-consuming character, the difficulty of carrying things, health conditions and physical factors that prohibit walking, the efforts necessary, susceptibility to the weather, and, last but not least, all the benefits connected to car use. The topography is unpleasant or challenging in many places. Poor design of traffic infrastructure is another great problem. Inadequate or absent pavements and badly working pedestrian crossings are criticised. Ramps and special infrastructure for the disabled are often missing. The connections of pedestrian networks and facilities with public transport are frequently sloppily planned. There is a lack of pedestrian information systems, of appropriate lighting of traffic signs, of telephone boxes, of litter bins, street furniture, trees, and cafés. Comfort for walkers is bad. The state of the surfaces of roads and footpaths is poor and so is cleanliness. There are long waiting times at crossings, and there is a lack of space available while waiting to cross. There are frequently barriers on the pavement and walkways, like parked cars, poles (also those carrying traffic signs for car drivers), rubbish bags, advertising signs, and construction material. Moreover, the authors identified the following research gaps with regard to walking:

- Because pedestrians are a very heterogeneous group, there are sometimes conflicting needs concerning infrastructure. Adaptations to make the pedestrian environment more accessible for one group can be problematic for other groups. For example, tactile paving helps blind and partially sighted people to navigate, but it constitutes a hazard for people who have problems lifting their feet. This demonstrates the need to consider the accessibility of the pedestrian environment in a more differentiated way.
- Data on pedestrians' needs relies too heavily on survey snapshots of asset-focused information; however, the pedestrian experience is fluid – familiarity with the environment, fitness, mood, and different activities and contexts can all play a role in how pedestrians find the experience of walking or of place – not just the state of the asset.
- A particular gap in the literature concerns the rural pedestrian. Studies focus almost exclusively on urban pedestrian environments. The need to increase physical activity in urban and rural communities remains both a priority and a challenge and is coupled with the need for better understanding of how different attributes of the environment in urban and rural areas may facilitate walking. Interventions to increase walking in rural and remote areas need to be tailored to accommodate the geographic location and, accordingly, the differing preferences of men and women.

5.1.1.4   *United States of America*

For decades, planners have designed American cities, towns, and suburbs with the primary aim of making car driving fast, cheap, and safe. The result of that policy is that more than 85% of Americans drive to work every day — while less than 4% cycle or walk (Stromberg, 2015). To change this, cities and towns will have to adapt their streets in order to make non-motorised travel safer and easier. These are some of the most effective ways to make that happen, according to Stromberg:

- Stop building culs-de-sac and bring back the grid: gridded streets make distances for pedestrians and cyclists shorter and allow them to reach a much greater number of destinations than *'culs-de-sac'* or similar types of street networks with fewer interconnections (Figure 5.1).
- Change zoning rules to allow for density and mixed use: regardless of street design, cities can dramatically alter an area's walkability just by making changes to their zoning requirements. Many municipalities have zoning laws that prevent businesses from operating in certain residential areas, as well as other sorts of restrictions that limit the number of residences that can be built in a given area. In practice, these rules can help to provide enough public space for active traffic modes and, generally, for making areas more liveable and friendly.
- Change the parking regime: many cities provide lots of free on-street parking or require all new residences to be constructed with off-street garages or lots. If you want a dense, mixed-use city, mandating off-street lots and garages for all new residences is one of the last things you should do.
- Put roads on a diet and make lanes narrower: a road diet involves modifying a road so that cars cannot travel as fast. Most often, a second traffic lane will be converted into a turning lane, bike lanes, or a parking lane (Figure 5.2). These changes give cyclists or pedestrians more space that used to go to cars. But the real goal is to increase safety for all the parties involved by slowing down traffic. A related concept is lane narrowing.

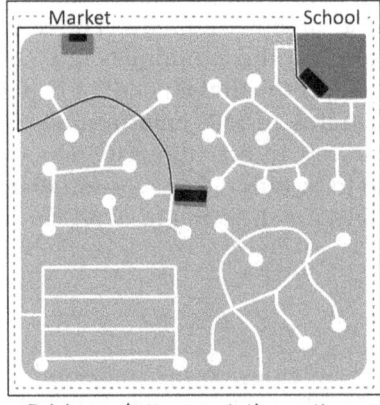
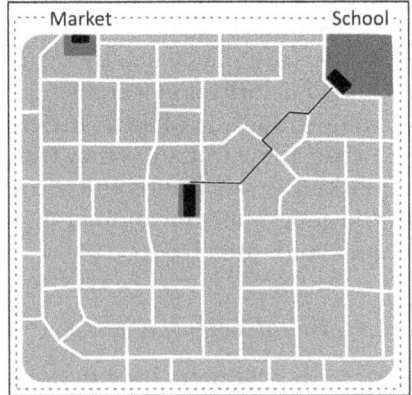

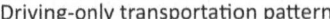

Driving-only transportation pattern   Walkable connected transportation network

Figure 5.1 Culs-de-sac and the grid street design (Stromberg, 2015).

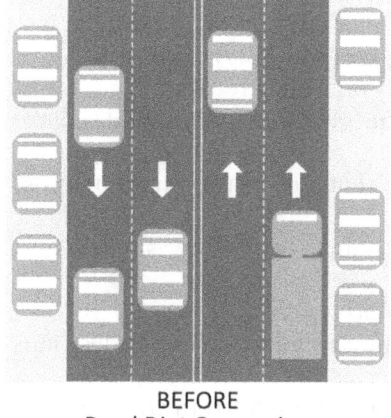
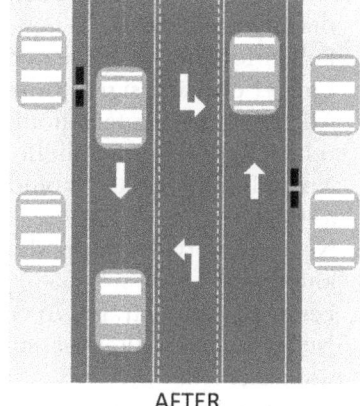

BEFORE
Road Diet Conversion

AFTER
Road Diet Conversion

Figure 5.2 Road diet conversion (Stromberg, 2015).

- Build protected bike lanes: build bike lanes which are blocked off by some sort of physical barrier (such as a kerb or a row of bollards), rather than just a stripe of paint. They are a little more expensive to build and take up more space than bike lanes demarcated by paint, but research consistently shows that people — especially those who are new to cycling — are much more comfortable riding in them.
- Connect bike lanes to create usable routes: bike lanes in most major US cities are a disconnected mess, forcing cyclists to mix in with traffic on the majority of journeys.

Another promising example is from Baltimore. City officials have propagated the idea that we do not have to wait years before important changes can be made and results are visible. Instead, they used 'tactical urbanism' and moved very quickly to make temporary adjustments to the streets. The approach of using paint, barrels, and timber ties to try out new traffic arrangements fits in very well with the idea of observing people to see what works, a really obvious approach. Tactical urbanism consists of a set of quick and simple solutions that act as experiments and can gradually be improved towards a final installation. In this way, Baltimore implemented measures that should be applied in any city that is truly pedestrian friendly. Many of them could be implemented 'tomorrow or the day after', because they are neither expensive nor 'rocket science' (Philipsen, 2017):

- No right on red anywhere in the central city or where pedestrian traffic is heavy
- No rush hour lanes directly abutting a pavement
- Well-marked and well-lit crossings everywhere, especially mid-block

- No pedestrian signals requiring push-button activation anywhere in the city centre area
- Full enforcement of the pedestrian right-of-way laws at crossings
- Longer crossing signal times, especially on wide streets
- All pedestrian signals should provide the 'go' signal two seconds before vehicles get the green light
- No pedestrian phase should be so short that it takes two phases to cross a street
- No inner-city bus stop should be without extra space, shelter, and amenities
- Fewer parking garages in city centre areas
- No construction sites that simply close the pavement, saying 'Pedestrians use other side'
- Fewer kerb cuts across pavements with a high pedestrian volume
- No pavements with less than 160 cm of actually usable space, free of obstructions
- A general maximum speed limit of 40 km within the city limits, except designated expressways, and 30 km in residential streets and near schools
- No crossings without kerb ramps
- No large car parks or garages without marked pedestrian routes and refuges
- Reinstate the red light and speed camera system
- Each city centre block must have some visual interest points for pedestrians
- Install pedestrian rest areas and trailblazing throughout the city
- Reduce the number of one-way streets

In this section, a variety of measures focused on support for active traffic modes were presented. Most of the measures presented deal with infrastructure, and we can see these as preconditions to boost walking or, more generally, active traffic modes. Measures based on 'tactical urbanism' are particularly useful, because they can be implemented very quickly and give us an opportunity to discuss the pros and cons with citizens and evaluate the impact of measures and thus to prepare a solid basis for more general and more complex changes to support walking and other active modes.

5.1.2 Data

Policy makers rely on mobility statistics, including data on personal travel behaviour, to formulate strategic transportation policies and to improve the safety and efficiency of transportation systems. A substantial amount of pedestrian activity and, consequently, the importance of walking are underestimated under the current data collection practices. The majority of pedestrian trips are quite short. The distance travelled, however, should not be used as a measure of the importance of walking relative to other modes of transport because it results in a gross underestimation. For example, in Switzerland 28% of all trips are pedestrian trips (entire trips on foot), but 45% of all trip stages are pedestrian stages. Stage data from other countries is not available, but the example of Switzerland illustrates that the real share of walking is much higher than reported in the statistics. Statistically, the amount of walking is a reflection of car use. In general, as the share of walking increases, car use declines (Berge & Peddie, n.d.). Distance is not a measure of importance. Expressing pedestrian mobility in terms of distance travelled should not be used as a measure of the importance of walking relative to other modes of transport, because it represents a gross underestimation of the overall walking undertaken. When important factors such as the time spent travelling and the number of trips are considered, one can see that walking has a much more prominent place in the modal mix than measures of distance would suggest.

5.1.3 Walkability evaluation

Walkability can be broadly defined as the extent to which an environment, usually the built environment, enables walking and is pedestrian friendly. The Walk Score index has become increasingly applied in studies of walking and walkability. The index assesses the 'walking potential' of a place through a combination of three elements: the shortest distance to a group of preselected destinations, the length of the block, and the intersection density around the origin. The Index is best understood as a surrogate measure of the density of the built environment of a specific neighbourhood that indicates its walking potential. It has to be noted, though, that the Walk Score measure cannot be used as a single measurement for walkability, but it can provide important information on the walking features of a place. Furthermore, the analysis shows that the socio-demographic profile of walkers must be taken into consideration when trying to promote walking, together with greater attention to the purpose of walking (recreational or purposive) (Hall & Ram, 2018).

5.1.4 Gender-sensitive walking interventions

As already discussed in Chapter 2.7, the need to adopt a gender-sensitive perspective is emerging as a challenging and impending task in support of making more people walk more. Women travel differently than men with regard to the transport modes used, distance travelled, the daily number of trips and their pattern, and, not surprisingly, they also travel for different purposes. Women's travel patterns differ from men's in many ways (Figure 5.3): women are likely to travel shorter distances than men, are more likely to use public transport, engage in more non-work travel outside rush hours and make more multi-stop trips, run household errands and escort other

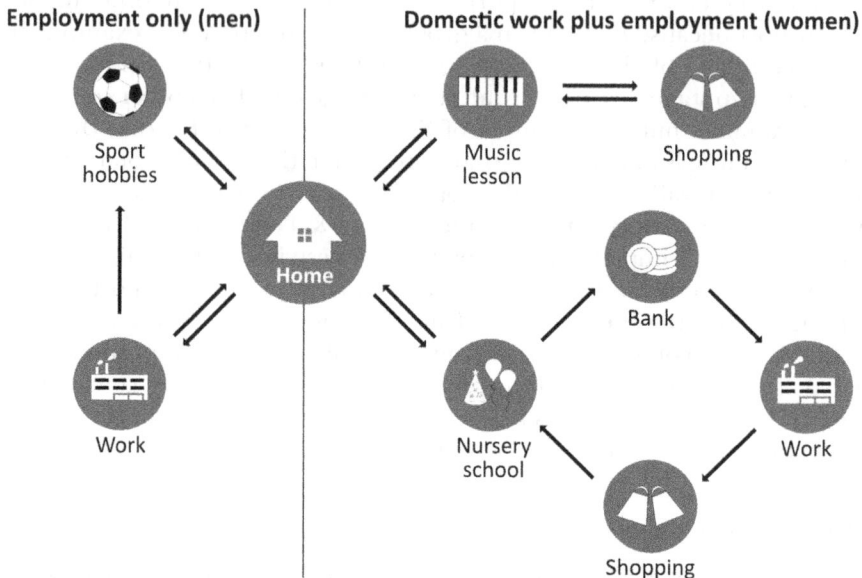

Figure 5.3 A normal day (for a woman from Western Europe) (Civitas, 2014).

passengers (usually children or dependent elderly persons), and tend to be safer drivers than men. Some of these differences are going to become less relevant once gender differentiation in parental models, the labour market, and so on becomes less relevant, but others will continue to play a role (Civitas, 2014).

To tackle these different needs, a gender-sensitive policy has to be applied. The availability of public transport outside rush hours and the physical and financial accessibility of transport facilities for women accompanied by children or disabled people, as well as safety conditions, are the main aspects to be considered in designing women-friendly transport systems. A gender perspective in transport policies is important, not only to reduce the inequality of gender mobility, but also to support a more environmentally friendly development. Women's lower rate of motorisation forces them to use more public transport, as well as to walk and cycle more, and this should be honoured (although it would be even better if more men adopted similar behaviour – and also took over more of the female 'duties'). Indeed, women are more willing to reduce their car use, more positive towards reducing the environmental impacts of travel, and more positive towards ecological issues. Examples of gender-sensitive mobility measures include:

- close proximity of public transport stops to buildings or entryways and combination with commercial use;
- day passes for multiple trips for women;

- convenient access to well-lit and safe bus or rail stops with good visibility and protection from the elements, equipping stops with communication devices for guard services;
- underpasses and transit places (metro) with mirrors or other devices in order to eliminate the 'blind spots' (it is necessary to see and to be seen);
- lifts in addition to flights of stairs and escalators;
- areas where children can be cared for in railway stations;
- low-floor vehicles that reduce the gap between the ground and the vehicle;
- interiors with appropriate space for transporting strollers, shopping carts, and so on;
- in-vehicle seats reserved for women near the driver;
- parking for women nearest to the exits, checkouts, and so on;
- 'pink taxis' with the intention being to provide safe conditions for women in the evening and at night (e.g. after 10 p.m.) when the public transport service becomes less frequent or non-existent;
- discounted fares for car sharing at night for women;
- while public transport services (public or private public transport as well as taxis, etc.) are, in most cases, designed for travel towards the city centre during rush hours, women also need transport services in their local neighbourhood outside rush hours, which will allow them to make short but linked journeys.

In order to gain a better understanding of gender differences in mobility patterns, gender-based statistical data and research should be adapted and improved. Supporting women's participation in decision-making would help women's needs to be taken into account more thoroughly. It is essential to involve women in consultation, transport planning, and decision-making processes. This would definitely help to improve the accessibility, safety, and comfort of modes of transport in a way that suits the target group.

5.2   Success stories and good examples

There is an abundance of lists of 'the most walkable cities' around the globe, usually presented from visitors' point of view. For example, Insider (14 cities around the World That Are Better for Pedestrians Than for People with Cars, 2019) names the following 'best walkable' cities: New York City, Copenhagen, Amsterdam, Paris, Venice, Madrid, Hamburg, San Francisco, Florence, Dubrovnik, Helsinki, Philadelphia, Boston, and Washington, DC. Other sources list other cities. But what makes these cities walkable? And how can we measure the success of measures to make cities more attractive for walkers? The cases which are listed subsequently deal with specific towns and locations (e.g. streets) and with specific approaches and measures that aim to boost walking. Many measures refer to walking *and* cycling, because improvements for both groups often come in combination. For instance, car speed-reducing measures improve preconditions dramatically for both groups.

5.2.1   *The Norwegian national walking strategy*

At the Walk21 conference in September 2013, Guro Berge introduced *the Norwegian national walking strategy*. The main goals were that walking should appeal to everyone and to make more people walk more. The specific goals were:

- The share of journeys entirely on foot shall increase – from 22% to ~30%.
- More children shall walk or cycle to school – national goal: at least 80%.
- The share of people who do not walk at all shall decrease – from 16% to less than 10%.
- The share of people who regularly walk 1500 metres or more shall increase from 19% to more than 25%.
- Demographic differences shall be reduced: especially male professionals, parents with children, and people with high incomes shall walk more.
- The risk of traffic accidents for pedestrians shall go down.
- The number of pedestrians killed and seriously injured in traffic shall be reduced.

The policy areas which should be dealt with in order to reach these goals are responsibility and cooperation, the physical environment, service and maintenance, traffic interplay, walking culture, and knowledge and communication (see Figure 5.4 subsequently).

According to this strategy, the most important things to start with were to draw up action plans in order to reinforce the walking strategy and communication plans to engage relevant players. Moreover, the necessity of promoting cooperation between the state, counties, and municipalities was underlined, so that at least 50 cities would actively pursue local walking

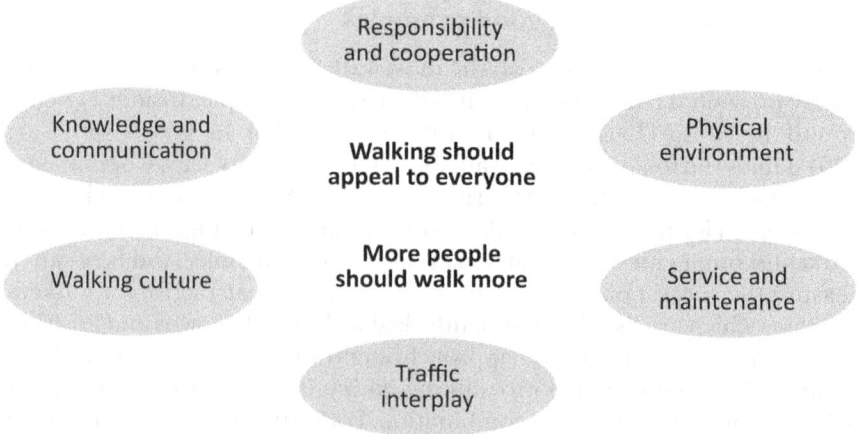

Figure 5.4 Policy areas to be dealt with within the strategy (Berge, 2013).

strategies. Last but not least, the necessity of investing in the development and dissemination of knowledge was pointed out.

This strategic plan provides figures for the envisaged changes and thus allows the rather exact measurement of whether goals have been achieved. At the moment of the production of this book, it was not possible, though, to get any information concerning the implementation of the recommended measures, and neither could we find out what results have been achieved.

5.2.2   Strøget, Copenhagen, Denmark

Strøget – a pedestrianised zone in the heart of Copenhagen – has set a standard as a successful and charming pedestrian-only throughway. What makes this inspiring car-excluding endeavour a success? Strøget, possibly one of the best-known examples of a successful zone, originated when Copenhagen experimented with this concept throughout the 1950s by closing the four-block area to cars for two days during the Christmas holidays. Later, in October 1962, the Copenhagen City Council decided at a council meeting that the area should be tested as a pedestrian street from November 17th, 1962, on. After a successful two-year trial period with much cleaner air and many happy pedestrians, the city council decided to transform the zone that had been tested into a permanent pedestrian street in February 1964. This new pedestrian street was the first one in the world and is still the longest one (The World's Longest Pedestrian Street 'Strøget', 2019). But the start was not easy. Like many measures with the goal of reducing accessibility for cars, the project was controversial, and it took time for people to see the benefits. The original opposition to shutting down this street was the same as the arguments that come up today in similar contexts: shop owners feared that shoppers would forget or not go to local stores without the opportunity to drive by them. There were dramatic warnings that traffic would become congested on the streets surrounding the car-free zone. It was predicted that the local community would not be interested in gathering in these public spaces.

All those worries disappeared as the car-free area became one of the top destinations for shoppers and tourists. Local businesses found their sales rising by 25%–40%. Many of the city's most famous and expensive stores are located along the strip, as well as some of the most famous and expensive chain stores in the world. It also features a multitude of souvenir shops and gastronomic outlets. It catalysed the economy of the surrounding areas and helped define the walking and cycling culture that helped earn Copenhagen the title of 2013's most liveable city (Returning Streets to People: 5 Tips for Going Car-Free, 2015).

About 80,000 people use Strøget every day at the height of the tourist season in summer, and about 48,000 do so on a winter's day. On the last Sunday before Christmas, as many as 120,000 may use Strøget. Strøget is by now reaching its handling capacity on a summer's day, given its width of 10–12 metres, with space for roughly 145 people/minute (Gehl & Gemzøe, 1996).

5.2.3   *Vienna's Mariahilferstraße, Austria[1]*

Another success story is the redesign of Vienna's Mariahilferstraße, the Austrians' most important shopping street, which now consists of a pedestrian zone and shared spaces. The success of Mariahilferstraße is reflected in, for example, the significant increases in pedestrian volume (up from 25,000 to 70,000 per day). There are now longer opening hours, a more attractive retail offer, and more people coming not only on foot but also by bicycle and public transport. Two adjoining districts of Vienna decided to *redesign the street* and transform it into a pedestrian zone and Vienna's first 'Begegnungszone' (shared space) with an overall budget of ~€25 million. The transformation was accompanied by a large-scale information campaign and opportunities for civic engagement through a dedicated *website*, newsletter distribution, expert round table discussions, resident surveys, feedback boxes, and finally – after a fiercely debated trial (interim redesign) period – decided with the support of a public referendum among the 48,642 residents of the two adjoining districts, which brought a narrow 53.2% approval rate at an unusually high participation rate of 68.1%. The construction began in May 2014, immediately after the positive outcome of the referendum, and was completed in November 2014. A second phase of construction took place from February to July 2015. On the basis of qualitative observations during the trial period and after the first construction phase, it can be seen how the street already acts as a catalyst for urban transformation, with pedestrians now walking in the middle of the street and claiming more space once the differences in surfaces and surface levels were removed. As Mariahilferstraße allows us to directly compare a shared space and pedestrian zone approach, it can also be observed that this effect is noticeably more predominant in the pedestrian zone than in the shared space zone where cars are present. Nonetheless, Mariahilferstraße supports the argument that streets with mixed-use buildings and a high desire of pedestrians to cross the street – such as shopping streets, old city centre areas, or railway station forecourts – are well suited to shared space approaches. While Mariahilferstraße is Austria's largest shopping street, it should be remembered that the shared space approach can also be applied to smaller streets but might have disadvantages compared to pedestrian streets (Vienncouver, 2015). A systematic evaluation of the effects of the changes is still lacking, but it can be stated that traffic accidents have gone down considerably. Cyclists, who were considered a nuisance at the beginning of the new regime, have started adapting their behaviour according to studies by the Austrian traffic club, the VCÖ.[2] The number of people visiting the area both for shopping and sojourning is constantly increasing. The general notion in Vienna is that Mariahilferstraße is a complete success.

5.2.4   *Vienna, Austria, and Tehran, Iran*

In this study, Oberlader et al. (2015) show examples of good practices from two very different settings, one in Vienna, in Europe, and the other one from Tehran, in Western Asia. According to discussions with experts and citizens in both cities, among other things, elements of pedestrian-friendly infrastructure should include 'consumption-free' zones (areas where people can sit and relax without having to buy food or drinks) and appealing street furniture (for the more sensory, aesthetic aspects of walking), as well as a well-accessible, well-connected, and safe network of routes.

To limit the walking challenges in *Tehran*, a campaign called 'White Line' was launched in 2014, with the aim being to encourage the regulated movement of people and goods, especially in the central business district, where the traditional crowded market (the bazaar) is located. As one of the most important measures related to walking safety, pedestrian crossings were clearly marked. It was decided to convert certain zebra-type crossings into 'white line' crossings at signal-controlled junctions. These crossings clearly indicate the spot where drivers must stop their vehicles. The measure is intended to minimise the encroachment on the walking path when the traffic light is red (Oberlader et al., 2015).

However, an evaluation of the measures is missing and the authors conclude and stress that if we want to promote walking, we need to improve the data situation. For this to happen, we need good indicators and adequate (data) collection methods. Some of the known difficulties of the planning and designing process are (Oberlader et al., 2015) very often related to the fact that necessary data is lacking: trip length, starting time, ending time, trip chains, trips below 1 km, trips with only walking. Thus, walking is systematically underestimated. Moreover, different types of pedestrians (age, gender, etc.) have different needs concerning infrastructure design, information systems technologies, and technical innovations. We need to know more about the different subgroups of people who walk. It is also necessary to carry out a constant and systematic assessment of vulnerable road user needs (pedestrians, cyclists, etc.) for reliable and comparable analysis. Not least, there is a lack of systematic assessment of pedestrian accidents, especially when cars are not included (falls), and this is not only the case in Tehran. Finally, concepts such as the comfort or easiness of mobility (the 'usability' of the infrastructure for walking) for vulnerable road users are missing more or less completely.

5.2.5   *Seville, Spain*

When the Mayor of Seville polled residents in 2006 on whether cycling infrastructure would benefit the city, 90% of the respondents agreed. Sevilla then built an 80-km network of segregated bicycle lanes in just 18 months, mostly by repurposing 5000 on-street parking spaces. Segregation – separating bikes by a physical barrier such as a raised kerb or fence – is something of a holy grail for campaigners, who argue that it makes cycling accessible to people of all ages, allowing them to trundle along at slow speeds in everyday clothes. Crucially, this was done within a single mayoral political term. The cycle network was immediately popular. The net result is not Dutch or Danish levels of cycling, but nonetheless impressive. The average number of bikes used daily in the city rose from just over 6000 to more than 70,000. The last audit, about a year ago, found that 6% of all trips were made by bike, rising to 9% for non-commuter journeys. The number of trips taken by bike per day increased by over 11 times in just a few years. The city is now one of the best in Europe for cycling. The effects are arguably greater than the 6% share of cycling would indicate. For instance, there has been a small but appreciable mini-boom in a bike-related economy, a particular benefit in a city with an unemployment rate of about 30%. Before the lanes were built, Seville had about 10 bike shops. Now it has around 50 (How Seville Transformed Itself into the Cycling Capital of Southern Europe, 2015).

This case refers only to cycling, but we postulate that similar procedures can successfully be applied for boosting walking.

5.2.6   Barcelona, Spain

Cerdà's design for Barcelona is perhaps the most famous large-scale urban master plan in the world and is often cited as a model for modern mixed-use neighbourhoods. When Ada Colau campaigned to be Mayor of Barcelona in 2015, the city was suffering from congestion, pollution, and a lack of green spaces. She focused her transportation policy platform on reclaiming Barcelona's streets as enjoyable and healthy places to walk. Since her election, Mayor Colau has begun implementing an innovative plan based on the city's historic street layout, with the goal of reducing car and moped use by 21%. The famed L'Eixample, the district designed by Ildefons Cerdà in the 1850s, would be transformed into a network of so-called superblocks. Cars would be virtually eliminated from within the superblocks, 'liberating' 70% of the city's land for public use. Without demolishing buildings or undertaking massive redevelopment, superblocks will create pedestrian-centric neighbourhoods while addressing the health, sustainability, and pollution problems facing Barcelona. The mechanics of superblocks are relatively simple. A typical superblock will consist of a three-by-three-block square made from nine existing blocks. Circulating traffic will be limited to the streets on its perimeter. Intersections at every 400 metres will maintain steady traffic flow and allow the development of nodes to intersect with the bus and bicycle networks. Within the superblocks, cars will be limited to ten kilometres per hour and restricted to one-way lanes. Barcelona has a successful experience with traffic calming from the past. In the Gràcia neighbourhood, where cars were eliminated in 2006, cycling trips have increased by 30% and driving is down by 26%. Superblocks will increase the number of neighbourhoods with acceptable air quality from 56% to 94%. The number of green districts within the city will increase by almost 300%. After years of debate, Barcelona was poised to turn the superblocks concept into a reality. The concept was adopted as a centrepiece of the city's mobility plan in 2015, and a test case was instituted in the neighbourhood of Poblenou in September 2016. The city hopes to reduce auto traffic in the city by 21% in the next two years. 'The idea is not to eliminate cars but to change the system of mobility. The superblock strategy moves the focus away from private cars and toward public systems, which can mean anything from buses to autonomous cars, supporters say. The future of mobility is not having your private car. Proactive and transparent communication with residents and business owners, as well as investment in designing new public spaces in the intersections and streets formerly occupied by roads, have been central to its success' (Brass, 2017). As can be understood easily, walking should profit considerably from all of these measures. The goal was that 75% or more of all trips or trip segments should be done by walking, and less than 25% of the trips in the area should be by car.[3] More detailed evaluation results can be expected during the next two or three years.

5.2.7 Fredericton City, Canada

One of the success stories of redesigning small to middle-sized city centres to make them better walkable is the city centre of Fredericton in Canada. In September 2013, the Planning Partnership presented to the city council the 'Fredericton city centre plan', with the goal of preparing a comprehensive urban design concept. The key objectives were to create a vision and urban design framework for the city centre area that would aid future decision-making. Accessibility for all users should be improved, including pedestrians, cycling, transit, and traffic. Tourism initiatives should be enhanced, and a city centre should be created that demonstrates sustainable design excellence in built form in the public realm. As a first step, in-depth consultations with the public and relevant experts were held. The main conclusions of the experts concerning the status quo were that here there is a younger generation of residents open to a city centre lifestyle and living. There is a desire for more cultural attractions and events. Those needs are not fulfilled at the moment. The existing heritage stock is important but is often neglected. Significant areas are occupied by surface car parks. Generally, there is a need for greater emphasis on achieving good urban design and architectural excellence. In more detail, within the frame of the evaluation of the 'state of the art' in the city centre, experts and city officials identified the following key issues:

- some details of the transportation infrastructure and even some 'improvements' are at odds with factors for the success of the city centre and can often serve as barriers – too fast, too busy;

- more can be done to cultivate and nurture an active transportation culture. There is a need to make walking or cycling an easier, safer, and more convenient and appealing choice;
- outdated parking structure designs, surface lots, and blank walls undermine the quality of the public realm and the pedestrian experience;
- the quality and the standard of streetscapes vary greatly from block to block and from street to street;
- where the city centre begins and ends is mostly unclear.

As a theoretical background, a list of attributes of outstanding small and mid-sized city centre areas, defined within the frame of research work conducted in 2005 at Cornell University, was used. In this study, 11 cities were identified as having national reputations for successful city centres: State College, Burlington, Providence, Northampton, Portland, Madison, Ann Arbor, Boulder, Charlottesville, Chapel Hill, and Wooster. Altogether, 11 common characteristics of successful city centre areas were identified, keeping in mind that no single organisational model exists:

1. They have multiple traffic generators within a short walking distance.
2. They are much appreciated by the citizenry.
3. They have been, and still are, overcoming challenges and obstacles.
4. They are walkable and are scaled for pedestrians.
5. They demonstrate a commitment to mixed-use development.
6. There is broad public/private investment in their future.
7. The nature of city centre retailing appears to be in flux.
8. Entertainment is a driving market segment.
9. There are adjacent residential neighbourhoods within walking distances.
10. City centre housing is prevalent or underway.
11. Universities help with research.

5.2.8   Oklahoma City, US

Many cities around the world were designed after the advent of the car, with the convenience of vehicles first in mind. This is particularly true of US cities, with sprawling suburbs and eight-lane highways. But one great example of a city that has switched its point of view from behind the steering wheel to the pavement is Oklahoma. Mayor Mick Cornett started an ambitious campaign when he found his home on a list of America's fattest cities (These Streets Are Made for Walking: How Oklahoma City Overturned Car Culture, 2015). Cornett asked citizens to vote for a tax to fund a series of public works that would encourage less sedentary lifestyles. 'And so the citizens have funded more sidewalks, more jogging and biking trails, senior wellness centres, new gymnasiums for kids', says the mayor. 'Perhaps most notably (we now have) a completely different infrastructure that is built to be more pedestrian-friendly, where life revolves around people instead of cars'.

A new park is about to break ground in the centre of the city, and a tram system is being installed. 'In 20 years (the) downtown's come from a place where virtually no one lived to a vibrant mixed community', he says. 'Streets have been narrowed, more highly landscaped; it's designed now to be walkable, as opposed to seeing how fast we can move cars around'. Cornett says that the main difference between Oklahoma City and other places around the world that have recognised this challenge is that 'we've figured out a way to pay for these changes'. Citizen buy-in was key and secured by the initial awareness campaign asking its residents to go on a diet. The campaign has transformed the city. 'Highly educated 20-somethings that are moving to Oklahoma City are fuelling an incredibly vibrant economy', he says (These Streets Are Made for Walking: How Oklahoma City Overturned Car Culture, 2015).

5.2.9 New Orleans, US

'Connect the Crescent' (2018), a three-month transportation network demonstration in the year 2018, made travelling to and through the centre of New Orleans safer and easier for people cycling, walking, and riding the bus. At its heart was 2.5 miles of protected bikeways, which create physical separation between people cycling and driving, and are proven to be effective in improving safety and increasing ridership across the country and in countless cities across the globe. With increased options comes the benefit of healthier communities and increased economic activity.

'Connect the Crescent' came together as a private-public collaboration between Bike Easy and a range of community partners working with the City of New Orleans. Over 200 community residents gave their time as volunteers to make it a success. Because community residents and organisations were in the lead, 'Connect the Crescent' was able to be executed quickly and flexibly, while the city's involvement guaranteed that all the renovations were fully accountable to the citizens of New Orleans.

Follow-up evaluation showed that the project was successful and met its goals:

- Bike ridership increased by 20%–84% over the baseline numbers during the demonstration
- Helmet usage increased
- Illegal pavement/wrong-way riding decreased
- New Orleans' bicyclists are demographically diverse, especially in areas underserved by infrastructure
- Vehicle speeds: median speeds held steady but *max speeds dropped by up to 26%*
- Crashes and safety – 12% fewer crashes on Baronne Street during the demonstration compared to the rest of the city

- Vehicle travel time on Baronne: no change during off-peak; increases only at peak hour
- Reduction in illegal lane usage on Baronne
- Transit ridership increased and on-time performance improved
- 85% of the cyclists rated their experience as improved
- 50% of the pedestrians rated their experience as improved, 50% as 'about the same'
- 76% of everyday drivers support the project or say safety was improved
- 57% of the businesses surveyed were neutral about the installations. Of those who indicated an opinion, 73% were positive
- 87% (719 out of 826 respondents) of residents were supportive of the project overall; the majority would like to see the changes made permanent

5.2.10   Other measures in US cities

The use of car-free shopping streets in city centres is another good example of how to improve walking in American cities (and not just there). With the return to traditional walkable areas and modern suburban mixed-use developments, there has been a revival of car-free shopping streets. The following trends and benefits of car-free shopping streets are summarised by Lee Sobel in the article 'Six Reasons for the Resurgence of Car-Free Shopping Streets' (Build a Better Burb, 2019).

The suburbs are changing: walkable areas have become more attractive, and people in the places where they already live, work, and play are looking for additional shopping choices. In fact, if the retail avenue is well incorporated into a street network with numerous transit options, the opportunity for attracting new customers is enhanced.

Size (and scale) matters: car-free shopping streets have a better chance of succeeding when smaller, and their limited scale makes them easy to implement. Their more intimate settings offer retail on a human scale, with sufficient points of interest and places to linger, encouraging customers to browse at their own pace and make connections with shop proprietors.

Flexibility: to serve pedestrians does not necessarily exclude the automobile: *Shared Streets* are designed for both people and cars (e.g.: Pennoyer Street in Portland, OR, and Palmer Street in Cambridge, MA), *Intermittent Streets* are regular streets that are closed to automobile traffic at certain times (for instance: Ellsworth Drive, in Silver Spring, MD, closes to traffic in the evenings and at weekends), and *True Pedestrian Streets* primarily provide access only to people—they vary in scale from alleys and passageways to more traditional streets (e.g. Palmer Alley in Washington, DC).

These different configurations reject the one-size-fits-all model and maximise a street's function. Also, many car-free shopping streets are privately owned and operated, sometimes as part of a larger development project, for example Bethesda Lane, the addition to Bethesda Row in Bethesda, MD.

Car-free shopping streets create a new market choice for retail activity: they respond to market trends for additional places to shop. City planners have also developed strategies to activate retail along existing streets, lanes, and alleys, and so there is no need to build from scratch, such as, for example, Winthrope Street in Cambridge, MA.

It is all about the experience: the smaller street offers a more intimate and inviting feeling. With their pop-up shops, al fresco dining, and repurposed spaces, these car-free shopping streets put a modern twist on an ancient concept.

5.2.11   Good examples in the field of gender equality and mobility

Subsequently, based on the policy note by Civitas, 'Gender Equality and Mobility: Mind the Gap!' (Civitas, 2014), gender-sensitive experiences of some cities that have started embedding gender mainstreaming in urban and mobility planning are presented. Examples of both implementation and data collection are included. These recommendations deal in a broader sense with mobility and gender equality, including walking issues.

5.2.11.1   Malmö (Sweden)

The city of Malmö has decided to gender-mainstream the process of developing the city's system of public transport. The result was a series of 'dialogue meetings' arranged with high school students, commercial employees, and participants in various free-time activities. Most of the users involved in the project declared that they felt unsafe using public transport at night. Many municipalities have started to work on safety issues, taking measures such as removing bushes and shrubbery adjacent to bus stops and eliminating dark access ways, such as tunnels, to the stops. Another relevant aspect emerged from travel surveys: the need to focus on men (both middle-aged and older men) in order to convince them to start travelling more like women, who have been proven to exhibit more sustainable travel behaviour.

In 2010, the City of Malmö started another large project to develop new 'socially friendly' pedestrian and cycle paths connecting the central areas of Malmö with the socio-economically less advantaged suburb of Rosengård. A main component of the project was to engage inhabitants through active dialogue with citizens in order to provide opportunities for residents to take part in and influence their local environment. It was decided that with regard to the new activity area of Rosengård, an effort would be made to make it a more gender-balanced area. Other priorities were a focus on sustainability and the improvement of the participation processes to allow citizens to get involved.

A focus group of young women was then established to contribute ideas on activities that could be organised in the space. The group called for more cultural activities related to music and dance rather than other physical activities. As a second step, a group of stakeholders composed of local associations and small businesses became involved. The idea was to build upon the engagement mobilised through the planning processes so that the activities offered in the area would be managed and maintained by the users themselves (i.e. the residents of the neighbourhood).

Moreover, the name for the space, 'Rosens Red Carpet', was the winning proposal in a competition organised in the suburb as a further way for inhabitants to take ownership of the space. The contribution from the group of young women was acknowledged by the media and generated a public debate on the importance of including gender equality in urban planning.

5.2.11.2   Bolzano (Italy)

In 2005, the City of Bolzano set up the Time and Schedules Plan to help citizens in the reconciliation of family time and working time.

* 'Taxi Rosa' (Pink Taxi) – a dedicated taxi service available to all women in the evening hours and at night between 10 p.m. and 6 a.m., with an extension, from 8 p.m. to 6 a.m., for women over 65, at rates with a €3 discount per ride.
* Parking areas dedicated to women, 'Parcheggi Rosa' (Pink Parking), are reserved around the city: they are easily accessible, well lit, and near exits in garages.
* Greater flexibility of times and schedules of activities which tend to be more women related, such as kindergarten opening hours, in order to distribute women's travel demands better throughout the day.

5.2.11.3   Berlin (Germany)

The city of Berlin decided to implement gender mainstreaming in the updating of the local public transport planning. A Gender Check was carried out in 2006 and has been carried out regularly since then in order to identify the gaps and the need for further action in supply and infrastructure. The following main criteria for better public transport planning are applied:

* Accessibility (stops/stations/vehicles). The catchment radius should be between 300 and 400 m, according to the population density of the area, with a specific focus on social trouble spots. Accessibility is a prerequisite for disabled people; the provision of properly designed vehicles is an impending need.

- Ample space in vehicles. Access to transport has to be made easier for mobility-impaired people and those in wheelchairs, as well as those with prams and children. Multipurpose compartments – for wheelchairs, prams, and so on – have to be provided or kept.
- Security. Security in public spaces and in public transport areas and vehicles is one of the central quality requirements of local public transport from a gender perspective.

SUMMARY

General recommendations for successful projects describe key factors which we identified in good examples for enhancing walking. These include topics such as *Measures to support walking, Data about pedestrians and efficient use made thereof, Walkability and its evaluation,* and *Gender-sensitive walking interventions.* It is crucial to have detailed data on pedestrians and their behaviour and needs. On this basis, one can design and implement relevant measures and evaluate the impact of these measures, if possible in a standardised way. A gender-sensitive approach in the design of interventions must be considered. Success stories and good examples should be characterised by an empirical evidence background, successful implementation or at least successful steps in that direction, and indications or evidence that the wished-for impact is achieved. The latter should be evaluated in a scientifically sound way. Unfortunately, these examples are so rare that we decided also to present cases which lack some of the previously mentioned qualities. Thus, we also include as success stories those cases where the municipality asks for the advice of experts concerning how to enhance walking, which might show the problem awareness of decision-makers.

In this sense, we present good examples from *Norway (The Norwegian national walking strategy), Denmark (Strøget, Copenhagen), Austria (Vienna), Tehran (Iran), Spain (Seville and Barcelona), Canada (Fredericton City)* and *the United States of America (Oklahoma City, New Orleans, US shopping streets), Sweden (Malmö), Germany (Berlin),* and *Italy (Bolzano).*

Notes

1. https://www.wien.gv.at/stadtentwicklung/studien/pdf/b008433.pdf (December 16th, 2019)
2. https://www.google.com/url?sa=t&rct=j&q=&esrc=s&source=web&cd=1&cad= rja&uact=8&ved=2ahUKEwjc-uaVi7rmAhVBwMQBHTDpAiIQFjAAegQIBxAB& url=https%3A%2F%2Fmobilitaetsprojekte.vcoe.at%2Fmariahilfer-strasse-neu&us g=AOvVaw0khORavMMm9o3GKHBGrllK (December 16th, 2019).
3. http://archiv.la21wien.at/mehr-wissen/fundgrube/superblocks_Gracia_BCN_ Echave140911_kl.pdf (December 16th 2919).

6   Instead of conclusion

The story of Walkington

6.1   How it all started

My name is Aristoteles Perpatimenou. I live in the city of Walkington. I am 42 years old. I own a small shop and workshop where I sell and repair bicycles. I live on the outskirts of the city. My shop is some three km away from my apartment. I usually cycle to work, which takes no more than ten minutes, but sometimes I walk when the weather is fine or when I am meeting friends in the city centre in the evening or maybe to get to the theatre or the cinema. I sometimes take the bus or the tram home, with a five-minute walk for the last bit from the tram stop.

Some people do not like Walkington, but many people do like it, especially those who are not frequent car users but prefer to travel in other ways. The main reason is that the city provides perfect conditions for these alternative ways of getting about. People who like walking are particularly enthusiastic because it is so easy and pleasant to walk in Walkington, and has been for many years now. How could the city have developed in this way? The reason is quite simple: 20 years ago, the mayor asked if anyone knew where the name Walkington came from. Nobody knew. The mayor then expressed the opinion that, no matter where the name came from, people should think of the Brundtland report, which said that people should strive for sustainability because otherwise the ecological system of the world would be endangered. (Today we would say that we live in times of global warming. Some maybe do not believe that, but there is growing evidence that global warming is, in fact, taking place.)

The mayor announced that all kinds of measures should be taken in order to counteract this development. It was decided that all modes of transport which were sustainable and had the least impact on the environment, especially walking, should be supported. As the city had the name that it had, they (the leaders of the city) should follow the Latin phrase 'nomen est omen' and make the nomen – Walkington – an omen, a really symbolic place that would provide optimal conditions for walkers. Of course, many measures should be taken to support cyclists, and public transport of good quality would have to be provided – and using a car should not become totally impossible – but the main efforts should focus on walking. This would mean that everybody except those with major disabilities who could not travel would benefit.

6.2   A city that is friendly to walkers

But how was this process of making the city friendly for walkers, cyclists, and users of public transport to be started? And what would 'friendly' mean? The mayor explained to the other delegates of the municipality that 'walker-friendly' should not just be an idea or a concept that everybody would find desirable without taking any further action than simply talking about it and paying lip service to it. No, the city should be 'friendly' in the sense that people would be keen to start walking, and so on.

Maybe not everybody could be encouraged to walk, but many could. After much debate, the majority of the delegates agreed. And thus, a goal was formulated: let us take action to get (many) more people to walk or cycle and/or use public transport (more). It was clear to everybody that in order to achieve this goal, the more unusual forms of transport would have to be made much more normal in the future. And it should be rewarding. Giving up using your car should make you feel good. There should be pleasure when you do it. The delegates realised that people should not feel pressured or shamed into doing this and it should be made as hassle-free as possible for everyone. It should not feel punitive in any way.

The delegates did not underestimate the difficulty involved in weaning people from using their cars. They realised that making the city more walking friendly might cause problems for car drivers but decided not to make this concern their main or initial focus. They decided to begin by looking at how to make walking and cycling much more rewarding for the people of their city and to try to remove any barriers that prevented people from using these means of transport. What could encourage the population to consider walking a pleasure rather than a punishment? Even though they wanted to get people to cycle and use public transport, too, it was decided to start with walking, especially as this was the activity their city name would suggest! So, how could walking be made rewarding so that people would do it more? It is blindingly obvious that many people do not even walk very short distances and may use their car to pop out to their local shop maybe only 100 metres away to buy milk or bread.

6.3   Walking can be a pain in the neck

There is a saying that 'people are different but they are all the same'; I do not know who coined this, but if it is correct, it means that one can ask oneself what one finds frustrating or rewarding to start with. Maybe an obvious way to make the city more inviting for walking is to find out what we find annoying ourselves and to eliminate it and thus improve things.

And we should also find out what makes walking a pleasure, interesting, and rewarding, the mayor said. He realised that even the delegates did not walk much! 'Honestly speaking, we do not walk too much ourselves', he announced. 'So why do we not, as a first step, figure out what keeps us from walking, and where and under which circumstances we enjoy walking or even want to walk instead of any other way of getting about?' The mayor suggested to the delegates that everybody who volunteered should write down what they considered pleasurable when walking and also what they found frustrating. He would also walk more and more conscientiously himself and make notes during the coming weeks and months, in order to register what he, personally, found disturbing on the one hand and when and where walking was a pleasure on the other. He invited everybody to join in these activities, and he asked the assembly whether he was allowed to ask the municipality's employees whether they would volunteer to take part in this project. The majority supported this, and thus the process started.

Long lists of what made walking 'a pain in the neck' were produced, as well as extensive summaries of things and circumstances that made walking a pleasure: materials for a perfect start to a project that they later called 'make Walkington walkable Walkington – mWwW'. But the mayor and the assembly did not confine themselves to following the mayor's idea just by their own observations. Although the mayor's arguments sounded convincing and inspiring, it was thought necessary also to provide some evidence that investing in walking would pay and was really worthwhile. Therefore, to start with, a scientifically educated mobility expert was employed by the municipality, who was to search for and collect all the materials that analysed the consequences of substantially increasing walking: how shops and business were developing according to studies, how people's health was affected, how satisfied citizens were with such changes in the end. One had heard noises that all these things would develop positively, but a more systematic and comprehensive investigation was considered wise. The hired scientist should also elaborate, with the help of relevant literature, on how to achieve this goal: what to do in order to achieve a substantial increase in walking.

He/she would be expected to summarise the written observations of the volunteers in a way that would provide a detailed overview. The expert should be somebody who knew how to make people talk openly and honestly about their experiences. In interviews, people may exaggerate or say things that are not correct, and maybe they do not observe things very thoroughly. After all, many are probably not used to observing certain things and to writing down what they see. People may also say the same things in many different ways, and it is up to the expert to recognise this. For all these reasons, a social psychologist who had been working with transport matters in her own small research institute was appointed. An assistant was also appointed, who was to help with the organisational work. There were meetings where all the volunteers were instructed. They were asked to either write down their observations – what they saw, what they liked, what they disliked – or use a voice recorder. Later, everybody would be invited by the assistant to help him go through all the materials on three or four occasions. This was to ensure that he had read and understood everything correctly. It would also allow for additions and corrections.

Everybody attended their meetings with the assistant, including the mayor. This was very unusual, but this was a large project to which the municipality had given high importance. Therefore, the necessary resources, time, and money were provided and everybody who had volunteered cooperated. Even though not everything written down by the volunteers would really be relevant, most of the information gathered was going to be of use in deciding the future steps to be taken. If there were similarities in the observations, these would, it was hoped, reinforce the evidence to be found in books and articles on the subject. Fine-tuning by asking representative samples of the citizens could be done later.

6.4   Really disturbing preconditions in many respects

So it happened. A large part of the municipality's delegates, and, of course, the mayor himself started walking longer or shorter distances regularly. At that time, many bodyguards who usually went in big black cars used their legs more often, too. Many of the municipality's employees volunteered as well, perhaps more than anybody had expected. And what resulted within a rather short time?

Of course, one wants to be safe as a walker. It is always more pleasant to walk in places where the drivers of motor vehicles cannot endanger you as a pedestrian. When they go slowly, do not restrict your space, and do not force you to wait or to be cautious all the time, things are fine. Walking is much more pleasurable when you do not have to look around constantly and be always on your guard in order not to get knocked over. In a similar vein, level and smooth surfaces without holes, kerbs, or other low obstacles on the ground are much appreciated. Walking is really pleasant only if you do not have to look down at the ground all the time in order not to stumble and fall. Streets and places where you have room to move are good, where pedestrians can walk side by side or in small groups – families, for instance – and where one can pass by pedestrians walking side by side or in small groups coming from the opposite direction without squeezing, stopping, or pushing. Bicycles are fine where there is enough space for both walkers and people on their bikes to be able to move rather freely without proving a nuisance to each other.

Another point was raised by the volunteers. They noticed that there were sometimes items of street furniture such as lamp posts or bollards that got in their way. The placing of dustbins and the tables outside street cafés could also prove to be a problem.

Places that are pleasant for walking are also characterised by their aesthetics, of course. The planners and architects, along with the garden designers, had done a good job there. There were trees providing shade and green patches, benches, alongside delightful façades of houses, some newly painted and attractively decorated. It is always difficult to specify exactly what 'looks nice', what is aesthetically 'well done', but involve artists of all kinds; they know how to do it. Architects and garden planners are often artists, and their artistry was evident in Walkington.

The places that the female volunteers really valued were those where you could walk outside without the slightest hint of fear that anybody would bother you: well-lit open places, paths without hideouts behind bushes or columns, areas that were always full of life. It was noted that being among other people made the female volunteers feel safe.

Parents of children would point out that they loved those places and roads where they did not have to worry that their children would be knocked over by a car. There, car drivers either went slowly or could not go at all; the infrastructure was such that it forced car drivers to be attentive all the time, and those who walked there had the feeling that they could communicate with the car drivers, by eye contact, gestures, and so on. Not many places of that type could be found then, but some did exist.

The conclusions drawn from the investigation carried out with the volunteers revealed that there were indeed things that the municipality of Walkington could do to make walking a more regular and pleasurable experience. There were already some places where walking was good, and these were readily identified. Photographs were taken as well, and some of the comments written down were quite enthusiastic.

The discussion went on to the question of what it was that disturbed or frustrated people when they were outside walking on the roads and about the city, especially when they moved away from the centre towards the outskirts. One answer that came had nothing to do with infrastructure and the design of the public space but was connected to a barrier within people. It was the fact that the comfort of their cars meant that it almost felt stupid to walk. The car stood in front of their door and could take them anywhere easily and without any effort. There were the added comforts of the radio and air conditioning or heaters. There was no need to think how to carry your shopping or how to organise your meetings and obligations at different places in the city. One fact was clear, they said. As a novice pedestrian, you had to use your brain more than usual and you had to spend some time planning and organising your journeys. This was a side issue, of course, though an interesting one: it seems that the comfort and ease of use of the car keep people from walking. Many of the other obstacles to walking more were the flip side of the things that people said made it attractive.

An outstanding concern that would keep people from walking, or from letting their children walk, was that of personal safety. Danger came mainly from car and lorry drivers who drove fast even when pedestrians had to cross the road. On busy pavements, there was always the risk of being pushed into the road by others walking alongside you. The voluntary walkers could not say whether people drove above the speed limit with their cars, but the feeling expressed was that drivers were going 'too fast'. Because of their speed, it seemed that drivers also had difficulties in slowing down and stopping where walkers wanted to cross the road, causing them severe safety problems and long waiting times in places where there were no traffic lights. When there was heavy car traffic, it was almost impossible to cross the road halfway down a block, which made distances for walkers much longer in many cases, because they had to move to the next intersection where there was a pedestrian crossing which would give them the obvious right to cross. But even there crossing was not safe, even though the right of way, at least theoretically, belongs with the pedestrian there.

One would assume that things were better where there were traffic lights. However, those traffic lights were obviously programmed completely to the advantage of drivers. Pedestrians had to wait far too long until the lights turned green, and once they did, the system would allow only a very short time before the lights turned red again. This happened regularly when people were still crossing and even though they knew that they still had the right of way at this time, it made them feel very nervous and afraid. 'Do not get old and slow', it was said, because then crossing becomes impossible in many places. And what should you tell your children? They should not cross when the lights are red, but then they find themselves in the middle of the road when the lights have changed to red. Of course, our children have to differentiate. But parents appreciated that the advice was confusing: 'You may start crossing when the lights are green and you may also finish it when they are already red'.

All of these issues – long waiting times, a short time for crossing, and the lights changing midway through a crossing – caused problems for the pedestrians. These problems need to be solved in a fair way. The volunteers, who by now were beginning to feel like 'walkers', felt very strongly that they were being treated like second-class citizens.

Another issue that was raised was that, as in many other countries and cities, there were problems with car drivers turning right or left at intersections. They frequently had the 'green light' at the same time as the pedestrians trying to cross a road. As a consequence, not even the short time that one had to cross the road remained inviolate. On the contrary, some of the turning drivers did not stop fully but let their car roll on slowly, 'crawling forward' when there were many walkers about. Even at zebra crossings, drivers could often be found encroaching on the crossing as pedestrians crossed the road.

There were many comments regarding safety. The comment of one female employee of the municipality was particularly interesting and reflected the views and comments of others. She lived about 800 m from her workplace.

It would take her about 10 minutes to walk to the office, which she in fact did regularly, she said, because it was a nice walk, partly through a park with trees and flowers and lawns. But when she knew that she would be working late, having dinner in a restaurant near her workplace, or going to a cinema in the vicinity, she would take the car in the morning. The friends whom she met in those evenings had their way home in other directions, and she did not want to walk through the dimly lit park when it was dark. She obviously felt uncomfortable and unsafe about walking home in the dark. She even commented that she would not 'dare'.

Another issue that was often raised was that of ease when walking. There were complaints saying that more space was given to parked cars than to walkers. You walked along rows of vehicles parked recklessly while your own pavement was so narrow that you could not even walk side by side with a colleague. Sometimes you were lucky if there was a pavement at all. People also complained that often lamp posts, traffic signs, rubbish bins, sloppily parked cars, and the like would obstruct their way. Maintenance of pavements was considered poor, and holes and unevenness were frequent. As the period of collecting impressions stretched into wintertime, they also observed that the car lanes were always free from snow, while it took much longer until the pathways were cleared, if that happened at all.

There were also complaints that the layout of roads made walks unnecessarily long in many cases. For instance, there were intersections with no pedestrian crossing provided on one or two branches, and if you were unlucky, you had to cross two or three roads at those intersections in order to reach a destination on the other side. To avoid illegal but direct crossing that would make the route considerably shorter, railings had often been installed. It was observed that sometimes people – especially children – climbed over these in order to reach the other side the shorter way instead of 'walking around in circles' and losing a lot of time waiting at a series of traffic lights.

One delegate reported that in the past, there had been a couple of footpaths leading through courts midblock, thus providing a rather tight network of walks in parts of the city. To his knowledge, many of those passages through the courts were now closed. He had recently tried one and found out that you could not walk there any more. He asked his assistant to find the caretaker and ask him about this matter. The assistant was informed later that the walkways had been closed to the public for safety reasons.

Many of the volunteers, in fact most of them, were not used to walking and so it is no wonder that they had some difficulties finding their way, especially if the trip that they were making was new for them. Either you had to learn using maps (because 20 years ago there was no navigation system for pedestrians on smartphones) or you had to ask somebody, which was only possible when there was someone to ask. By the way, asking people was actually considered quite pleasant by some; it was thought good to have some interaction with other people. In rare cases, the signs that had been put up for car drivers would indicate the way to your own destination. But for car drivers, it would not matter if the way was two or three kilometres longer because such distances are easily covered by car. For a walker, this was definitely not a good solution. Another important point concerning signage for drivers was that there were dead-end streets announced by a traffic sign that in fact were not dead ends for pedestrians. They could pass there. But usually only residents would know of the existence of these short cuts. It would obviously have been a great boon to pedestrians if there had been signs showing that although there was no through way for cars, pedestrians could shorten their journey considerably by using this route.

Some of the volunteers noted how much more affected they were by noise, bad air, or ugly surroundings when they were moving more slowly, which you do as a pedestrian. The constant noise of motor vehicles would really be annoying. This was obviously much more disturbing when the traffic was flowing faster. Streets and places that could look nice lose a lot of their attractiveness with all those parked cars standing around, and as soon as they move, they smell. People realised that all these things looked and felt different when you were sitting in your car, with only short walks to and from it. For those of them who were walking longer distances than others, benches or other seating facilities were lacking. Some had decided to test what a 3-km walk to work would feel like, and especially on their way home, when there was no particular hurry, it would have been pleasant and comfortable to sit down now and then. A male colleague who had broken his hip in a sports accident and had to walk with a cane for a long time particularly emphasised this.

Another topic that is not talked about frequently is toilets. When you walk, you are sometimes out in the street for a longer time, and moving also seems to boost the digestive system. So what to do when you have to use a toilet? People realised that public toilets were lacking or there were too few of them, and when they went into restaurants or bars, they were almost forced to buy a coffee or something else because shop owners obviously disliked people just walking in, using the toilet, and then leaving.

The colleague who walked with a cane had strong opinions concerning the smoothness of surfaces on walkways, the heights of kerbs, flights of steps, pedestrian bridges, tunnels, and the like. When you had difficulties raising your feet – or one of them in his case – you wanted smooth surfaces, kerbs that were as low as possible or no kerbs at all, and road crossings where there was no need to use a tunnel or bridge. If a bridge or a tunnel were absolutely necessary, it should be possible to use them without having to climb steps. He could list a large number of places where people like him had problems. And imagine that there were many people in the city with much worse conditions than him.

Quite a number of observations of the volunteers concerned the weather. Of course, there is nothing you can do to change the weather. But you can protect yourself, and those who govern the city can provide conditions so that citizens can protect themselves, at least better than is the case now. For instance, there could be stands with roofs at all bus and tram stops, and around metro stations there could be more well-covered areas. Some have heard of the tradition – was it in Japan? – of having umbrellas in shops which could be used by everybody. It would be possible to take one and give it back in another shop or in the same shop on the next occasion you were there and it was not raining. Anyway, there are no limits to creativity. Ways to make life more comfortable for people who did not go around protected by a vehicle could certainly be found.

6.5   The psychologist, the engineer, the scientific team

All this work lasted for more or less six months. At the beginning of the year 2000, the psychologist asked to be allowed to address the municipal assembly. There she explained that one could now consult the population of Walkington in order to find out how many of them agreed with the observations of the volunteers. She explained that this was a way to show the relevance of what the mayor, the delegates, and the employees of the municipality had noted. However, she was quite confident that what she held in her hand already gave a clear picture. The results of the experiment were supported by the books and articles on the topic that she had studied extensively since the beginning of the project. So, in her opinion, one could skip asking the citizens at this point. This would take at least another half year and she felt that nothing really new would result from it. If the assembly agreed, she would proceed to summarise the results in a way that allowed for suggestions which could be put to the assembly for action. For this, the experience of an engineer would have to be utilised. The decision taken by the majority of the assembly was to contract an engineer to join in as a member of the scientific expert team.

During the weeks that followed, the engineer, who had extensive experience working in the traffic and transport area, was briefed on the findings of the volunteers' activities by the psychologist and her assistant. Together, they then discussed what the most important issues raised by the 'test pedestrians' were. They were hopeful that they could tackle several of these issues together and find ways to solve a substantial number of problems simultaneously.

6.6   Speed and space

The result of their discussion was that two aspects had to be addressed: speed and space. It appeared obvious that walkers need more space in almost all places and in almost all the streets of the city. At this point, much of the space was taken by parked motor vehicles. At the same time, the vehicle speeds permitted at this time made it necessary to have rather broad car lanes. With lower speeds, the lanes could be narrower. It was clear to them that removing all parked cars from the streets and reducing vehicle speeds would provide a great deal of increased free space for pedestrians and would also allow bicycle lanes to be added, where necessary, as well. This would help to solve one problem that had arisen in recent years. More people had started cycling, but as there was often no space allocated to them, cyclists sometimes used the pavements, or mixed foot and cycle paths were installed that left everybody dissatisfied. Sometimes the space for cycle lanes was taken from former pedestrian walkways. This was obviously unsatisfactory.

The scientific team agreed that suggesting a reduction in vehicle speeds all over the city, removing parked cars from the streets, and taking away space from vehicle traffic to allocate it to walkers and cyclists were really radical steps. If they did not want to fail, they would have to produce a list of arguments, as many and as detailed as possible, that would convince the assembly. And even if the mayor and the delegates were convinced, they would need good arguments when they addressed the citizens in order to explain why such measures had to be taken. The scientific team would have to demonstrate what the advantage of reducing vehicle speeds could be. But they also needed to be very aware of what would be considered disadvantages by many. This was especially important because they expected resistance and obstruction from parts of the population and from certain interest groups, even if the majority of the municipal assembly had approved their proposals. The same opposition would be felt about the reallocation of space, as some would argue that 'it was to the disadvantage of road users', with 'road users' meaning car drivers.

What could be said about speed that sounded convincing? First of all, speed had to do with safety. Everybody who was not sitting in a vehicle would feel less endangered if vehicle speeds were lower. Parents of children would be more confident if people drove more slowly, and they would be less of a danger for their kids. Crossing the street, both at intersections and midblock, would be safer because there would be more time to do so with vehicles moving more slowly. If a car was being driven more slowly, one also had a better chance to see the person in the car and to establish a kind of dialogue. From research literature, the expert team had learned that drivers were more prepared to yield and to stop for pedestrians at lower speeds. Walkers could not only feel safer if car speeds were lower, they would in fact be safer. The experts argued that fewer pedestrians would be hit by cars. Their regular accident statistics would show this. Moreover, if there were a crash, it would happen at a lower speed, causing less damage. Fewer pedestrians would die in such accidents.

Something that was linked to the concept of improved safety was the matter of comfort. At that time it was easy for pedestrians to feel uncomfortable whenever car drivers passed very close by at high speed or when they had to negotiate with them when crossing roads. Lower speeds would provide more comfort in this respect.

The experts were not so sure whether air quality would improve when speeds were reduced. They surmised that it would probably depend on the way a car was driven at a lower speed. People were not so used to driving continuously at 30 km/h or below. Instructions on which gears to choose, how to accelerate, and the like were probably needed. Concerning noise, the experts were positive that its level would be reduced and – with good police enforcement – peak noise levels when people drove their cars very fast would vanish.

Then the possibility of gaining a considerable amount of space was raised. If the limits were reduced to 30 km/hour everywhere in the city and if the police enforced this appropriately, vehicle lane widths could be reduced to the extent that two buses could pass each other at walking speed. On existing roads, this could be done whenever repairs were needed; the pavements could be broadened at the same time and bicycle lanes could be inserted. 'We are talking about square kilometres here that can be made better use of', the engineer was quoted as saying. In addition, pedestrian bridges could be replaced by crossings at surface level, because walkers disliked those bridges. Tunnels/subways for pedestrians could be complemented by zebra crossings on the surface so that everybody who did not want to buy anything in the shops in the subway could cross there. People who had physical difficulties with walking would be grateful. Road maintenance costs could go down with lower speeds on narrower lanes, helping the city to save money.

I do not know in which way these arguments were presented to the city council. It was certainly done in a professional and detailed manner. We citizens would read about those things in the newspapers which were involved in the public discussions of the city's plans from the beginning. Luckily, the journalists of the most important media were not biased in any direction and they reported both the pros and the cons of the development that the city was taking with regard to its transport policies in a balanced way. This was also the case with the issue of space as far as cars parking on the road were concerned. The experts argued that parked cars took up more space than all the areas dedicated to walking and the few bicycle lanes and paths together. It was therefore suggested to take measures to change this situation.

According to the law, one garage per apartment or per house had to be provided. Maybe in the past the idea had been 'one garage per family' for the family car. The problem was that by now many families had more than one car. One of them would stand in the garage when not being used. The others would be parked on the road somewhere. Car parks did exist, but not so many in the areas where people had their houses and flats, away from the centre. In the centre and near the centre, the multi-storey car parks were half empty because parking on the roadside was allowed. It was not always easy to find a space, but drivers spent time in order to find a place that would get them as near as possible to their goal. Walking distance should be kept to a minimum.

6.7 Opposition and arguments

As expected, strong objections regarding all these arguments came from those who opposed the changes in their municipality's transport strategy. Generally, the minority in the city council that was against the changes argued that they were not objecting to improvements for walkers. But they were against achieving such a goal 'to the disadvantage of working people who needed to go about their jobs'. Without those hard-working citizens, the economy of the municipality would not flourish. They considered the two main suggestions 'crazy'. The plan of a general speed limit was considered outrageous. The time losses would be atrocious, the media wrote. And to consider taking away all parked cars from the road network lacked logic in their eyes. Where would everybody who had to come to work by car park it? And where should the families with more cars leave vehicles when everybody came home and there was only one garage in their house or in a few places two, while the mother, father, and the grown-up children all needed their cars for their daily lives and had to park them somewhere?

The experts were well prepared for most of these arguments. They responded to them in detail and had also produced leaflets reiterating what they were saying. Those leaflets were distributed to the newspapers in order to make sure that there were no misunderstandings when they were quoted. Concerning speeds, they argued that if one measured all days and nights and in all the streets and places in the city, an average speed of motor vehicles of below 30 km/h resulted. The reason was that the streets were often congested and stop-and-go traffic was the norm as a result. Dense queues moved slowly or very slowly during peak hours, often way below 30 km/h. As soon as people had a chance, they pushed their accelerator hard in order to 'regain time'. This means that the speed was then often far above the permitted limits. This driving behaviour led to many of the problems the team had already outlined.

There was also something mathematical about the different speed levels that the prevailing speed limit – usually 50 km/h – allowed. As far as I could understand, the heterogeneity of speeds had negative effects on the capacity of the road network. They wrote in their leaflet that a strictly enforced maximum speed of motor vehicles of 30 km/h would lead to net time gains, that is, time advantages for the total population of the vehicle drivers. This was due, not least, to the fact that many vehicles from side roads would need less time to join major traffic routes. Not many citizens would understand these arguments, but the engineers referred to sound mathematical models that had been tested in practice, and they explained things plausibly. On the other hand, if a single car driver had 10 km of free road ahead of him or her – a total illusion, of course – and could only drive at 30 km/h instead of 50, how much time would he or she lose? The result was a mere eight minutes. This was in an ideal situation, and even there the damage caused by a lower speed was obviously not overwhelming. Of course, the opponents argued, 'yes, but calculate eight minutes × 300,000 drivers and you will arrive at a tremendous time loss of 40,000 hours'.

The experts countered that this assumed time loss was based on an unrealistic assumption of everybody having free roads ahead, and in reality it was the net effect that counted. If a net gain in time for the total population of vehicle drivers was to be expected, then this should be the fact that determined the assembly's decision. Concerning the individual loss that every individual driver had in mind, the experts claimed that there would also be benefits for the drivers, such as reduced stress with more relaxed attitudes. As soon as a habit had developed, everybody would find it normal to drive more slowly. The problems were always there before such a measure was implemented and during the first weeks or months. After a year or so, and if the plans were really enforced, nobody would complain any more, and the advantages of the change would become visible, not least when vehicle drivers became walkers themselves after having parked their cars.

The opponents did not believe all these arguments and went on criticising the plan to make parking in the streets impossible even more vehemently. Even in this case, the expert team had prepared arguments which they presented to the assembly and also in leaflets to be distributed to the media. The issue was complicated and solutions to this problem would cost money, they said. Mainly, more multi-storey car parks would be needed. But the costs would partly be covered by the fees car owners would have to pay for parking, although it was suggested that those should be moderate. In addition, the experts assumed that local shops and retailers would sell more because more people were walking from the parking space to their destinations and vice versa. They had found several pieces of research and documentation from other places that indicated that local business improved when there was more footfall in the area. This would lead to an increase in tax income, including municipal taxes.

6.8   The test site: Acatia

However, one could never say for sure whether experiences from other cities and other countries would be good predictors of exactly how things developed in one's own city. Therefore, the expert team came up with an interesting suggestion. In the city district called Acatia, extensive road maintenance works were planned for the upcoming months. In addition, a larger shopping mall and a hotel were going to be built. This was a perfect test site to decide whether mWwW – remember: make Walkington walkable Walkington – could work in the way expected. The people of the department in charge should get in contact with the consortia of the shopping mall and the hotel. After lengthy discussions, they received permission from the city council to offer some financial support – tax reductions – if they added areas, one or two floors, for parking, or even more if planning and architectural preconditions allowed it. They could install an electronic system that made it possible to differentiate between customers of the hotel and of the mall, who would park for free, and others, who would have to pay a charge. Thus, a considerable number of parking places would be provided. At the same time, the road maintenance work in the district should be seen as an opportunity to redesign the roads. Car lanes could be narrowed or even, in some cases, removed where a traffic census showed this was possible. The pedestrian areas could be enlarged and refurbished. The delivery areas would need to be preserved and, where necessary, cycle lanes could be inserted. When car speeds were low, cyclists could use the car lanes in those streets where car traffic was not that dense. During the construction works, parking was not possible anyway, and by the end of the year, both the hotel and shopping mall and maintenance work were to be finished.

Even if, as the optimists expected, things worked out nicely in the end, it was clear that there would be chaos in the meantime. It was obvious that the business of local retailers would suffer during the construction. People who worked or had other business in the area would have considerable difficulties in reaching their destinations. But the greatest effect would be on the local residents. So once the decision to proceed with this scheme had been made and in order to use Acatia as a sort of a large guinea pig, the psychologist and his assistant started an information campaign. They had been allowed to employ more personnel for one year to meet the demands of this campaign. These helpers were students from the Institute for Communication of the University of Walkington. They would collect practical experience and earn an acceptable sum of money. It was also negotiated with the University of Walkington that they should get points towards their degree courses for this practical work. All of the local media, newspapers, and the radio station were provided with the necessary background information to help them to promote the campaign. On top of this, every household, company, shop, and institute in the Acatia district received leaflets outlining the reasons for the disturbance and detailed explanations of why all this was happening. So much fuss only to support walking? Yes, but a number of advantages should result for everyone, in the end: improved business in the area, more places to relax, more cafés, more green patches, and even some small parks would be forthcoming. This should lead to a better quality of life for everyone in the area. There was no doubt that there would be short-term disruption, but in the end there would be huge improvements. The psychologist and the communication students put a lot of work and effort into formulating their campaign and explaining things in a most convincing way. I can remember that I read some of the letters to households, although I am not resident in Acatia and don't work there. But as some of those letters were printed in the newspapers, everybody could see them, and I thought that the texts were top quality and convincing, and so did many of my friends.

I heard that the students produced prototypes of the leaflets they were going to distribute and then invited comments from members of the public as to how effective and informative they were. The campaign materials were also sent to their university lecturers for their input. All this explains why the information forwarded to the public was so well accepted and worked effectively.

During this time of chaos and explaining the chaos, one aggravating event took place: the elections for most of the local governments in the country, that is, the municipal elections. The opposition shouted out loud that the existing city council should be voted out because of all the mess it had caused. Earlier, some members of the ruling parties had recommended that the work should be postponed until after the elections. They did not do this in public, but the media were informed by sources that they would not reveal that it had happened. In any case, the municipal government did not change its decision and decided to go ahead with the project. They firmly believed that what they planned was good for the city, and they did everything to convince the citizens that this was the case. In the end, right in the middle of all the construction work, with all the dirt and dust and lack of parking space, the government was returned, but with a much-reduced majority, while the opposition achieved an all-time high. A lot of explanations followed as to how this could have happened, but whatever, the project to mWwW was able to continue.

6.9   The first round of measures and their effects

The engineer and two colleagues who had been employed in the meantime worked closely with the department of the municipality responsible for road planning, construction, and maintenance. They saw to it that the comments made by the volunteers in the first phase of the project were taken into account as far as possible. The involvement of the city architect made sure that all the aspects concerning aesthetics would also be taken into account and acted upon. Walkway surfaces should be smooth without potholes, and the kerbs separating the walkways from the vehicle lanes or from the cycle path, where there was one, were to be kept low and should be reduced to almost zero where walkers crossed the road (I was told that there should still be a very small kerb so that visually impaired walkers could feel this either with their feet or with a walking stick.) Trees were planted in such a way that they would not reduce the space provided for pedestrians but would enhance the area. Also, lamp posts and traffic signs were placed right at the edge of the pavements so that they did not impede the pedestrians. Benches were put in between the trees, and green patches and flowerpots were positioned where this was considered feasible by the architect and by the garden department.

And toilets were also installed. It was not easy to find places for them and to decide on ways of maintaining them and keeping them clean. I read in the papers that there was quite some discussion about these things. In the end, the problem was solved. Some new toilets were built and contracts were made with some owners of cafés who would allow passers-by in need to use the toilets for a moderate fee, and they would also announce this outside so that people looking for a toilet would be aware if a café was part of this scheme. (Later it turned out that the 'toilet business' would draw some new customers. 'Have a coffee and a sh…' was the joke that was frequently heard at that time).

The engineer's team focused quite a lot on the intersections, which also had to be reshaped while the roads were being reconstructed. First of all, mini-roundabouts were installed at smaller intersections with lower traffic volumes, where they replaced traffic lights. According to what was known at that time and is still valid today, mini-roundabouts save waiting times for all traffic streams from every direction. They allow zebra crossings to be placed on all the roads without causing detours for walkers. They also had an additional speed-reducing effect, and there were aesthetic elements too, as they are much nicer to look at than traffic lights. Still, both at traditional intersections with or without traffic lights and at the mini-roundabouts, the problem of motor vehicles turning right, and thereby having to drive over the zebra crossing while pedestrians were using it, remained. It would, of course, be mitigated by the considerably lower speeds that were expected in the future, but additional measures were nevertheless thought necessary. What we eventually saw was a mixture of measures. In some places, they put humps before the pedestrian crossings; in other cases, they raised the pedestrian crossings; and at some smaller intersections, the intersection plateaus were elevated altogether. I do not know the principles that were applied in order to decide which measure should be chosen. What the whole city knows by now, many years later, is that these measures worked tremendously well. The number of pedestrians killed at intersections is zero now, and has been for many years, and everybody that you ask would say that it is really comfortable to cross roads nowadays. People old enough to remember how it was earlier say that 'nothing compares to the situation today'.

The roadworks in Acatia started in May or June 2001, approximately one year after the mayor's proposal to mWwW, and it took one year until everything was more or less finished, though in some places the work was not completely finished, because restructuring the road network the way it was planned in Acatia was obviously taking longer than regular maintenance work. They would not shut down all the roads at the same time, and in many places they had to keep temporary vehicle lanes and walkways open while working. Life in Acatia had to go on and citizens had to move about for their daily errands. A lot of people parked their cars outside Acatia during that time, and many of them had to walk longer distances than usual and under rather poor conditions. But as Acatia is a small district, most of the distances could, in fact, be covered rather easily by walking. The neighbouring districts suffered under the burden of increased parking pressure. Perhaps this also had a paradoxical effect, namely that citizens undoubtedly became more aware of how much parked cars interfere with a good quality of life in the city.

Anyway, both in Acatia and in the neighbouring districts, there were many complaints. In the neighbouring districts, citizens were annoyed by the fact that the streets were more full than ever with parked vehicles, and in Acatia, they complained about long walking distances, about 'murderous' walking conditions, about dirt and dust everywhere, and about noise from the workers and all the machines, starting at seven in the morning and ending at six in the evening. In many places and on many occasions, work went on during the night, so that traffic on the provisional facilities was possible during the day. However, there were not as many complaints as many had feared. There was no 'revolution' by the citizens which some of the opposition parties had predicted and hoped for.

In the summer of 2002, most of the work was done, the hotel parking and the parking at the shopping mall were also completed, and life could go back to almost normal. But what is normal? There were no parked cars in the streets any more; they had to be left in the new parking facilities in the hotel and the mall, and the two multi-storey car parks that existed formerly were now full. Many people working in Acatia and many residents hurried to get yearly parking passes and place reservations so they would not have to bother to find a place and they could save some money as well. The speed limits were rigorously kept to by car drivers; speed cameras and police officers who were visible in the streets saw to that. Walking distances were longer now for many people, but even under the not fully finalised conditions, walking, even for 15 or 20 minutes, was not really a burden now, I heard people say. It was interesting that folks from other parts of the city came to Acatia, many of them by bus, tram, or metro, because 'you cannot park your car in Acatia'. They came in order to see and experience this 'city with a totally new quality', as it was labelled by the media.

6.10 Countings are necessary; the opinions of the citizens need to be reflected quantitatively

Some comments by the opposition parties or by citizens who were against the changes criticised the media and the information materials provided by the municipality. They said that they reported only the positive comments, but in reality there was strong opposition to all those 'ridiculous changes'. Now it turned out that it had been a mistake not to ask the citizens, and especially those of Acatia, beforehand to assess the conditions for walkers in the same way as had been carried out in the first phase of the plan. But fortunately, between the decision of the city council to use Acatia as a 'pilot city' and the start of the roadworks, there had been time for thorough recording of the number of pedestrians. They were counted along streets, at road intersections, on the squares, and at the main public transport stops.

They were also counted at two metro stations and several bus and tram stops. These censuses took place in March and April 2001. The main bulk of the work was completed in the summer of 2002, with minor tidying up and the addition of some aesthetic parts continuing into the autumn. The 'new' traffic system flowed quite well from the beginning of August. It was agreed that a second pedestrian census to compare with those from the year before should be carried out in September and October 2002. It was hoped that the weather in September and October would not be too different from the weather in March and April the year before and the results at that time would already be starting to reflect a positive change in the attitude of the citizens to the new situation.

The census in September and October took place. There were also face-to-face interviews with people at the roadside, and questionnaires were sent to all the households in Acatia. The team of experts realised that they had made a serious mistake by not distributing such forms before the changes that were implemented during the last year. In the media, the expert team explained that at that time they felt confident that they would not miss important points, as they felt that the information gathered by the test walkers was more than adequate. They did admit, however, that it would have been a good move if they had had information and opinions from the people of Acatia before they began the work there. This would have made it possible to compare the conditions for walkers from before and after all those changes directly.

However, they did find a way to compare them indirectly. They asked who had been walking regularly in Acatia before the restructuring and who had not. Then, those who had not walked previously should simply answer questions concerning all the positive and negative aspects which had been listed. The questions were formulated in such a way that one could easily express the degree to which one agreed or disagreed that observation X made by the test walkers really was positive or that critical aspect Y really was negative. Those people who had walked there before the changes were asked to answer additional questions which expanded on these points. Did they think that the things which had been commented upon originally had changed for the better or the worse, and by how much?

The results of the censuses revealed that there were more people walking in Acatia than before the changes. The increase was not huge, though, and this left both the expert and the city council a little disappointed. The media reports were fairly positive about this increase, but they did question whether all the efforts made in Acatia were 'much ado about little', citing Shakespeare not quite exactly. The results of the evaluation of the questionnaire, which were published some weeks later, were more satisfying, however. Those people who had not walked before – not very many, it was said – had not encountered many of the problems that the test walkers initially reported. For example, feeling unsafe when crossing the road at an intersection was considered a minor problem. At the same time, the elements that had been mentioned in a positive sense by the test walkers were recognised and appreciated by them as well.

6.11 Media involvement is essential

The majority of the interview sample that responded to the questionnaire had been walking in Acatia before. They said that they walked more and longer distances now and that, overall, walking was much more pleasant after the changes. In their opinion, all the aspects that the volunteers had highlighted had improved. Although many of the respondents had walked before, there were no regular longer-distance walkers. Most of them referred to shorter walks to and from their car or from their workplace to a lunch venue or the like. They were usually car drivers. Thus it was a nice surprise that a majority, even if a small one, appreciated the two most radical measures – reducing the speed limit and eliminating parking cars on the street. The media reported the result of the questionnaire survey and printed the questionnaire form. I heard that there were people from other parts of the city who came to Acatia for a visit and filled in the questionnaire just for themselves. Residents of Acatia were asked to write down stories of their own experiences of walking in Acatia and to send those stories to the newspapers. Many stories came in, and a lot of them were printed. The media stressed that there was no bias when they selected these stories. In general, most of the stories were positive, and only a few were really critical. The critical ones mainly complained that using the car had been made very difficult and they could not understand why the municipality could not find other ways to enhance walking. Some even questioned the value of walking in the first place.

But among the positive comments and friendly stories in the newspapers, there was still also some criticism. People still wanted further improvements to be made. Some people pointed out in their questionnaire responses that it was still difficult for women if they were out in the evening because in many places there were no other people walking about. During the day, it was OK but after office hours, in many places, hardly anybody took a walk. Where there were cafés, restaurants, and shops with long opening hours, or other places that people would go to in the evening and where there were lights and signs of life, women felt safe. But where there were none of these facilities, the streets were quiet and one was often alone when it became dark. Moreover, so far, the municipality was focused on restructuring the roads, reducing speeds, and providing more space for walkers by eliminating parked cars from the streets. But the buildings along the roads had not been touched. Corners, columns, and other structures where someone could hide had remained unchanged. Gardens and parks could also make people afraid that somebody was hiding. Some men thought that the women were overreacting. But the fact is that women expressed feelings which would probably keep some of them from walking in the evening and make them take the car in the morning when they had plans for what to do after work. There were discussions about this issue in the media, and the city council made it clear that the experiences from Acatia would be made use of and solutions would be looked for during the next steps of the mWwW project.

Other comments referred to schoolchildren. The impression seemed to be that not much had changed concerning what was called the 'mama-taxi'. Many children were still brought to school by car. So the arguments why this was not good were repeated. By this time, it was generally accepted that children had too little physical exercise and were sitting about too much. Walking or cycling to school would provide a very good opportunity for schoolchildren to have some daily exercise. The counter-argument to this was that even though car speeds were lower now, motor vehicle drivers still constituted a severe danger for children who came to school on foot. In reaction to the comments that the situation in front of schools had not changed, the media asked the public for their comments on this issue, and citizens commented quite extensively. It was agreed that it was still too easy to drive one's car right up to the front of the school. Some arguments also referred to the organisation of daily activities and errands based on the use of the car that had become a habit for some people over many years. You would drop your child at school, continue to your workplace and, after work, drive to the supermarket to buy food and other essentials, then fetch your children from afternoon care and drive home. It seemed difficult to solve this problem. To let the children walk to school by themselves when you drove to work with the car, often even passing the school, would be a strange thing to do, wouldn't it? Of course, starting a discussion with the children that physical exercise was essential and that walking to school was the easiest way to get physical exercise was a step in the right direction. However, it was also pointed out that many parents were not really good models in this case. They would not walk but go by car in spite of needing exercise themselves. Lots of adults did use a gym but travelled there by car!

There was an interesting issue concerning the supermarket. Why would one have to drive to the supermarket? The answer to this question was that there were hardly any shops in the vicinity of where people lived, or at least not so near that they could easily be reached by walking. Most corner shops had vanished over the years and had been replaced by a few bigger supermarkets with parking facilities in front of them. Therefore, it was much more convenient to travel by car.

There was also another question around the disappearance of the corner shops. The fewer shops there were, the less lively the streets became. Or had it been the other way around? Could it be said that as fewer people moved about in the streets as walkers, those shops had fewer customers? Anyway, their vanishing contributed to the fact that the streets looked darker in the late evenings, as quite a lot of those shops had stayed open until late in the past. Less light and fewer walkers in the evening and at night made some women abstain from walking when it was dark. At the same time, the lack of shops for daily groceries probably made quite a lot of residents use their car instead of walking.

There you have one of the factors that lie both behind the increasing use of the mama-taxi and the avoidance of walks by women when it was dark. For some time, this was also pointed out in the media, which reminded readers of the third group that was affected by the lack of shops, among other things. In spite of the huge improvements made to the ease of walking, people continued to comment on this. It was much more comfortable to be outside now for older people and for people with disabilities, and even to walk longer distances. Even when you had to use a walking aid, life outside was much easier now. But the question was, where you should go? Of course, being able to leave your apartment and to go out is great and walking for pleasure is fun. But many older people argued in their letters to the media that in former times you could get 'everything' in the vicinity of your home: food, clothes, tools for the household, even washing machines, refrigerators, vacuum cleaners, and the like. Bookshops were also usual. There was also the local hairdresser, the beautician, and, quite importantly, there were all the cafés and restaurants. There were often several to choose from and none of them were far away. Both the physical and the social necessities of life could be found 'around the corner'.

Once again, there was a good deal of discussion in the media. Some opined that since everybody went by car now, there were no more customers for the local services. Others thought that the opposite was true; since there were no more suppliers in the vicinity, people had to use their car. Whatever, the lack of shopping, service, and entertainment facilities in many of the streets and places of Acatia was obvious. The further away from the city centre you got, the fewer the facilities. The people from the municipality acknowledged that this was a real problem. That was one of the many things they had learned by using Acatia as a guinea pig. It would not be so easy to find solutions, but the search for them started immediately. As many of the buildings in Acatia belonged to the city, they started offering sites that could be used for setting up small businesses for a reduced rent so that people would dare to start such businesses. House owners were contacted and asked whether they would be prepared to allow small shops or businesses to be opened in the ground floors of their buildings. When these were officially dedicated for housing only by law, such laws could be changed. Also, and most importantly, empty properties, which often looked ugly with their windows and doors boarded up and looked dark and foreboding at night, should be revitalised. The city supported such activities by helping those who started businesses to get cheap loans and to negotiate for sensibly low rents, at least for the first year or the first two years of their business. Within half a year or so, quite a lot of shops, cafés, bookshops, hairdressers, and shops that sold smaller household items reopened.

During the same period of time, the gardening department worked on trees and bushes along the streets, with the intention of reducing hiding places and blind spots. Bushes were cut down so that one could see over them, and the lower branches of some trees were removed. The municipality could not, of course, remove all the corners and other possible hiding places around buildings. However, they did improve the lighting in dark places.

6.12 Another census and the conclusions drawn

After more or less half a year, a new round of questionnaires were sent out and the media again asked the citizens to comment. At the same time, pedestrians were counted. That was in March or April 2003. The questionnaire results showed that the assessment of all the changes was positive and even better than that in the autumn of 2002. The measures to boost local business were commented on positively, both in the questionnaires and in the newspapers. The general consensus was that things were 'not perfect but much better'. Even the most radical measures – reducing the speed limit and taking away the parked cars from the streets – were regarded significantly better now than in the autumn of 2002. A very clear majority of the citizens of Acatia supported the municipality's activities. The census showed a further increase in the number of walkers in all the places where counting was done. One disappointment was that the number of children brought to school by car did not really go down.

There were long discussions in the city council at that time. Were the results achieved in Acatia by all the measures to enhance walking good enough? Did the council feel sufficiently sure about what to change in the rest of the city and how to proceed in this? Was everybody positive that there would be support for all the envisaged changes from a substantial majority of the citizens of Walkington? Were the experiences regarding the boosting of local business and gastronomy clear enough, or was the time period of half a year too short and was what had happened only a strawfire? The conclusion was that the results achieved in Acatia were good or very good, in fact. What had been learned would help enormously when the municipality started activities in the rest of the city.

The problems with the 'dark corners' and with lighting could be solved. As far as the trips to school were concerned, in no way did the results indicate that the general measures to enhance walking were useless. In fact, those parents whose children walked or cycled to school by themselves assessed what had been done quite positively. The psychologist who convened the expert team said in an interview at the local radio station that in the future, cooperation with the schools would be started and that experiences from other cities and countries showed that this brought about good results. However, it would also be necessary to be patient. Many people, in fact, 'most of us', she said, had developed routines and habits. Especially those habits concerning more complicated daily routines, like those including taking and fetching children, going to work, and looking after all the supply activities for our households help us to do these things without too much effort. Thus, it is not easy to change habits. 'Habits are like steel ropes, both in a positive and in a negative sense', the psychologist said.

All the measures that had been taken so far had positive results. There was no doubt that reducing vehicle speeds and eliminating parked cars from the streets were prize-winning measures. But in addition, it was necessary to address the citizens using campaigns and other contacts, she said, and also to ask them for their opinions, needs, and expectations more regularly from now on.

To start with, all the citizens of the rest of the city of Walkington were asked to fill in the same questionnaire as the one used in Acatia to assess the conditions for walking in their part of the city. I do not remember any figures, but the media wrote that 'many' had answered the questionnaire and that the situation in the rest of the city was perceived as being much worse than in Acatia, where the questionnaire had been answered twice after measures had been taken. However, citizens in the rest of Walkington had not been asked yet what they thought of the measures taken in Acatia. The reason was that the mayor and the city council wanted to have support from the citizens for what they planned to do. The mistake of not involving the citizens at an early stage was not to be repeated.

6.13   The referendum: The city says Yes

So in the spring of 2003, a referendum was carried out in Walkington, and the city council announced that this referendum should be binding. The text that accompanied the referendum described very simply, but clearly, what had been done in Acatia, outlining the radical measures concerning speed and space. The text also explained that these measures had been assessed positively in Acatia and even more so after a certain time during which the citizens there had become accustomed to the new situation. The question that was asked in the referendum was whether the respondent was in favour of the same measures being taken in the rest of the city. There was a simple question to which one could only answer yes, no, or undecided.

Before I tell you the result, I have to remind you that the local radio station and the local newspapers are, of course, not 'local' just for Acatia but for all of Walkington. Thus, the whole city had followed what happened there. They knew about the measures even without reading the text of the referendum thoroughly. They were aware of the criticisms that had been sent to the newspapers, but they had also learned that the citizens in Acatia generally approved of the changes that had been made. All this explains the result, which was a narrow 'Yes'. It was as narrow as it could be, by half a percentage point or so. I myself was, as many others were, convinced that the citizens would reject the plans. When it comes to walking, I was neutral because I am a cyclist and thus belong to the group that has to rely the least on walking. But as the planned activities promised also to bring about some improvements for cyclists, I voted 'Yes'. But I had heard many critical comments in my own area, and especially during the final weeks, the opposition left no stone unturned in order to prevent a 'Yes'. They commented in broadcasts and other media and placed wall posters everywhere. They painted a very black picture of what would result. It would take longer to get to work, organising one's day would be much more difficult, the costs of the car would increase dramatically because of the fees that had to be paid for parking, shopping would become much more complicated, business would suffer, and so on and so forth. The discussions among those in favour and those against the measures became very lively and somewhat aggressive. There were even serious quarrels within families, as I experienced myself. Anyway, 'It is a Yes', the mayor was able to announce happily. On the television, one could clearly see the relief on his face. Asking the citizens had been a risk, but it had paid off. Not asking them could have been an even bigger risk in the long run, some said.

6.14   Measures: Finalise the plans

By the end of the year 2003, as a Christmas gift to the city, the decision to move on to measures to mWwW according to the original plan was taken by the city council. During the first phase of the work, the expert team should develop an agenda together with the responsible institution of the municipality: how to start, where to start, how to organise the work, and how to manage the traffic during the inevitably long transition phase during which chaos would prevail in many respects. Life had to go on during this time.

At the beginning of 2004, with the whole project in front of them, it felt like the task of Sysiphos. After some weeks of the year had passed, the municipality finally came up with some information as to how they planned to manage this task. Two to three districts of those remaining should be adapted per year. Together with Acatia, there were 14 of them. So it was calculated that all the work would be finished within five years (in a little more than four years, there would be elections again). The same principles should be applied in all districts, the two leading ones being to eliminate the parking of cars in the streets, thus providing space for walkers (and cyclists), and to reduce speed limits to a rigorously enforced maximum of 30 km/h all over the city. The psychologist and her team explained in a number of media interviews that at the beginning, every infringement of the limit had to be punished immediately because only then would car drivers develop the habit of driving slowly.

Concerning the 30-km/h limit, a new discussion arose very soon, this time with respect to the larger roads with heavy traffic, such as those leading out of the city to the highways which connected Walkington with other towns. Wasn't it ridiculous to force all those many car drivers to drive at 30 km/h on those larger roads that, for many, were the starting point for a long journey? The first answer of the city council's spokesperson on the television was a question. Did everybody know how many people lived along those roads? The answer to this rhetorical question followed immediately, and I hope that I remember correctly that between 15% and 20% of the citizens of Walkington (and also of other cities), depending on how you count it, lived there. Often there were smaller apartments there; the housing was cheaper and people with lower incomes resided there. Heavy traffic along those roads reduced the quality of life, which led to lower prices of land and to lower rents. Thus, leaving the situation there as it was now meant that large numbers of citizens with lower incomes would be excluded from the improvements provided for the other roads and places in Walkington. Some people argued that traffic moving more slowly could increase the levels of pollution in these areas. The logic of their thinking was that if cars moved more slowly, they would be driving there for a longer time and thus produce more polluting gases. Various differing and often quite complex arguments followed. According to what was known at that time, air pollution would be reduced in spite of the cars driving along those streets at a lower speed being there for longer. This had something to do with pollutants that increased exponentially with the speeds of vehicles. Many people, like me, did not fully understand all those arguments. But the plan of the city was to measure air quality over a longer period and at many spots and thus to make sure that they did not produce new problems by something that was originally planned to be done in order to reduce them.

Some other things were also clear: the noise level would definitely go down on those larger streets when nobody could drive faster than 30 km/h; and what was more, safety would be improved significantly. It was hoped that traffic fatalities could be eliminated. Lane width would be reduced, and the space originally used for parking cars would now provide more room for pedestrians to move more freely and allow bicycle lanes to be introduced. Moreover, this new space would also give the municipality the opportunity to make the areas more aesthetically pleasing.

The lane widths on larger roads were intended to be somewhat broader, though, than the absolute minimum that had been used in the pilot scheme, as these roads were used by more lorries and buses and it was necessary for them to pass each other whilst still maintaining their speed. The only exception to the 30 km/h limit was the motorway that crossed the city coming from the west and splitting into two branches, one leading to the north and the other one leading in a southeasterly direction. There, the limit would be 80 km/h. The restructuring of all roads should otherwise be similar to Acatia. Where possible, traditional intersections were to be replaced by roundabouts, and where they remained, with or without traffic lights, measures should be taken to allow pedestrians to cross both, comfortably and safely.

These plans caused a discussion about 'loss of time' for road users again. Not only would the speeds be limited, but at intersections, one would lose further time because of 'all those barriers'. The municipality, together with the expert team, produced information materials for all of the media. They repeated their arguments from earlier that those who drove in a straight line without turning off would take more time, of course. However, it was likely that the traffic lights being replaced by roundabouts would mean that some of the lost speed could be made up. On the other hand, according to all of the evidence gleaned from the changes to Acatia and other studies that looked at speed reduction, the use of mini-roundabouts, elevated zebra crossings, and the like showed that there was a net gain for all road users. For instance, vehicle drivers from minor roads would take less time to enter major ones, as already stated. Most importantly, though, walkers would lose less time when crossing roads. 'Pedestrians are road users' and 'The time of walkers is as valuable as the time of car drivers', they declared.

The kerbs of pavements were to be reduced to a minimum at intersections, making it possible for people with walking difficulties, with walking aids, or with prams to move over them easily, while some structures still remained that helped people with visual impairments to find their way. In order to give additional help to these citizens, traffic lights were equipped with sound signals, indicating when it was safe to cross.

The interactions with schools started immediately in the year 2004, and the plans concerning students' journeys to schools were drawn up together with representatives of schools. Where possible, all through traffic in front of schools should be excluded. If parents brought their children by car, they would have to stop and let them get out some 100 or more metres away from the entrance. Maps displaying safe walking and cycle routes to the schools would be produced and distributed to households. As most children under ten lived within a kilometre of their school, it was possible to have these tailor-made to fit local schools. In addition, information was prepared that was addressed to all car drivers and that, it was thought, should not wait until the changes in the districts or in all of Walkington were implemented. It asked all citizens of Walkington who drove a car whether they 'agree that it is ridiculous that children have to take care of grown-up car drivers in order to be safe. Shouldn't that be the other way round?' Those car drivers who thought that traffic education courses were needed should attend one. Especially this last comment was seen as provocation by many, and there was a heated discussion again. It was said that the municipality was discriminating against car drivers. But the answer was that it was unacceptable that every year children who were walking to school – an ever-decreasing number anyway – were injured and even killed by car drivers. Moreover, more children were injured and killed as passengers in cars than as pedestrians and cyclists, another reason to address drivers and not the children.

Women who were uneasy when being out in the evenings as walkers were reassured by the promise that all existing know-how would be applied in order to make the lighting in the city more efficient so that there were fewer dark corners. Trees and bushes along walkways would be cut in such a way that they could not easily serve as hiding places. New buildings should be constructed in such a way as to provide open and free views and perspectives for pedestrians. The regulations for buildings and constructions allowed the authorities to impose such regulations. But I think that the details of those regulations were less important than the fact that a lively discussion had started about the question as to why such measures were necessary at all and that women felt that their fears and feelings concerning the use of the public space were taken seriously.

With respect to the goal of boosting local businesses, especially gastronomy and shops open until late, the same policy as in Acatia would be applied. There the development looked promising, although not even a year had passed since steps had been taken. It was still possible that the success stories of Acatia were only a flash in the pan and would not last. But, 'while working we will learn', they said, and if things did not turn out well, the plans could be changed on the way. One difficult thing to do was to reopen courtyards for pedestrians to walk through them. In former times, many of those courtyards could be entered and exited from more than one side, thus contributing to a tight network of walkways. Then most of them had been closed to the public step by step. People there wanted their privacy; it was argued that 'you do not know who goes there'. Maybe people were afraid of theft and harassment. Anyway, things had worked without many problems in former times, so why shouldn't it be possible to reinstate those courtyards in the walking network nowadays? This had not been done in Acatia, and thus there were no experiences from there to indicate how to proceed. It was decided that this matter should not interfere with the other work in the districts. The team of experts were going to have to break new ground in this respect and work out a plan to reinstate the courtyards. They would have to decide how to address the owners or the people responsible for them and what to offer them as an incentive to reopen the pathways. They would also need to consider what to do to make those places attractive, both for the people who walked through and for those who lived there, once they had been reopened. The newspapers pointed out that there were very good experiences from other cities. Photographs with attractive-looking passages through building blocks with shops and with flowers and interviews with happy residents were published.

Other steps to make the network of walkways tighter were easier and included in the plans right away: there should be more ways to cross both the motorways and the railway lines in the city (there are five of them). This should be done by raising bridges that had steps, spiral ramps to be used by cyclists, and lifts for people who had difficulties with walking or could not walk. There were complaints by the opposition about the 'tremendous costs of all this nonsense'. The clever move on the part of those responsible for the municipality at this point was to let economists compare the price of all those 'goodies for non-motorised citizens', as some of the papers called them, with the price of one kilometre of motorway. The economists showed that the motorway was more expensive. There were also many comments about the fact that it was the car drivers who paid taxes, whilst the cyclists and walkers did not. As a reaction to that, the economists came up with a detailed list of the costs connected to the organisation of car traffic. I do not remember in detail what this list contained, but the astonished public learned that only a small part of those costs was covered by the dedicated taxes paid by car drivers, while the rest had to be borne by all taxpayers, including those who never used a car, and that the money came from budgets that were not specific for car traffic. In other words, car traffic costs society a lot, we learned. The opponents were not convinced, of course, but the decision to build those bridges for pedestrians was now bolstered with more facts and good arguments.

Although the pedestrians did not like bridges, it was decided that they were the only way to allow them to cross the motorways or railway lines, so they were necessary. This should mitigate the 'barrier effect of formerly insurmountable obstacles'.

Another important issue was the matter of parking. In Acatia it had been learned that in addition to the car parks belonging to big hotels and the shopping mall, there were also some smaller supermarkets and some restaurants with areas for parking. Most of them had, of course, placed signs saying 'for customers of XY only', but the fact was that quite a lot of car drivers used those areas for parking without permission. Some bought some items in the shop or a coffee in the restaurant and left their car all day. Others parked without buying anything. The municipality concluded that in all districts, all businesses that had areas for parking attached to them should either see to it rigorously that those areas could only be used by customers or introduce systems that allowed others to park there too, but they should have to pay a comparable price to the one in the multi-storey car park. To organise these things was complicated. The municipality did not want the businesses to have to incur a great deal of expense to do this, and the team of experts worked on ways of helping the owners to come up with schemes to solve this problem in the future. All the other activities that were planned should go on unimpeded.

In contrast to this, some issues that had to do with public transport could not wait. These involved the stops and stations. The municipality wanted bus and tram stops to include certain features: all of them should have a roof to provide protection from wind, rain, and snow and to provide shade on hot summer days. There should be benches to sit on at all stops. Getting on and off buses and trams should be as safe as possible. On smaller streets, buses would simply stop and the cars behind them should not pass them. On streets with more car traffic, there should be bus bays. Tram stops in small streets would work in exactly the same way as bus stops. On larger streets, where the tram tracks are normally in the middle of the road, elevated zebra crossings should lead to the waiting areas for passengers, protected by traffic lights that were activated as soon as trams arrived at the stops. In front of metro stations and around them there should also be some weather protection and seating facilities. There were other matters to be negotiated with the public transport companies, but the measures I mentioned here were to be instigated right from the beginning within the frame of the planned reconstruction and restructuring activities.

6.15 To implement measures takes time and needs strength

It took until May 2004 for an agreement to be found and 'real work', as some called it, could start. Discussions with the transport companies, however, went on for a longer time. They concerned primarily the integration of public transport policies into the concept of the mWwW project. According to the arguments formulated by the expert team, walking in a larger city was only a really good option if you could combine it easily with good public transport. To seamlessly combine public transport and walking first of all means that it should be easy to get a ticket. If someone who is walking decides for any reason, for instance, because they get tired, that they want to go on by public transport, it should be easy for them to do so. Bus or tram drivers will sell tickets, and payment can be in cash or with a debit or credit card. There is also a ticket machine, which makes it even easier to buy a ticket. There are single tickets and blocks of five or ten prepaid ones. There are also one-, two-, or three-day tickets or weekly tickets, which are appropriate for tourists. And, of course, there are cheap monthly or yearly tickets and special offers for children and seniors. Especially during a phase where – it is hoped – more people start using public transport because of a change in transport policy, single-ride tickets and prepaid tickets that can be bought from the driver are most important, and they should be cheap and as easily accessible as possible: people should not even need to think about where they can get a ticket. Everywhere. What if I have no cash? Use cards. Shouldn't I check and calculate before buying a single ticket in order not to spend too much on a ride? You could, but the difference from blocks of tickets is small. Will I be able to buy a ticket from a machine with a queue of people behind me? The machines are easy to use, but there are also counters where you can buy from people, and, as already stated, you can get tickets from the drivers of buses and trams.

The expert team knows that this goes against the trend, but unlike other cities, in Walkington, they asked larger samples of people what the most important things were that would motivate them to use public transport, both spontaneously and when planning a trip. The most relevant issues are the ease of getting tickets and their price. Other important things are the quality of the network, frequency of the service, punctuality, cleanliness, and the like. Visitors to Walkington who were also asked agreed with all of these, but they added that clear information on how to get from A (say the airport or the train station) to B (a hotel or any other place) is at least as important. Such information should be displayed on leaflets and maps that can easily be obtained in the dedicated shops of the transport companies, in supermarkets, in all metro stations, and in all buses and trams, and all public transport stops should be equipped with information too. Information will, of course, also be distributed via the internet so as to be found on your smartphone or tablet, but this would not suffice. Finally, all hotels should have such information and employees should be trained to give advice on transport around the city. At the airport, at train stations, and at all metro stations, there should also be staff who can provide information. All these things are, of course, expensive, but they should help to acquire more customers and to keep them satisfied.

It is too difficult for me to report all the arguments put forward by the public transport companies concerning the 'problems' connected with an increase in passengers, that this increased costs, that more people being transported meant that it would be necessary to buy more buses and trams, services would need to run more frequently, more staff would be required, and so on. One could get the impression that those negotiating for the transport companies were not interested in increasing their market shares and that they were not prepared to fight against their competitors – motor vehicles – as they seemed to spend a good deal of time outlining the problems that would accompany increased use of their services rather than seeing it as a positive move. They seemed to lack creativity and to be not really prepared to invest either brain power or material resources. One can understand that under these conditions, the negotiations with the public transport companies took a long time. The problems were aggravated by the fact that different transport companies saw the other companies as their competitors and were reluctant to cooperate. To achieve a unified ticket regime and customer information policy was the 'job of the century', as one spokesperson of the municipality put it. 'Technical problems are peanuts compared to dealing with people with different interests and to motivating them to find solutions together'. But if they wanted to make people walk more, this job had to be done.

The people responsible for the metro also had to be informed that it was necessary to install lifts at all metro stations. There were a considerable number of people who could use neither the stairs nor the escalators. In the longer run, when new stations were being built, the design should also include elevators. Some of the stations that already existed were architecturally noted and had won several prizes for their aesthetic design, but the issue of hiding places had not been considered when they were being designed and built. Last but not least, toilets that could be used for free had to be installed at all stations. The company protested that the costs of cleaning and maintaining the toilets were very high. But the municipality insisted and the company gave in because they realised that citizens really got angry at their attitude and accused the companies of failing to provide a good service by always using the argument of high costs.

To settle many of these things with the public transport companies took a long time, while other things had been finalised when the restructuring work in May 2004 started. Bars, cafés, restaurants, and shops had been contacted and there was a complete list of those which were prepared to provide a toilet service to the public. It was also clear where new toilets would be installed by the municipality. It had been agreed that every district should have some totally pedestrianised areas where everybody could walk freely and meeting points where cyclists were allowed, too, but were asked to ride slowly. Within these areas, bars and restaurants could place tables and chairs in the street during the warmer season. They should also be present where there were cinemas or theatres or other attractions in addition to the usual local businesses. This scheme had been very successful in Acatia. The idea that those pleasant, attractive places should not be limited to the city centre was well received by the inhabitants of Walkington. It was known that sometimes such concepts failed. The municipality and the experts had studied the documentation about this topic thoroughly, though, and they obviously knew which mistakes to avoid. When I look back today, I can only say that they did a good job.

Another way to make life more comfortable for walkers and for residents was to close a number of smaller streets to through traffic by cars. People who lived there could reach their garages but there were no through roads. By May, there was a complete city plan with those places where such restrictions should be carried out where it was not going to be too costly to implement. In the beginning, in Acatia, the residents were not too happy with the new layout. But the campaigning of the municipality was convincing enough to make people accept them without too much opposition. When the residents there were asked about their experience after some months, support had increased considerably. This helped to put a more positive spin on the public discussion.

Later, when work in the streets had started and had already been finalised in some districts, they came up with a new invention: pillars that could be lowered to street level and raised again with the help of a remote control which was only issued to residents or that reacted automatically to vehicles that were equipped with a chip. This allowed residents to gain access to their houses and garages, while other motorised traffic was kept out. Later, such solutions were also used to allow only public transport buses to drive through certain areas.

It was intended that the restructuring work should start in the outer districts and not in the centre. When the work first began, another difficult issue came up that the previous experience in Acatia could not help solve, nor were there any good solutions to be found in other cities: large industrial and trade establishments covered huge areas in some of these districts. They created a barrier between the residents and the rural environment outside the city, and they were very unsightly. A team from the Department of Design from the University of Walkington had already started dealing with this issue during the test activities in Acatia, and they came up with some plans for how to improve these ugly areas. These plans were presented to those responsible for the city and the expert team. At an international symposium held in Walkington, they were also shown to architects and city planners from other countries and cities. Although the response was not overwhelmingly enthusiastic, it was generally agreed that the proposed measures could work.

6.16   A subdepartment is installed at the municipality

The work lasted a little longer than originally planned, into the year 2012. A subdepartment for transport of the Department for City Planning and Development had already been established in 2005. The psychologist and the engineer who had steered the scientific work and two or three other members of that team were employed to form this subdepartment. There were rumours that they earned less money there than in their former jobs but that in the meantime they had started to get a great deal of job satisfaction from the work for the municipality. This group was to take care of all issues connected to walking, and soon others joined in who specialised in cycling. The goal was to organise and to promote all non-motorised transport within the framework of cooperation, but with the greatest emphasis on walking. There was to be no competition between these teams and they should work cooperatively to achieve their goals.

They supervised all the restructuring work, from the outer districts to the very centre of the city, districts 1 and 2. All the time they had an eye on No. 7, Acatia, and what had been learned there and how things were developing. For instance, they constantly reviewed the issue of local business and its performance. They also continued to follow and to study documentation from other places both inside and outside the country in order to be able to fine-tune and, if necessary, even redirect ongoing work. Although it transpired that little fine-tuning was necessary, the team considered it important to maintain a continuous dialogue with the citizens. Every year a questionnaire was distributed to evaluate the development. After some experimentation, the team came up with a format that was effective and the questionnaire became routine for the citizens. One got used to filling in that questionnaire by the end of the year. It ended with an open question asking for suggestions. Many citizens commented on improvements to the scheme, often suggesting additional measures or even some things that they felt were unnecessary.

Over the years, satisfaction with the measures taken in order to enhance walking grew. People reacted more positively. Suggestions became less fundamental, and comments such as 'kill the whole business' were not made any longer. I would say that things became normal. Walking had become an important but normal issue; it had started being part of our identity. The letters to the media showed that the citizens had started becoming experts. They 'knew' how to improve this and how to change that and suggested what the municipality should do. The ethos of walking became something that the city found normal and was even proud of.

6.17   Normality

And what does this normality look like today? First of all, you do not see any cars parked in the streets. A really radical change. Every city should try this. There is plenty of space for walking and also for cyclists like me. Walking feels comfortable and safe; I too take to walking sometimes. The yearly censuses, the results of which are reported in the media, show that more trips than ever are made on foot now. Women do not seem to be so worried about their safety when they are out walking in the dark. Old people and those with all kinds of impairments live an easier life today. Many more of them leave their homes now and go for a walk or go out shopping for food and other things that one needs for a living, including mixing socially and having fun. The number of children and youngsters travelling to school on foot or by bike alone or accompanied by their parents or other grown-ups has gone up slowly but steadily. They don't use 'mama-taxi' any more. Car trips within the city have decreased radically, and so has the number of those entering and exiting the city by car. But there are more visitors today, and the number of commuters – people who live outside the city and work or have other business within it and, to a lesser degree, vice versa – has increased. This means that public transport is used much more often. In fact, the public transport companies have improved both their service and their image considerably. Local business did not die, as many predicted; on the contrary, it exists better than before in all parts of the city. In those districts where there are many office complexes and few residential buildings, companies leave the lights on in their offices so that those areas do not appear completely dead. The municipality has successfully seen to a 'mix of functions', as they call it. They dedicated a certain number of buildings there to housing and hosting. The result is that there is life everywhere. There is life because people not only live there in their homes but also in the streets. They make use of the city. Thus they also make use of the local shops and bars and restaurants and cinemas. You can now find plenty of green areas in all districts, quite a few of them with playgrounds for children, which can safely be reached by parents with prams or with small children taking their time to get from their homes to the playground because they want to walk by themselves. There are benches everywhere. If you get tired, you sit down. Thus, just spending time there is more fun.

But the most fundamental improvement, in my eyes, is the change in the behaviour of people driving cars. One may say that literally no one drives faster than 30 km/h today; this obviously makes it easier for them to reduce their speed even more when circumstances make it necessary. In recent years there have been accidents, of course, but there is a steady decrease and if I am not totally wrong, nobody has died in an accident during the last five years or so. In the questionnaires, it becomes obvious that people experience this change in an overwhelmingly positive way. In their open answers and in their letters to the media, they write about comfort, about politeness, about 'peaceful coexistence', really. However, the number of such comments has decreased lately, but there is no increase whatever in the number of negative comments, if there are any negative comments at all. Things have become normal.

Since the start of the mWwW project – make Walkington walkable Walkington – there have been four elections. The ruling parties, those responsible for the project, suffered slight losses in the first two of them but still remained in power. The last two of them, especially the last one a year ago, they won with a comfortable majority.

References

ADAC. 2019. Die 10 günstigsten Autos der Mittelklasse im ADAC Autokosten-Check. Retrieved on 9 October 2019, from https://www.adac.de/rund-ums-fahrzeug/auto-kaufen-verkaufen/kostencheck/guenstigste-mittelklasse-autos/

Ajzen, I. 1991. The theory of planned behavior. *Organizational Behavior and Human Decision Processes*, 50, 179–211.

Alfonzo, M. A. 2005. To walk or not to walk: The hierarchy of walking needs. *Environment and Behavior*, 37(6), 808–836.

Amann, A., Reiterer, B., Risser, R., and Haindl, G. 2006. *Life quality of senior citizens in relation to mobility conditions (SIZE)*. University of Vienna, Institute of Sociology and FACTUM Chaloupka & Risser OG.

Ampofo-Boateng, K., and Thomson, J. A. 1986. Children's perception of danger and safety on the road. *British Journal of Psychology*, 82, 487–505.

Appleyard, D., Gerson, M. S., and Lintell, M. 1981. *Livable streets, protected neighborhoods*. University of California Press.

Ausserer, K., Braguti, I., Füssl, E., Höfferer, G., Risser, A., and Risser, R. 2009. *Bef(w) usst unterwegs: Fußgängerstudie in Wien*, geförderte Studie des BMVIT, Wien.

Ausserer, K., Füssl, E., and Risser, R. 2013. *NutzerInnenbefragung: Was gefällt am Gehen und was hält davon ab?* Endbericht, FACTUM Chaloupka & Risser, Im Auftrag der Magistratsabteilung 18 - Stadtentwicklung und Stadtplanung.

Ausserer, K., and Risser, R. 2018. Assessing the Influence of Greenery on the Behaviour of Road Users. *Transactions on Transport Sciences*, 9(2), 67–75.

Ausserer, K., Risser, R., and Röhsner, U. 2011. Once a walker always a walker or "You can't teach an old dog new tricks": *Results of a mobility study of preschool children, presentation at the WALK21 conference*, The Hague, 17–19 November, Vienna: FACTUM & makam.

Ausserer, K., Röhsner, U., and Risser, R. 2010. *Zufußgehen beginnt im Kindesalter. Wege zum und vom Kindergarten*. Vienna: FACTUM & makam.

Ausserer, K., Sumper, E., Reindl, I., Röhsner. U., and Risser, R. 2012. *Gemma weiter. Auswirkungen von Mobilitätsmanagement im Kindergarten auf das Mobilitätsverhalten von Eltern und Kleinkindern*. Vienna: FACTUM & makam.

Banas, J. A., and Rains, S. A. 2010. A meta-analysis of research on inoculation theory. *Communication Monographs*, 77(3), 281–311.

Baumgartner, F. R., Berry, J. M., Hojnacki, M., Leech, B. L., and Kimball, D. C. 2009. *Lobbying and Policy Change: Who wins, who loses, and why*. University of Chicago Press.

Beenackers, M. A., Kamphuis, C. B., Mackenbach, J. P., Burdorf, A., and van Lenthe, F. J. 2013. Why some walk and others don't: exploring interactions of perceived safety and social neighborhood factors with psychosocial cognitions. *Health Education Research*, 28(2), 220–233.

Bein, N., Petrjánošová, M., Plichtová, J., Risser, R., and Ståhl, A. 2004. Final Report of the EU-Project HOTEL: How to analyse Life Quality, an accompanying measure within the EU fifth Framework Programme, Key action "Improving the Socio Economic Knowledge Base". *HPSE-2002-60057*, Bratislava & Vienna.

Bell, D., Füssl, E., Ausserer, K., Risser, R., Wunsch, D., Braguti, I., Oberlader, M., and Friedwagner, A. 2010. *Scenarios of the future mobility of elderly people. Life transition points and their impact on everyday mobility of elderly people; future mobility developments and necessary support measures with special regard to retirement and loss of partner. Final project report, ERA NET TRANSPORT, ENT14 Keep Moving,* Vienna: FACTUM Chaloupka & Risser OG.

Bell, D., Risser, R., Morris, A. et al. 2013. VRUITS: Improving the Safety and Mobility of Vulnerable Road Users Through ITS Applications. In: Dorn L. (Ed.), 2007, *Driver Behaviour and Training.* Vol. III, Aldershot: Ashgate Publishers.

Benz, J., Blakey, C., Oppenheimer, C. C., Scherer, H., and Robinson, W. T. 2013. The healthy people initiative: Understanding the user's perspective. *Journal of Public Health Management and Practice*, 19(2), 103–109.

Berge, G. 2013. Walking forward on a national level: The Norwegian national walking strategy. Munich: Walk 21.

Berge, G., and Peddie, S. (n.d.). Walking pattern in OECD/ITF countries.

Bian, Z., and Andersen, G. J. 2008. Aging and the perceptual organization of 3-D scenes. *Psychology and Aging*, 23(2), 342.

Brass, K. 2017. Redesigning the Grid: Barcelona's Experiment with Superblocks. Retrieved on 7 December 2019, from https://urbanland.uli.org/planning-design/barcelonas-experiment-superblocks/

Brehm, J. W. 1966. *A Theory of Psychological Reactance*. Academic Press.

Brunswik, E. 1956. *Perception and the Representative Design of Psychological Experiments*. Univ. of California Press.

Bryan, F. R. 1997. *Beyond the Model T: The Other Ventures of Henry Ford*. Wayne State University Press.

Build a better Burb. 2019. Six reasons for the resurgence of car-free shopping streets, Lee Sobel. Retrieved on 21 November 2019, from http://buildabetterburb.org/six-reasons-resurgence-car-free-shopping-streets/http:/buildabetterburb.org/six-reasons-resurgence-car-free-shopping-streets/

Carr, K. E. 2019. When did people start riding horses? *Quatr.us Study Guides, June 20, 2017. Web. September 16, 2019.*

Cauzard, J. P. 2004. European drivers and road risk. SARTRE 3 reports Part 1, INRETS, Arcueil.

Chaloupka, C., and Risser, R. 2004. *"… bis dass der Führerschein …" - Mobilität in Kindheit und Jugend*. Kröning: Asanger Verlag.

Chaloupka, C., and Risser, R. 2016. Walking in the city – Infrastructure Developments for Pedestrians in Vienna. Vienna: Factum OG Traffic and Social Analysis.

Civitas. 2014. Gender equality and mobility: mind the gap! Retrieved on 13 November 2019, from https://www.eltis.org/sites/default/files/trainingmaterials/civ_pol-an2_m_web.pdf

Connect The Crescent. 2018. Retrieved on 12 December 2019, from https://connectthecrescent.com/overview

Creswell, J. W., and Plano Clark V. L. 2018. *Designing and Conducting Mixed Methods Research*. London: SAGE Publications.

Croft, P. 1986. *Nature Diary of a Quiet Pedestrian, Madeira Park*. BC: Harbour Publishing Federal Highway Administration 2006, Federal Highway Administration University Course on Bicycle and Pedestrian Transportation, US Department of Transportation.

DaCoTA. 2012. Children in road traffic, Deliverable 4.8c of the EC FP7 project DaCoTA.

Damjanovic, D. 2005. *Women and Men on the Move in Hermagor – Presseggersee. Landscape planning for transport networks in the rural areas with a gender perspective.* Vienna, Hermagor: Planungskooperative Architektur/Freiraum/Landschaft.

Delhomme, P., De Dobbeleer, W., Forward, S., and Simões, A. (Eds.). 2009. *Manual for designing, implementing, and evaluating road safety communication campaigns: Part I*. Institut Belge pour la Sécurité Routière (IBSR).

Donovan, R. J., Fielder, L., and Ouschan, R. 2011. Do motor vehicle advertisements that promote vehicle performance attributes also promote undesirable driving behaviour? *Journal of Public Affairs*, 11(1), 25–34.

Dorn, L. 2012. *Driver Behaviour and Training (Human Factors in Road and Rail Transport)*. Ashgate Publishing Group.

Elvik, R. 2009. *The Power Model of the Relationship between Speed and Road Safety: Update and New Analyses*. TØI Report 1034/2009. Oslo: Institute of Transport Economics TØI.

Elvik, R., Christensen, P., and Amundsen, A. 2004. *Speed and road accidents. An evaluation of the power model*. TOI Report 740/2004.EPRS 2014, Mapping smart cities in the EU, study requested by the European Parliament's Committee on Industry, Research and Energy, Policy Department A: Economic and Scientific Policy.

European Commission. 2018. Traffic Safety Basic Facts on Pedestrians. European Commission, Directorate General for Transport.

FARS. 2018. Fatality Facts 2017 Pedestrians. Retrieved on 30 September 2019, from https://www.iihs.org/topics/fatality-statistics/detail/pedestrians

Federal Highway Administration. 2014, Nonmotorized Transportation Pilot Program: Continued Progress in Developing Walking and Bicycling Networks – May 2014 Report

Festinger, L. 1950. Informal social communication. *Psychological Review*, 57(5), 271–282.

Festinger, L. 1954. A theory of social comparison processes. *Human Relations*, 7, 117–140.

Festinger, L. 1957. *Theory of Cognitive Dissonance. Stanford*. CA: Stanford University Press.

Fietkau, H. J., and Kessel, H. 1981. *Umweltlernen. Veränderungsmöglichkeiten des Umweltbewußtseins*. Königstein: Hain.

Fleming, M. 1999 *Safety Culture Maturity Model*. UK HSE Offshore Technology Report OTO 2000/049, Norwich: HSE Books.

Freeland, A., Banerjee, S., Dannenberg, A., and Wendel, A. 2013. Walking associated with public transit: moving toward increased activity in the United States. *American Journal of Public Health*, 103(3), 536–542.

Frey, H. 2015. *Wien zu Fuß 2015. Daten und Fakten zum Fußverkehr.* Mobilitätsagentur Wien GmbH.

Funk, W., and Fassmann, H. 2002. *Beteiligung, Verhalten und Sicherheit von Kindern und Jugendlichen im Straßenverkehr.* Bericht der Bundesanstalt für Straßenwesen, Bergisch Gladbach, Heft M 138.

Füssl, E., Jaunig, J., and Titze, S. 2019. ROUTINE: Development of a Physical Activity Promoting Journey Planner Web App, in: *MDPI Journal of Social Sciences,* Special issue Public Transport and Social Psychology.

Fyhri, A., Hof, T., Simonova, Z., and de Jong, M. 2010. *The Influence of Perceived Safety and Security on Walking, COST-project PQN,* Final report part B: Documentation.

Gärling, T., and Schuitema, G. 2007. Travel Demand Management Targeting Reduced Private Car Use: Effectiveness, Public Acceptability and Political Feasibility. *Journal of Social Issues,* 63(1), 139–153.

Gehl, J., and Gemzøe, L. 1996. *Public Spaces, Public Life. Copenhagen:* The Danish Architectural Press and the Royal Danish Academy of Fine Arts.

Gifford, R. 2007a. *Environmental Psychology: Principles and Practice.* Colville, WA: Optimal Books.

Gifford, R. 2007b. Environmental psychology and sustainable development: Expansion, maturation, and challenges. *Journal of Social Issues,* 63(1), 199–212.

Givoni, B. 1998. *Climate Considerations in Building and Urban Design.* New York: John Wiley and Sons Inc.

Gobster, P. H. 2005. Recreation and leisure research from an active living perspective: Taking a second look at urban trail use data. *Leisure Sciences,* 27(5), 367–383.

Gössling, S., Choid, A., Dekker, K., and Metzler, D. 2019. The Social Cost of Automobility, Cycling and Walking in the European Union. *Ecological Economics,* 158, 65–74.

Groeger, J. A., and Rothengatter, J. A. 1998. Traffic psychology and behaviour. *Transportation Research, Part F,* 1, 1–9.

Hakamies-Blomqvist, L., and Jutila, U. 1996. In Hydén, C., Nilsson, A., and Risser, R. (1998). Walcyng – How to enhance walking and cycling instead of shorter car trips and to make these modes safer, Final report, Transport RTD Programme of the 4th Framework Programme, Lund & Vienna.

Hakkert, A. S. 2010. Based on data from ETSC. (1999). *Exposure Data for Travel Risk Assessment: Current Practice and Future Needs in the EU.* Brussels, Belgium: European Transport Safety Council.

Hall, C., and Ram, Y. 2018. Walk score® and its potential contribution to the study of active transport and walkability: A critical and systematic review. *Transportation Research Part D: Transport & Environment,* 61: 310–324.

Hall, C. M., Ram, Y., and Shoval, N. (Eds.). 2018. *The Routledge International Handbook of Walking.* Abingdon: Routledge.

Hansen, A. 2019. *Hjärnstark. Hut motion och träning starker din hjärna.* Stockholm: Månpocket.

Hanson, S., and Jones, A. 2015. Is there evidence that walking groups have health benefits? A systematic review and meta-analysis. *British Journal of Sports Medicine,* 49(11), 710–715.

How Seville transformed itself into the cycling capital of southern Europe. 2015. The Guardian. Retrieved on 7 December 2019, from https://www.theguardian com/cities/2015/jan/28/seville-cycling-capital-southern-europe-bike-lanes

Hydén, C., Nilsson A., and Risser, R. 1997. *Walcyng – How to enhance WALking and CycliNG instead of shorter car trips and to make these modes safer,* Final report, Department of Traffic Planning and Engineering, Lund University, Sweden & FACTUM OHG, Austria.

International Transport Forum ITF. 2011. *Research Report – Summary Document,* OECD/ITF.

Johanson, D., and Edey, M. 1981. *Lucy: The Beginnings of Humankind.* New York: Simon and Schuster.

Johanson, D., and Shreeve, J. 1989. *Lucy's Child: The Discovery of a Human Ancestor.* London: Viking.

Kagge, E. 2019. *Walking: One Step at a Time.* New York: Pantheon Books.

Knoblauch, R. L., Pietrucha, M. T., and Nitzburg, M. 1996. Field Studies of Pedestrian Walking Speed and Start-Up Time. *Transportation Research Record,* 1538, 27–38.

Knoll, B., and Szalai, E. 2008. *Frauenwege - Männerwege. Entwicklung von Methoden zur gendersen sib len Mobilitätserhebung,* Wien: Forschungsarbeiten aus dem Verkehrswesen, Bundesministerium für Verkehr, Innovation und Technologie, Band 175.

Kotler, P., Armstrong, G., Harris, L. C., and Piercy, N. 2016. *Principles of Marketing.* 7th European Edition. Harlow: Pearson Education Limited.

Kubitzki, J., and Fastenmeier, W. 2019. *Sicher zu Fuß. Mobilität und Sicherheit von Fußgängern.* München: AZT Automotive GmbH & Institut Mensch-Verkehr-Umwelt, sowie Wien: MAKAM Research.

Laakso, S., and Heiskanen, E. 2017. Good practice report: Capturing cross-cultural interventions. Report D3.1 of the EU-project ENERGISE.

Langford, J., Methorst, R., and Hakamies-Blomqvist, L. 2006. Older drivers do not have a high crash risk – A replication of low mileage bias. *Accident Analysis and Prevention,* 38(3), 574–578.

Lawton, M. P., and Nahemow, L. 1973. Ecology and the aging process. In: Eisdorfer, C., and Lawton, M. P. (Eds.), *Psychology of Adult Development and Aging.* Washington, DC: *American Psychological Association,* pp. 132–160.

Levasseur, M., Généreux, M., Bruneau, J. F., Vanasse, A., Chabot, É., Beaulac, C., and Bédard, M. M. 2015. Importance of proximity to resources, social support, transportation and neighborhood security for mobility and social participation in older adults: Results from a scoping study. *BMC Public Health,* 15, 503.

Le Vine, S., and Polak, J. 2009. The Car in British Society. Working Paper 1: National Travel Survey Refresh Analysis.

Litman, T. 2007. *Developing Indicators for Comprehensive and Sustainable Transport Planning. Transportation Research Record: Journal of the Transportation Research Board,* 2007, 10–15.

Luft, J., and Ingham, H. 1955. The Johari window, a graphic model of interpersonal awareness. In: *Proceedings of the Western Training Laboratory in Group Development.* Los Angeles: UCLA.

Maffii, S., Malgieri, P., and Di Bartolo, C. 2016. Smart Choices for cities. Gender equality and mobility: mind the gap! CIVITAS Policy Note.

Mander, U., Brebbia, C. A., and Tiezzi, E. 2006. *The sustainable City IV: Urban Regeneration and Sustainability.* Wit Press.

Maring, W., and Van Schagen, I. 1990 Age dependence of attitudes and knowledge in cyclists. *Accident Analysis & Prevention,* 22, 127–136.

Martin-Puerta, S. 2014. *Commuting Mode Choice: Motivational Determinants and Road Users Profile*. Paris: Transport Research Arena.

Maslow A. H. 1943, *A theory of human motivation. Psychological Review*. 1943, 50(4), 370–396.

Mechakra-Tahiri, S. D., Freeman, E. E., Haddad, S., Samson, E., and Zunzunegui, M. V. 2012. The gender gap in mobility: A global cross-sectional study. *BMC Public Health*, 12(1), 598.

Mehta, V. 2008. Walkable streets: pedestrian behavior, perceptions and attitudes. *Journal of Urbanism: International Research on Placemaking and Urban Sustainability*, 1(3), 217–245.

Methorst, R., Monterde, I., Bort, H., Risser, R., Sauter, D., Tight, M., and Walker, J. 2010. Pedestrians' Quality Needs PQN, European Cooperation in Science and Technology (COST), Action 358.

Methorst, R., Schepers, P., Christie, N., Dijst, M., Risser, R., Sauter, D., and Van Wee, B. 2017. 'Pedestrian falls' as a necessary addition to the current definition of traffic crashes for improved public health policies. *Journal of Transport & Health*, 6, 10–12.

Meyer, W. U. 2003. *Einige grundlegende Annahmen und Konzepte der Attributionstheorie*. Universität Bielefeld.

MiD (Mobilität in Deutschland). 2019. BMVI; available from www.bmvi.de/SharedDocs/DE/Artikel/G/mobilitaet-in-deutschland.html

Monheim, H. 2010. Efficient mobility without private cars: A new transport policy for Europe. In: Ramos, M. J., and Alves, M. J. (Eds.), *The Walker and the City*. Lisbon: ACA-M.

Morar, T., and Bertolini, L. 2013. Planning for pedestrians: A way out of traffic congestion. *Procedia – Social and Behavioral Sciences*, 81, 600–608.

New Zealand Transport Agency NZTA. 2018. The pedestrian experience. A literature review from www.nzta.govt.nz/assets/resources/the-pedestrian-experience/The-pedestrian-experience-literature-review.pdf

Niebuhr, T., Junge, M., and Rosén, E. 2016. Pedestrian injury risk and the effect of age. *AAP*, 86, 121–128.

Oberlader, M., Barker, M., and Zavareh, M. F. 2015. *Walking in Growing Cities: Infrastructure Developments for Pedestrians in Tehran (Iran) and Vienna (Austria)*. Vienna: Factum.

Ogilvie, B. W. 2008. *The Science of Describing: Natural History in Renaissance Europe*. University of Chicago Press.

Oxley, J., Fildes, B., Ihsen, E., Charlton, J., and Day, R. 1995. An investigation of road-crossing behaviour of elderly pedestrians. *Road Safety Research and Enforcement Conference, 1995*, Fremantle, Western Australia.

Panter, J., Guell, C., Humphreys, D., and Ogilvie, D. 2019. Can changing the physical environment promote walking and cycling? A systematic review of what works and how. *Health & Place*, 58, 102161.

Pasanen, E. 2001. *The risks of cycling*, Helsinki City: Planning Department. Traffic Planning Division.

Patek, G. C., and Thoma, T. G. 2013. Pedestrian Fatalities—A Problem on the Rise. *Annals of Emergency Medicine*, 62, 613–615.

Patterson, I., Pegg, S., and Omar, W. R. W. 2017. Walking to promote increased physical activity. In: Hall, C. M., Ram, Y., and Shoval, N. (Eds.), *The Routledge International Handbook of Walking*. Routledge, pp. 274–287.

Pelssers, B. 2019. Pedestrians. Thematic File Road Safety N 7, VIAS Institute. Retrieved on 17 November 2019, from https://www.vias.be/publications/ Themadossier%20verkeersveiligheid%20n°7%20-%20Voetgangers%20(2019)/ Thematic_file_road_safety_N_7_-_Pedestrians_(2nd_edition).pdf

Petty, R. E., and Cacioppo, J. T. 1986. The elaboration likelihood model of Persuasion. In: Berkowitz, L. (Ed.), *Advances in Experimental Social Psychology*, 19, pp. 123–205. New York: Academic Press.

Philipsen, K. 2017. 21 Easy Measures to Promote Pedestrianism and Complete Streets. Smart Cities Dive. Retrieved on 7 December 2019, from https://www. smartcitiesdive.com/ex/sustainablecitiescollective/21-measures-pedestrian-safety-baltimore-or-anywhere/1074306/

Precht, R. D. 2011. *Who am I? And if so, how many?* London: Constable and Robinson.

Prochaska, J. O., and DiClemente, C. C. 1982. Transtheoretical therapy: Toward a more integrative model of change. *Psychotherapy: Theory, Research & Practice*, 19(3), 276–288.

Pucher, J., and Dijkstra, L. 2000. Making Walking and Cycling Safer: Lessons from Europe. *Transportation Quarterly*, 54(3).

Ramos M. J., and Alves M. (Eds.). 2010, *The Walker and the City*, Lisbon: Associaçao de Citadaos Auto-Mobilizados.

Rauh, W. 2001. *Mobilitätsmanagement für Schulen – Wege zur Schule neu Organisieren.* VCÖ 1/2001.

Rehbein, P. 2014. Welche Faktoren beeinflussen die Gehqualität? *Mobilogisch!, der Vierteljahres-Zeitschrift für Ökologie, Politik und Bewegung*, Heft 4.

Returning Streets to People: 5 Tips for Going Car-Free. 2015. Landscape Infrastructure, Landscape Urbanism. Retrieved on 8 December 2019, from http://www.ideas.swagroup.com/tag/pedestrian-only-success-stories/

Risser, R. 2000. Measuring influences of speed reduction on subjective safety, *Workshop on Traffic Calming in New Delhi in March 2000, ICTCT.*

Risser, R. 2010. Pedestrians are second class road users. In: Ramos, M. J., and Alves, M. J. (Eds.), *The Walker and the City.* Lisbon: ACA-M.

Risser, R., Bein, N., Plichtová, J., Sardi, G. M., and Ståhl, A. 2004. *Pilot Study Report Kristianstad. EU-project HOTEL – How to Analyse Life Quality*, Vienna: FACTUM Chaloupka & Risser OG.

Risser, R., Månsson Lexell, E., Bell, D., Iwarsson, S., and Ståhl, A. 2015. Use of local public transport among people with cognitive impairments – A literature review. *Transportation Research, part F: Traffic Psychology and Behaviour*, 29, 83–97.

Rosén, E., Stigson, H., and Sander, U. 2011. Literature review of pedestrian fatality risk as a function of car impact speed. *Accident Analysis and Prevention*, 43(1), 25–33.

Rosenbloom, T., Shahar, A., Elharar, A., and Danino, O. 2008. Risk perception of driving as a function of advanced training aimed at recognizing and handling risks in demanding driving situations. *AAP*, 40(2), 697–703.

Rosenbloom, T., and Wolf, Y. 2002. Sensation seeking and detection of risky road signals: A developmental perspective. *AAP*, 34, 569–580.

Rosenkvist, J., Risser, R., Iwarsson, S., and Ståhl, A. 2010. Exploring Mobility in Public Environments among People with Cognitive Functional Limitations – Challenges and Implications for Planning. *Mobilities*, 5(1), 131–145.

Rosenstiel, L. 2003. *Grundlagen der Organisationspsychologie. Basiswissen und Anwendungshinweise* (5th ed.). Stuttgart: C. E. Poeschel Verlag.

Rudner, J., and Malone, K. 2011. Childhood in the Suburbs and the Australian Dream: How has it impacted children's independent mobility? *UK: Global Studies of Childhood*, 1(2).

Rundmo, T. 2014. *Traffic Safety Attitudes and Risk-taking Behaviour, Temporal and Cross-cultural Differences (Invited talk)*. Japanese National Traffic Safety and Environmental Laboratory; NTNU.

Rye, T., Mingardo, G., Hertel, M., Thiemann-Linden, J., Pressl, R., Posch, K. H., and Carvalho, M. 2015. Push & Pull. 16 good reasons for parking management available from https://www.europeanparking.eu/media/1279/12122014 _push_pull_a4_en.pdf

Santos, A., McGuckin, N., Nakamoto, H. Y., Gray, D., and Liss, S. 2011. *Summary of Travel Trends: 2009 National Household Travel Survey*. Federal Highway Administration FHA.

Saunders, R., Weiler, B., and Laing, J. 2017. Life-changing walks of mid-life adults. In: Hall, C. M., Ram, Y., and Shoval, N. (Eds.), *The Routledge International Handbook of Walking*. Routledge, pp. 264–273.

Sauter, D. 2010. Walking, time and public space: Perceptions. Policies and perspectives. In: Ramos, M. J., and Alves, M. J. (Eds.), *The Walker and the City*. Lisbon: ACA-M.

Schneider, R. J. 2013. Theory of routine mode choice decisions: An operational framework to increase sustainable transportation. *Transport Policy*, 25: 128–137.

Schulz von Thun, F. 2001. *Miteinander Reden 1–3*. Leipzig: Verlag Rowohlt Taschenbuch.

Shannon, C. E., and Weaver, W. 1949. *The Mathematical Theory of Communication*. Urbana: University of Illinois Press.

Silva, M. F. P. 2011. Road Safety – Driver from the Customer Satisfaction Rating. Public Defense Title of Specialist in the area of education/training 347 – Placement in the organization/company. Polytechnic Institute of Coimbra.

Skynner, R., and Cleese, J. 1993. *Life and How to Survive it*. New York & London: Norton and Company.

Solnit, R. 2001. *Wanderlust: A History of Walking*. New York: Penguin Books.

Stromberg, J. 2015. Fewer than 4% of Americans walk or bike to work. Here's how to change that. Vox.

Šucha, M. 2019. The Human Factor in Traffic – Possible Ways of Influencing People's Behaviour. *Habilitation Thesis*. Charles University in Prague.

SWOV. 2012, *Fact Sheet: Road Deaths in the Netherlands*, https://goo.gl/CztZPL

Szegö, J. 2004. *Vorstadt-Spaziergänge: Das alte Wien zwischen Ring und Gürtel*. Wien: Wirtschaftsverlag Ueberreuter.

Tacken, M., Marcellini, F., Mollenkopf, H., and Ruoppila, I. 1999. *Keeping the Elderly Mobile: Outdoor Mobility of the Elderly: Problems and Solutions, TRAIL, The Netherlands Research School for Transport, Infrastructure and Logistics*. Delft: University Press.

Theeuwes, J., Van der Horst, R., and Kuiken, M. 2012. *Designing Safe Road Systems. A Human Factors Perspective*. Aldershot: Ashgate Publishers.

The Pedestrian Experience. 2018. *The New Zealand Government Policy Statement (GPS) on Land Transport*. New Zealand: Ministry of Transport.

These streets are made for walking: How Oklahoma City overturned car culture. The Guardian, 19 November 2015. Retrieved on 21 November 2019, from https://www.theguardian.com/public-leaders-network/2015/nov/19/ oklahoma-walking-car-culture-pedestrians-cities.

The World's Longest Pedestrian Street "Strøget". 2019. Copenhagen Portal. DK. Retrieved on 8 December 2019, from https://www.copenhagenet.dk/cph-map/CPH-Pedestrian.asp

Thoreau, H. D. 1994. *Walking*. New York: HarperCollins.

Tomasch, E., Hoschopf, H., Weinberger, M., Risser, R., Chaloupka, C., Haupt, J., and Bell, D. 2016. *ATTENTION-Entwicklung von geeigneten Maßnahmen zur Verbesserung der FußgängerInnensicherheit von SeniorInnen durch Verhaltensbeobachtung und Tiefenanalyse von Realunfällen*. Wien: Technische Universität Graz und FACTUM OG.

Tomschy, R., and Roider, O. 2015. *Österreich unterwegs. Mobilitätsverhalten im Wandel der Zeit*. Wien: BMVIT & ÖVG.

UITP. 2015. Mobility in Cities Database. From www.uitp.org/sites/default/files/MCD_2015_synthesis_web_0.pdf

Umweltamt Stadt Karlsruhe. 2003. *Agenda 21 Projekt "Kindergesundheit"*. Zwischenbericht 2002/2003, Karlsruhe.

Umweltbundesamt. 2019. Indikator: Belastung der Bevölkerung durch Verkehrslärm. Retrieved on 27 September 2019, from https://www.umweltbundesamt.de/indikator-belastung-der-bevoelkerung-durch#textpart-1

Umweltbundesamt (Deutschland). 2010. PKW-Maut in Deutschland? Eine umwelt- und verkehrs po li tische Bewertung.

United Nations. 2014. Department of Economic and Social Affairs, Population Division. World Urbanization Prospects: The 2014 Revision, Highlights. From http://esa.un.org/unpd/wup/Highlights/WUP2014-Highlights.pdf

Usability Metrics – A Guide To Quantify The Usability Of Any System. 2015. Usability Geek. Retrieved on 12 June 2019, from: https://usabilitygeek.com/usability-metrics-a-guide-to-quantify-system-usability/

Uteng, T. P. 2012. *World Development Report. Gender and mobility in the developing world*. Retrieved on 20 June, 2019, from https://siteresources.worldbank.org/INTWDR2012/Resources/7778105-1299699968583/7786210-1322671773271/uteng.pdf

Vanderbilt, T. 2008. *Traffic. Penguin Books*: London, England.

Várhelyi, A. 1996. *Dynamic Speed Adaptation Based on Information Technology – A Theoretical Background. Bulletin 142*. Sweden: Lund University.

VCÖ. 2009. *Gender-Gap im Verkehrs- und Mobilitätsbereich, Hintergrundbericht*. Wien: Verkehrsclub Österreich VCÖ.

Vienncouver. 2015. A Tale of Two Cities (1): Vienna's Mariahilferstraße combines Pedestrian Zone and Shared Space. Retrieved on 8 December 2019, from https://www.vienncouver.com/2015/01/viennas-begegnungszone-shared-space-program/

Walkability: Creating great cities by putting pedestrians first. 2015. The Discourse. Retrieved on 13 June 2019, from https://www.thediscourse.ca/scarborough/walkability

Walkspace. 2012. *Fußverkehr in Zahlen. Daten Fakten und Besonderheiten*. Vienna: Ministry of Transport, Innovation and Technology BMVIT.

Watzlawick, P., Bavelas, B. J., and Jackson, D. D. 2011. *Pragmatics of Human Communication: A Study of Interactional Patterns, Pathologies and Paradoxes*. W. W. Norton & Company.

Wegman, F. and Aarts, L. 2005. *Advancing Sustainable Safety. National Road Safety Outlook for 2005–2020*. Leidschendam: SWOV.

What would a truly walkable city look like? 2018. The Guardian. Retrieved on 19 September 2018, from https://www.theguardian.com/cities/2018/sep/19/what-would-a-truly-walkable-city-look-like

Wiles, J. L., Leibing, A., Guberman, N., Reeve, J., and Allen, R. E. S. 2012. The Meaning of "Aging in Place" to Older People. *The Gerontologist*, 52(3), 357–366.

World Development Report. 2012. Gender and mobility in the developing world, Uteng, T. P. Retrieved on 20 June 2019, from https://siteresources.worldbank.org/INTWDR2012/Resources/7778105-1299699968583/7786210-1322671773271/uteng.pdf

World Health Organisation. 2007. Global age-friendly cities project. Retrieved on 18 June 2009, from www.who.int./ageing/age_friendly_cities_network

World Health Organisation. 2011. Information sheet: global recommendations on physical activity for health 18–64 years old. Retrieved on 18 September 2019, from https://www.who.int/dietphysicalactivity/publications/recommendations18_64yearsold/en/

Yang, Y., and Diez-Roux, A. V. 2017. Adults' Daily Walking for Travel and Leisure: Interaction between Attitude toward Walking and the Neighborhood Environment. *American Journal of Health Promotion*, 31(5), 435–443.

Zivotofsky, A. Z., Eldror, E., Mandel, R., and Rosenbloom. T. 2012. Misjudging their own steps: why elderly people have trouble crossing the road. *Human Factors*, 54(4), 600–607.

14 cities around the world that are better for pedestrians than people with cars. 2019. Insider. Retrieved on 7 December 2019, from https://www.insider.com/best-walkable-cities-for-pedestrians-2019-6

Index